D1571083

The Thyroid Axis
and
Psychiatric Illness

The Thyroid Axis
and
Psychiatric Illness

Edited by

Russell T. Joffe, M.D.
Mood Disorders Program, Clarke Institute of Psychiatry
and the University of Toronto, Toronto, Ontario, Canada

Anthony J. Levitt, M.D.
Mood Disorders Program, Clarke Institute of Psychiatry
and the University of Toronto, Toronto, Ontario, Canada

Washington, DC
London, England

Copyright © 1993 American Psychiatric Press, Inc.
ALL RIGHTS RESERVED
Manufactured in the United States of America on acid-free paper.
96 95 94 93 4 3 2 1

American Psychiatric Press, Inc.
1400 K Street, N.W., Washington, DC 20005

Library of Congress Cataloging-in-Publication Data
The Thyroid axis and psychiatric illness / edited by Russell T. Joffe,
  Anthony J. Levitt.
    p.   cm.
  Includes bibliographical references and index.
  ISBN 0-88048-364-4 (alk. paper)
  1. Hypothalamic-pituitary-thyroid axis—Diseases—Psychological
  aspects.   2. Thyroid gland—Diseases—Psychological aspects.
  3. Mental illness—Endocrine aspects.   4. Psychoneuroendocrinology.
I. Joffe, Russell T., 1954–   . II. Levitt, Anthony J., 1959–   .
  [DNLM: 1. Mental Disorders—complications.   2. Thyroid Diseases—
  complications.   3. Thyroid Gland—physiology.   4. Thyroid Hormones—
  physiology.   WK 202 T54665]
  RC455.4E54T49   1993
  616.89—dc20
  DNLM/DLC
  for Library of Congress   92-22046
                                                                            CIP

British Library Cataloguing in Publication Data
A CIP record is available from the British Library.

For Jennifer and Lina

Contents

PART I: Basic Principles

PART II: Clinical Principles

Contributors

Betty L. Chan, M.D.
Resident, Division of Endocrinology
St. Michael's Hospital and the University of Toronto
Toronto, Ontario, Canada

Mary B. Dratman, M.D
Professor, Department of Medicine
Veteran's Administration Medical Center
Philadelphia, Pennsylvania

James C. Garbutt, M.D.
Associate Professor, Department of Psychiatry
    and Center for Alcohol Studies
University of North Carolina at Chapel Hill
Director, Clinical Research Unit
Dorothea Dix Hospital
Raleigh, North Carolina

Philip W. Gold, M.D.
Chief, Clinical Neuroendocrinology Branch
National Institute of Mental Health
Bethesda, Maryland

Russell T. Joffe, M.D.,
Head, Mood Disorders Program
Clarke Institute of Psychiatry
Associate Professor, Department of Psychiatry
University of Toronto
Toronto, Ontario, Canada

Allan S. Kaplan, M.D.
Director, Eating Disorders Centre, Toronto General Hospital
Associate Professor, Department of Psychiatry
University of Toronto
Toronto, Ontario, Canada

Anthony J. Levitt, M.D.,
Deputy Head, Mood Disorders Program
Clarke Institute of Psychiatry
Assistant Professor, Department of Psychiatry
University of Toronto
Toronto, Ontario, Canada

Julio Licinio, M.D.
Assistant Professor, Department of Psychiatry
Yale University School of Medicine and West Haven
    Veteran's Affairs Medical Center
West Haven, Connecticut

Peter T. Loosen, M.D.
Professor, Department of Psychiatry and Medicine
Vanderbilt University
Chief of Psychiatry, Veteran's Affairs Hospital
Nashville, Tennessee

Arthur J. Prange Jr., M.D.
Boshamer Professor, Department of Psychiatry
University of North Carolina at Chapel Hill
Chapel Hill, North Carolina

Victor I. Reus, M.D.
Professor, Department of Psychiatry
University of California, San Francisco School of Medicine
San Francisco, California

William Singer, M.D.
Associate Professor, Division of Endocrinology
St. Michael's Hospital
Department of Medicine, University of Toronto
Toronto, Ontario, Canada

Murray B. Stein, M.D.
Assistant Professor, Department of Psychiatry and Pharmacology
University of Manitoba
Winnipeg, Manitoba, Canada

Thomas W. Uhde, M.D.
Chief, Section on Anxiety and Affective Disorders
Biological Psychiatry Branch
National Institute of Mental Health
Bethesda, Maryland

Ma-Li Wong, M.D.
Assistant Professor, Department of Psychiatry
Yale University School of Medicine and West Haven
    Veteran's Affairs Medical Center
West Haven, Connecticut

D. Blake Woodside, M.D.
Staff Psychiatrist, Eating Disorders Centre
Toronto General Hospital
Assistant Professor, Department of Psychiatry, University of Toronto
Toronto, Ontario, Canada

Foreword

Wen Joffe and Levitt invited me to write a foreword for this book, I accepted with enthusiasm. As they note, 19 years have elapsed since anyone attempted to assemble a coordinated series of statements about the relationships between thyroid state and behavior. Although all interested people probably share the sense that remarkable progress has been made, no one heretofore has surveyed it. I anticipated reading the manuscript as an important aspect of my education, and I have not been disappointed. I came away with more notes than could ever be incorporated into the paragraphs that follow and with more research ideas than can likely be executed, let alone funded.

The first four chapters of this book are basic, in two senses: they pertain to basic science, and they provide a foundation for the six clinical chapters that follow. Throughout the book, the authors have given careful attention to what is new and what is relevant to clinical issues, while maintaining perspective about the many decades of psychothyroidology that have gone before. (Incidentally, if "psychothyroidology" is a neologism on my part, so be it. I think its meaning is self-evident, and it is exactly what this book is about.)

In the first chapter, Dratman focuses on the details of thyroid transactions as they can be studied in laboratory animals. The reader gains insight at the cellular and subcellular level and comes to realize the myriad points at which the thyroid economy, of brain or of periphery, can be influenced. The brain, it seems, enjoys a series of fail-safe systems. But do these brain-guarding and brain-sparing mechanisms always function without fault? Dratman thinks that, compared with other organs, the brain is exquisitely sensitive to changes in thyroid economy when finally they occur. Indeed, in neonatal life, nothing can spare the brain the disaster of cretinism except an adequate supply of thyroid hormones from the infant's gland or from medication.

Energy metabolism is as much a concern of clinical science as of basic science, and its consideration by Levitt and Joffe in Chapter 2 provides a graceful bridge between the basic principles chapters and the clinical principles chapters of this book. Although the case for studying energy balance in eating disorders would seem prima facie, the authors build a case for studying it in affective disorders as well. Just as in affective disorders, in matters of energy balance both thyroid hormones and catecholamines are involved, sometimes interactively. Thyroid state, it would seem, is poised between being a target of nutritional intake and an agent of energy expenditure. In the latter case, peripheral events seem to account for most observations. Thus whether a study of energy metabolism is more useful than other approaches in psychothyroidology remains uncertain, but surely the effort is justified.

Licinio, Wong, and Gold broaden the perspective of the book when they take up the matter of interactions between the hypothalamic-pituitary-thyroid (HPT) axis and other endocrine systems in Chapter 3. Attention to this is critically important to progress in psychothyroidology. To understand the thyroid state of a patient, however thoroughly it may have been described, we need two other orders of information: a sense of what went before in the thyroid axis (a plea for longitudinal studies) and a sense of the broader endocrine context.

It is in patients with affective disorder that psychothyroidology so far has found its major place, and it is also in this group of patients that disturbances of the hypothalamic-pituitary-adrenal (HPA) axis are best described. It should not be astonishing, then, that the HPT and HPA axes are closely fitted, as Licinio and his colleagues show. But they are closely fitted, I think, not only at instants of time, but also across time. So far as I know, John Mason was the first to emphasize that, when experimental stress is prolonged, there occurs a sequence of responses by the organism: an autonomic response, an adrenal response, and finally a thyroidal response. In my view, it would be an error—surely not one committed by these authors—to think that the thyroidal response is less important for being delayed. It is probably chronic stress, not momentary danger, that produces changes of clinical significance.

Licinio and his colleagues invite the reader's attention to relationships that otherwise might be overlooked. One is that the insulin response to β-adrenergic agonists is a function of thyroid state. In a later chapter, Stein and Uhde state, rightly I think, that there is a need for measures of tissue response to thyroid hormones. Although several are known, what would be ideal is a measure of the response of brain, but we have no such measure, unless it is behavior itself. Lacking a dependent variable from brain that is readily measured, one might do well to assess some response of a peripheral tissue that seems to have special pertinence to brain. In this way, the measurement of insulin response to a β-adrenergic agonist has special appeal. Whybrow and I (1) once developed the view that thyroid-β-adrenergic interactions might be especially important for brain and thus for behavior.

Overlapping somewhat with the Dratman chapter, as it should, Chapter 4 by Chan and Singer strikes just the right note. The authors describe the remarkable advances in basic science that have permitted the clinical progress that, in turn, has made this book both necessary and useful. They provide a broad biological orientation. Thyroid glands are as characteristic of vertebrates as are their back bones. Just as the thyroid economy of the brain is regulated differently from that of the periphery, so may fetal (and neonatal) thyroid economy be different from that of the adult. The thyroid gland possesses a huge storage capacity. One appreciates that with this structure we vertebrates have found means not only of storing but also of concentrating and even recycling precious iodine, which, of course, is found most abundantly in the ocean.

In the first of the clinical chapters, Reus attempts the unenviable task of presenting the mental changes of patients with thyroid disease. It is unenviable because it has received attention now and again for almost 200 years. The subject is one side of descriptive psychothyroidology, the other, of course, being the HPT changes in psychiatric patients. In any case, Reus manages to maintain historical perspective, provide a comprehensive and structured survey, and develop a fresh point of view. He writes that hyperthyroid patients often present with something like agitated depression. I agree. Lesser representation, I think, can be regarded as tense dysphoria. If this pair of phrases does not encompass the spectrum of disability, at least they may provide clinical reminders.

To paraphrase Reus, one ought to be as mindful of the *cause* of an endocrine state as of the hormonal endpoint itself when thinking of mental consequences. Thus it may not be enough to consider the mental state of hypothyroid patients, qua hypothyroidism. Some may have arrived at that endpoint by inadequate hormone replacement after surgical operation, some from overprescription of antithyroid medication, some by a still active autoimmune process, and some by an exhausted autoimmune process. Hypothyroidism, then, has several possible causes, of which autoimmunity is the most common, but which can be of variable subtype, severity, and course. If brain can be an autoimmune target (not to mention a participant in some autoimmune processes), consideration of the immune process might yield a more refined understanding of mental symptoms than consideration of the endocrine endpoint alone.

Reus also points out that, other things being equal, as thyroid state diminishes, the tendency for seizure disorder increases. This provides a nice theoretical connection between what we know about the thyroid state of depressed patients and current concepts about the possible role of kindling in the cause and recurrence of affective disorders.

In Chapter 6, Joffe and Levitt show the reader the obverse of the coin displayed by Reus. They discuss the thyroid state of patients with affective disorders, having consigned the thyroid state of patients with other mental disorders to later chapters. However, this is only one of the three matters that they discuss. The others are *1)* what I am pleased to call *therapeutic* psychothyroidology and *2)* the effect of antidepressant drugs on thyroid state. Like Dratman's contribution, this chapter could readily be expanded to become its own book.

Joffe and Levitt present a measured statement of where matters stand in therapeutic psychothyroidology. What is remarkable, I think, is that such a discipline exists. There seems little place for hormones, other than hormones of the thyroid axis, in the treatment of mental disorders. Of course, I except from this generalization the use of hormones as replacement for frank deficiency when such deficiency has been accompanied by mental disorder. Among the several facets of therapeutic psychothyroidology that need to be refined are relationships between faults in the HPT axis and therapeutic response to one or another hormone of that axis.

Joffe and Levitt also review what is known about the effects of antidepressant and related drugs on thyroid axis function. To my knowledge, this is unavailable elsewhere, and it is enormously valuable.

Joffe and Levitt briefly present both sides of a controversy: Given that thyroid activation is often seen in depressed patients, is it an attempted compensation (for the presence of depression) or is it a contribution of cause? Should one seek to augment or diminish the thyroid state of the brain? Attempts to resolve this issue may have immense heuristic value, and I subscribe to the author's suggestions. I would add as a strategy the use of lithium as an antidepressant, with placebo, triiodothyronine (T3), or thyroxine (T4). I think lithium would be a *better* antidepressant if it were not for its antithyroid effect.

In their chapter on thyroid state and the anxiety disorders, Stein and Uhde open for us almost unexplored territory. For me, their presentation begins to sort out several related clinical puzzles. By using T3, they tried to augment the response to tricyclic antidepressant drugs of panic patients. The effort failed. Indeed, there was a tendency toward *aggravation* of panic. This makes sense, if one views panic patients as somehow having a tendency toward *hyper*thyroidism and thus, unlike depressed patients, experiencing a worsening of their condition with the ingestion of a thyroid hormone. However, no one has been able to show a clear fault of any kind in the thyroid axis of panic patients. I do wish, however, that workers in this field would study patients *during* a panic attack or at a series of points some of which by chance would be followed by an attack. Probably the brain, through thyrotropin-releasing hormone (TRH), can command quick responses in the HPT axis, though such responses are probably not the usual occupation of the HPT axis. If this is so, then it is possible that in some panic patients an outpouring of thyroid hormones (probably T3) will cause (or potentiate) other events on which the symptoms of the attack depend. It is true that under usual circumstances the thyroid gland secretes mainly T4, the long-acting hormone that needs deiodination to T3 for its action, but it is also true that if one administers a bolus of TRH (perhaps imitating an emergency signal from the brain), for a few minutes the thyroid gland preferentially secretes T3. In some vulnerable people an attack might follow minutes or hours later.

Among their other subjects, Stein and Uhde consider two studies with seemingly opposite results and offer a rationalization that, I think, could help clarify relationships between affective disorders and anxiety disorders. The authors of the first study found that a blunted response of thyroid-stimulating hormone (TSH) to infused TRH was especially characteristic of depressed patients if they were among the third or so who also experienced panic attacks. The authors of the second study, on the other hand, found no blunting in patients with "pure" panic disorder.

Stein and Uhde suggest that it may be the *conjunction* of depression and panic that accounts for TSH blunting, while neither disorder alone is often sufficient. What comes to mind is the similar formulation of Bauer et al. (2) that it may be the conjunction of the tendency for thyroid disorder and for bipolar disorder that brings a patient to threshold for rapid cycling.

In Chapter 8, Garbutt, Loosen, and I outline some of the main themes that connect the HPT axis with alcoholism. I will recite three. First, quite a few utterly "dry" alcoholic patients with no evidence of transient hyperthyroxinemia show a blunted TSH response to TRH. One can conclude from this that not all blunting in, say, depressed patients needs be due to hyperthyroxinemia. Second, propylthiouracil, an inhibitor of the conversion of T_4 to T_3, has been used to prolong the survival of alcoholic patients with severe liver disease. Third, in animal preparations, TRH has both "proalcohol" and "antialcohol" properties (i.e., it acts like alcohol [and anxiolytics] in a conflict paradigm); it shortens sedation produced by alcohol or any of several other central nervous system depressants. This observation begs for clinical application.

Kaplan and Woodside bring the reader up to date on the subject of thyroid state and eating disorders in Chapter 9. One comes away from this chapter with a greatly enhanced appreciation of how thyroid state and nutritional state are intricately related, in both the short term and the long term. This renders plausible the notion that thyroid dysfunction could contribute to eating disorders. Perhaps it can, but there is presently little evidence to support this idea. Thyroid abnormalities abound in eating disorders, but they can generally be regarded as the consequences of altered nutrition. As I read this elegant presentation, I heard an echo from earlier chapters: studies of peripheral thyroid state may tell us little of brain thyroid state. Kaplan and Woodside end with a clinical admonition: confronted with a patient with an eating disorder, rule out the possibility of thyroid hormone abuse.

The book concludes with a brief chapter by Joffe and Levitt that provides as much as can be written, to my knowledge, about schizophrenia and the thyroid axis. In schizophrenic patients, HPT findings are not prominent and tend to be inconsistent. Furthermore, the effects of neuroleptic drugs on thyroid state tend to be variable. On a more positive note, the authors point out that for purposes of sorting out HPT findings, it may be more fruitful to think of psychosis versus no psychosis than to adhere to more usual diagnostic distinctions. They also offer a brief statement of some interactions between thyroid state and dopaminergic transactions. This is germane, of course, because of the prevailing concept that dopaminergic function is disturbed in schizophrenic patients. Some readers will think that this chapter could have been omitted. I would disagree. Null findings in schizophrenia, apart from suggesting the need for more research, serve a similar function as the sharpening of thyroid distinctions between affective and anxiety disorders. They lend an element of specificity, and specificity has never been abundant in psychoendocrinology.

Joffe and Levitt have assembled an enormously valuable book. Its value for clinicians is self-evident, and clinician-researchers cannot do without it. By "clinicians" I do not mean only psychiatrists. I think that psychiatry is prominent among several clinical disciplines that, along with basic science, have directed thyroidology to the brain.

Arthur J. Prange, Jr., M.D.

REFERENCES

1. Whybrow PC, Prange AJ Jr: A hypothesis of thyroid-catecholamine-receptor interaction. Arch Gen Psychiatry 38:106–113, 1981
2. Bauer MS, Whybrow PC, Winokur A: Rapid cycling bipolar affective disorder, I: association with grade I hypothyroidism. Arch Gen Psychiatry 47:427–432, 1990

Preface

The study of brain-endocrine relationships and their impact on behavior has long been a fundamental and central component of biological psychiatry. A concerted research effort and resultant vast literature have implicated a wide range of hormones in the modulation of emotions and behavior and in the pathophysiology of various psychiatric disorders. Among these hormones, those of the thyroid axis have received considerable attention. The classical descriptions of psychiatric sequelae of clinical thyroid disorders provided the early impetus for investigation of the role of thyroid hormones in the etiology, diagnosis, and treatment of various psychiatric disorders. Most attention has been paid to the mood disorders, but the potential importance of the thyroid axis in anxiety, eating disorders, alcohol abuse, and psychotic disorders, among others, has received increasing attention over the past years.

A rich and diverse literature now exists on the relationship between thyroid function and a variety of psychiatric disorders. Despite this, there have been few attempts to organize or consolidate this body of data. A chapter summarizing the role of thyroid hormones in psychiatric illness, particularly affective disorders, appears in many standard texts of psychiatry or psychoendocrinology. However, the last volume devoted entirely to this topic, *The Thyroid Axis, Drugs and Behavior* edited by Arthur J. Prange, Jr., was published in 1974. Since that time, there has been an overwhelming increase in studies, not only those examining the relationship between thyroid function and psychiatric disorder, but also those elucidating basic thyroid physiology as it pertains to psychiatric illness. In the last 10 years, there has been increasing evidence that thyroid hormones have an effect on mature brain function. Furthermore, animal studies also suggest that brain utilization of thyroid hormones differs from that of peripheral organs. These advances create exciting possibilities for further studies examining the role of thyroid hormones in psychiatric illness.

The purpose of this book is clear. It is an attempt to consolidate a vast literature into a single volume and is intended to serve as a reference book for both basic scientists and clinicians in the field of psychiatry and the behavioral sciences. To achieve this purpose, the book is divided into two parts. Part I, "Basic Principles," deals in depth with selected aspects of thyroid axis physiology. The aim of this part is not to replicate the information contained in standard textbooks of endocrinology nor to be comprehensive in discussion of the anatomy and physiology of various components of the thyroid axis; rather, it examines issues that are particularly pertinent to understanding thyroid function as it relates to various psychiatric disorders. We have, therefore, focused on brain-thyroid relationships, the interaction of thyroid hormones with other hormonal systems, and their relationship with nutrition and metabolism. Part II, "Clinical Principles," deals with current knowledge of the relationship between thyroid function and specific psychiatric disorders. Each chapter stands alone as a comprehensive review by experts in the area. The overlap in information between chapters reflects the overlap in psychiatric illness, and we hope this will lend a richness to the text.

Over the last 8 years, there has been an opportunity in both Bethesda, Maryland, and in our own clinics in Toronto to examine in detail the fascinating complexities of the psychoendocrinology of the thyroid axis. These years of academic and research work, together with the time involved in compiling this book, have given us a greater appreciation of the seminal contributions to the field made by Prange and those associated with him including Loosen, Garbutt, Whybrow, and the late Morris Lipton. Our own contribution, albeit small, has hopefully been made with the combination of academic rigor, personal integrity, and human compassion taught and exemplified by our mentors and colleagues, Dan R. Offord of McMaster University, Hamilton, Ontario, Canada, and Robert M. Post of the National Institute of Mental Health. As with the aim of this book, our debt to them is clear.

If this book succeeds in its aim, the credit should go to the various contributors. They have responded to our charge of providing a thorough, clinically relevant review of the data. In addition, they have presented the many controversies, ambiguities, and unanswered questions that will be left to the future to resolve. It is our intent that this book—as with any book designed as a reference text for students, clinicians, and researchers—will not only provide a source of information about the role of the thyroid axis in psychiatric illness, but will also provoke discussion and stimulate ideas that will promote further research and understanding of this complex subject.

Russell T. Joffe, M.D.
Anthony J. Levitt, M.D.

PART I

Basic Principles

Chapter 1

Cerebral Versus Peripheral Regulation and Utilization of Thyroid Hormones

Mary B. Dratman, M.D.

CONTENTS

Appreciation is expressed to my long-standing collaborators, Janice T. Gordon, Effie K. Erlichman, and Floy L. Crutchfield, and to Marie C. Tomlinson for her expertise in editing this text. Current support is provided by the Medical Research Service, Philadelphia VA Medical Center, Patricia Kind Fund for Brain Research, and National Institute of Mental Health Grants 44210 and 45252.

1. INTRODUCTION

All vertebrate organisms have the capacity to concentrate iodine and produce iodothyronines. Requirements for iodoamino acids increase in the evolutionary sequence from protochordate to primate. In humans, iodothyronine deficiencies produce major abnormalities in growth, development, reproduction, metabolic adaptation, and function of the central and peripheral autonomic nervous system.

Present-day experimental approaches to the problem of thyroid hormone action are heavily influenced by significant advances made in understanding the cellular site and mechanism of action of other hormones and by rapid changes occurring in both the technology and the philosophy of hormone research. The widespread application of methods of molecular biology to the study of hormone action has added to the field of biochemical endocrinology the kinds of new dimensions that the discovery of the microscope provided for the field of tissue morphology.

As a result of these advances, previously inviolate tenets of endocrinology have given way to more fluid concepts of the way hormones are produced and how they work. Distinctions among different kinds of chemical messengers have become more tenuous, and overlapping functions have become widely recognized. Not only do endocrine and neuroendocrine cells produce hormones, but individual amine precursor uptake and decarboxylation (APUD) cells, dispersed singly or in clusters throughout a variety of tissues, can store and release functionally active amines and peptides of an amazing variety. Whereas hormones were once thought to be disseminated only via the bloodstream, they are now known to travel through whatever channels are available to them. Their products may even be released into the surrounding extracellular fluid, allowing hormone to be conveyed from a secreting cell directly to other cells occupying a contiguous space. Because moment-to-moment changes in femtomolar quantities of hormone, as well as their functional consequences, may be measured by assays conducted at light- and electron-microscopic levels of resolution and tracked by freeze fracture and patch-clamp techniques, insights into cellular hormone kinetics are providing new levels of appreciation for the beauty and complexity of hormonal systems.

Many previously confusing aspects of hormone action have been clarified by recognition that hormone action and hormone metabolism are interdependent processes. Not all hormone metabolites are generated in or are available to all tissues and not all receptive tissues are responsive to the same metabolite. These principles have been dramatically illustrated by observations regarding some steroid receptors that cannot uniformly distinguish between glucocorticoids and the mineralocorticoid, aldosterone. It happens that in the tissues in which this distinction is crucial, there is an enzymatic apparatus for rapidly converting glucocorticoids to a molecular form that makes them inaccessible for binding to the mineralocorticoid receptor (e.g., through conversion of cortisol to cortisone). On the other hand, in other tissues, notably brain, where the distinction is apparently not relevant, no such glucocorticoid-metabolizing mechanism exists.

Hormone actions are now known to be limited not only by their rate, route, efficiency of dissemination, metabolism, and half-life in extracellular fluids, but also by the nature and availability of their cellular receptors. The biochemical transformations resulting from hormone receptor–binding interactions are being unraveled in intricate detail. These transformations in turn produce widely different cellular effects, depending on both the classification of the receptor and the nature of its ligand. Hormone receptor complexes can cause ion channels to open or close; they can incite the formation of second messengers; they can reorganize the distribution of calcium within the cell; and they can alter affinities of one cell constituent for another or change the nature of existing proteins through adding or subtracting substituents (via phosphorylations, amidations, hydroxylations, and glycosylations). Possibly most decisively, they can alter the nature of the protein assemblies that express the functional intentions of each cell, tissue, organ, and organism. Because these processes are better understood, new appreciation of interrelationships among hormones has developed through overarching classifications of hormones according to their shared transduction systems, their receptor families and hierarchies, their common DNA response elements, and the ability of different receptors bound to different ligands to form multimeric units that then act in concert to alter transcription.

Finally, a new way of understanding central nervous system (CNS) requirements for and response to peripheral hormones is emerging. Almost every somatically active hormone is represented in the brain, through de novo synthesis or controlled admission across the brain barrier systems. Receptors for biogenic amines, peptides, and steroid and thyroid hormones are concentrated within discrete neural networks in which they are in a position to influence both the development and the adult function of the brain. It therefore seems evident that further knowledge of the distribution, metabolism, receptor interactions, and fate of hormones in the CNS and their relationships with one another will help elucidate many currently obscure aspects of the functions of the two major information-transmitting systems: the endocrine system and the nervous system.

Presently, far too little is known about thyroid hormone actions in brain. Even so, a great deal has been learned recently. To review this knowledge and describe its unique features, in this chapter the course and vicissitudes of newly synthesized thyroid hormone molecules are tracked from their inception in the thyroid gland to the time of their irreversible loss from the body. Some of these molecules are followed as they enter what are considered their major somatic tissue targets: heart, liver, kidney, and skeletal muscle. A somewhat different fate awaits molecules entering tissues particularly rich in noradrenergic innervation. However, hormone molecules examined during their travels through the brain will receive the most attention. The presently known differences between thyroid hormone processing in brain and in periphery will then become apparent.

Throughout this chapter, emphasis is placed on often overlooked sources of problems related to thyroid hormone. Thus even subtle and, therefore, potentially unrecognized thyroid receptor abnormalities or thyroid hormone deficiencies or excesses during fetal and perinatal growth and development may underlie mild adult-onset manifestations of abnormal brain function. In other words, there are problems short of full-blown cretinism that may be caused by brain defects arising from unrecognized, transient, or mild hypothyroidism during fetal or early postnatal life. Further, recurrent exacerbations of chronic or relapsing thyroiditis may lead to sporadic changes in thyroid hormone availability or cyclicity without necessarily grossly altering thyroid function tests. Likewise, changes in the spectrum of carrier proteins, blood-brain barriers, or choroid plexus proteins may contribute to defects in supplying thyroid hormones to the brain. Many of these possible etiologies could exist without producing changes in circulating levels of thyroid-stimulating hormone (TSH) or the thyroid hormones themselves. As a result, reliable identification of brain–thyroid hormone dysfunctions may only come from discovery of methods for making direct measurements of thyroid hormone–processing activities in brain in vivo. In the meantime, astute clinicians proceeding with an open mind on a case-by-case basis, assembling detailed data relevant to developmental and family histories and currently available, though not necessarily routine, thyroid function tests (see Chapter 4), will help to identify patients whose mechanisms for maintaining brain–thyroid hormone homeostasis may be derailed. If we can learn to make these diagnoses, it seems likely that effective methods of treatment will follow.

However, there is no intention to suggest that thyroid hormones are themselves at the center of any particular functional disorders of the brain. Rather, emphasis is directed toward understanding the participation of these hormones as one set of instruments in the brain orchestra. As such, they may be involved in setting the keys, major or minor, for certain themes, and possibly their tempi, expressed as affective states, motor activities, autonomic functions, and cognitive processes, developed and recurring through the lifetime of the individual.

2. THE THYROID GLAND

2.1 Functional Properties and Control Mechanisms

The thyroid gland is a highly reactive tissue, organized to carry out a series of transport and enzyme-mediated steps that culminate in the formation and secretion of thyroxine (T_4) (1). Although under some extreme conditions of thyroid hormone deficiency, coinciding with abundant iodine availability, extrathyroidal synthesis of thyroxine may occur in minute amounts, the sites and control mechanisms for this purported synthesis have not been identified. It is generally, if tacitly, accepted in both the laboratory and the clinical setting that the ultimate source of endogenously available T_4 is the thyroid gland. Thyroid hormones are found in almost all animal tissues. Therefore, a certain amount will be obtained on a regular basis by individuals in the course of ingesting meat or fish. Coprophagia provides another source of (recycled) hormone.

2.2 Physiology

a. Thyroid hormone biosynthesis

Whatever the form of ingested inorganic iodine, it is eventually converted to iodide and absorbed as such into the circulation. An energy-dependent, high-affinity transport mechanism carries the iodide from the bloodstream into the thyroid follicular cells, resulting in a 1:20 to 1:200 gradient of serum to tissue iodide concentration (2). Normally, the transported inorganic halide is instantaneously transformed by thyroid peroxidase to an activated state that promotes conversion of accessible tyrosyl residues in thyroglobulin to iodotyrosyl residues. The mechanism of this conversion involves formation of a carbon-iodine bond at the 3 position of the aromatic ring of peptide-bound tyrosines, yielding peptide-bound iodotyrosines. This is the so-called organification step of intrathyroidal iodine metabolism, a process that occurs so rapidly that except in instances of inborn or acquired defects in thyroid hormone biosynthesis, little free iodide is found within the thyroid follicular cell cytosol. Abnormalities in the organification process can be detected through the use of the perchlorate discharge test.

The process of iodide organification and iodothyronine formation (Figure 1–1) is dominated by thyroid peroxidase (3), which requires (at least) two substrates: iodide and thyroglobulin. Thyroglobulin is the major protein product of the thyroid follicular cell; it is a heavily glycosylated globular protein that is stored in a carbohydrate-rich matrix known as the *colloid*, held within the extracellular lumen of the thyroid follicle.

Iodination of thyroglobulin (i.e., organification) takes place at the interface between the thyroglobulin-rich colloid and the apical membrane of the follicular cell, where strong peroxidase activity mediates the organification reaction (4). Because some of thyroglobulin's tyrosyl residues have been replaced by iodotyrosyl residues and the newly formed iodothyroglobulin now has a different primary structure, changes in thyroglobulin tertiary structure ensue, which brings intramolecular iodotyrosyl residues into closer proximity. Again, in the presence of peroxidase, formation of single iodothyronyl residues from varying combinations of two iodotyrosyl residues, with elimination of one alanyl side chain, proceeds, though rather slowly and sparingly. In mature iodothyroglobulin, the ratio of iodotyrosyl to iodothyronyl residues is approximately 4:1. The major thyronyl product is in the tetraiodo form, but some triiodo and reverse triiodo forms are also created. Genesis from coupled tyrosines has led to the suggestion that the secreted hormones, which, strictly speaking, are diphenyl aromatic amino acids, might also be seen as (di)peptides. Such molecular distinctions are obviously important in considering possible mechanisms of thyroid hormone action in brain (5).

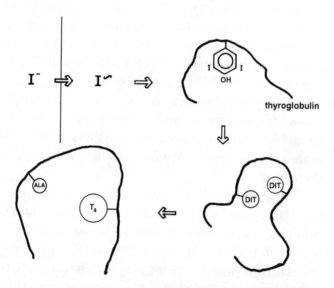

Figure 1–1. Biosynthetic route of iodothyronine formation in thyroid gland. *Following the arrows and reading clockwise from upper left:* Iodide ions (I⁻) are actively transported from serum across the plasma membrane of the thyroid follicular cells where they are converted by thyroid peroxidase to a reactive form capable of iodinating tyrosyl residues in thyroglobulin. Tyrosyl iodination promotes rearrangement of tertiary thyroglobulin structure, facilitating covalent coupling of two peptide-bound diiodotyrosine (DIT) residues with formation of one peptide-bound residue of thyroxine (T_4) and one of alanine (ALA). *Not shown:* Proteolysis of thyroglobulin releases the newly formed amino acid T_4, a hormonally active amino acid synthesized and released from a large protein precursor by means of directed proteolysis. *Source.* From Dratman MB, Crutchfield FL, Gordon JT: "Thyroid Hormones and Adrenergic Neurotransmitters," in *Catecholamines, Neuropharmacology and Central Nervous System: Theoretical Aspects.* Edited by Usdin E. New York, Alan R Liss, 1984, pp. 425–439. Used with permission.

As noted, the iodination state of extracellularly stored thyroglobulin depends on the protein synthetic potential of the gland (for synthesis of both thyroglobulin and peroxidase), as well as on iodine availability. The storage of a large pool of thyroid hormone precursor in the thyroid gland in the form of iodothyroglobulin is reminiscent of certain precursor-product relationships in the CNS. For example, peptides destined for neuromodulatory functions are initially peptide bound within the matrix of much larger protein molecules; the proteins must be attacked by peptidases before their active constituents can become available for their assigned roles in synaptic function. This storage function represents yet another control mechanism presumably designed to generate rapidly, on demand, active molecular species that might not otherwise be readily available for the millisecond-timed functional requirements of neural networks.

It appears that the thyroid gland also synthesizes hormone in two main stages: a relatively leisurely stage of collecting the rare element iodine and assembling large stores of peptide-bound hormone precursor (iodinated thyroglobulin) and a stage during which rapid release of hormone would be feasible if required. The latter process is accomplished when TSH or other secretion-inducing stimuli are brought to bear. In response, colloid droplets are taken up by reverse pinocytosis into the follicular cell cytosol where they are subject to proteolytic digestion by lysosomal proteases acting at an acid pH. The resulting lysis of peptide bonds leads to intracytosolic accumulation of free iodotyrosines and iodothyronines (6,7).

b. Secretory products of the thyroid follicle

The biosynthetic pathway that leads to the formation of thyroid hormones results in the formation of a novel series of amino acids: the iodotyrosines and their coupled products, the iodothyronines. Ordinarily, iodothyronines are the only iodocompounds released from the thyroid gland into the bloodstream. The iodotyrosine contents of thyroglobulin hydrolysates are intercepted before release by the enzyme iodotyrosine deiodinase, with resultant intrathyroidal release of tyrosine and free iodide. The latter is then subject to immediate recycling through the T_4 biosynthetic pathway. As products of colloid hydrolysis are being absorbed into the bloodstream, some intact thyroglobulin may also enter the venous capillaries or may find its way into the circulation indirectly, through uptake into the lymphatics draining the thyroid gland.

Although T_4 is the main secretory product of the thyroid follicle, some triiodothyronine (T_3) and reverse triiodothyronine (rT_3) are also released, the former in a molar ratio to T_4 of about 1:7. The molecular structures and main sources of these hormones are represented in Figure 1–2. The ratio of secreted T_3 to T_4 increases under circumstances that tend to increase TSH or TSH-like activity (e.g., iodine deficiency, hypothyroidism, and Graves' disease). The ratio may also change in response to autonomic nervous system activity, transmitted to the gland through the superior cervical ganglia (8). Proportions of T_3 to T_4 in the circulation are immediately changed as a result of differences in the distribution space of the secreted iodothyronines; the much more rapid serum disappearance rate of T_3 tends to lower the ratio, whereas the ratio is raised by T_4-derived T_3 (and rT_3), which is continuously exchanged between serum and tissues. Nevertheless, even in high T_3-forming states, T_4 is the predominant iodothyronine in the circulation, normally found at a concentration of about 100–130

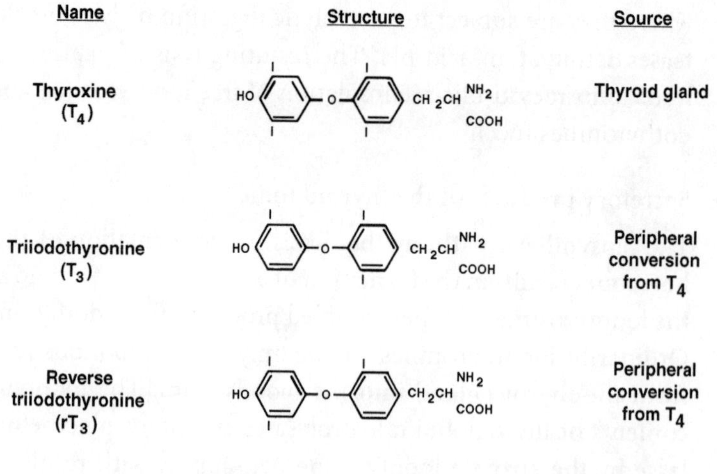

Name	Structure	Source
Thyroxine (T_4)		Thyroid gland
Triiodothyronine (T_3)		Peripheral conversion from T_4
Reverse triiodothyronine (rT_3)		Peripheral conversion from T_4

Figure 1–2. Molecular structures and major sources of the active iodothyronines.

nmol, whereas the concentration of T_3 is normally about 2–3 nmol. Because the distribution space for T_4 is much smaller than that for T_3 (170 versus 660 ml/kg), the total extrathyroidal T_4 and T_3 concentrations of a 70-kg person are approximately 1,200 and 55 µg, respectively, without considering the iodothyronyl residues stored in thyroglobulin (9,10).

A diurnal cycle of T_4 concentrations in serum has not been identified in human subjects, and, in healthy individuals, basal serum iodothyronine concentrations are remarkably stable from day to day, and even from year to year. At the same time, large changes in the demand for hormone occur constantly in response to the vicissitudes of daily life, such as carbohydrate ingestion (11), exercise (12), sleep deprivation (13), cold exposure (14,15), and photoperiod changes (16). The net stability of circulating hormones is therefore a testimonial to the sensitivity and efficiency of multilevel feedback mechanisms that detect and respond to changes in circulating and tissue hormone concentrations. Factors directly involved in both altering and stabilizing the serum iodothyronine pool include controlled thyroid gland secretion, tissue hormone uptake, metabolism, recycling, and irreversible disposal.

Thyroid hormone freshly secreted from the thyroid gland into the bloodstream is the source of iodothyronine renewal after previously secreted molecules have made their rounds through the organism and have been metabolized and finally excreted in feces or through the kidney. The penetration of secreted hormone into extracellular and intracellular fluid spaces and its rate of membrane and receptor binding determines its so-called space of distribution: the amount of volume the hormone would occupy if its concentration throughout the entire body were the same as that in the serum. Because the volume of distribution of T_3 (about 700 ml/kg body weight), for example, approaches that of the body volume, it is evident that most of the extravascular hormone has been instantaneously *1)* concentrated in bodily tissues, *2)* sequestered in an extracellular space (e.g., gut lumen), or *3)* excreted. By comparison, the distribution space of T_4 is much smaller than that of T_3 (about 175 ml/kg), reflecting both its higher affinity for serum

binding proteins and its relatively lesser affinity for cellular transport carriers or mechanisms of entry into cells. These measured
differences between these thyroid hormones have led to the loose
but convenient concept of T_4 as the extracellular and T_3 as the intracellular thyroid hormone (17).

2.3   Common Factors Adversely Affecting Thyroid Gland Function

a. **Iodine deficiency**

Goiter and hypothyroidism occur frequently, particularly among
females, even in iodine-sufficient regions of the world, where
these abnormalities can rarely be attributed to lack of dietary
iodine. Nevertheless, in searching for an underlying cause of presumed thyroid dysfunction, the possibility of dietary iodine deficiency (currently, or more importantly, during early childhood)
may be worth considering; enclaves of iodine insufficiency may
exist in isolated communities in the midst of an iodine-sufficient
region.

In contrast with the situation in most developed Western soci-
eties, large segments of the earth's population experience moderate to severe iodine deprivation (18,19). On this basis, they are
strongly goiter prone and may develop hypothyroidism at any age
and any stage of development. The consequences are tragic for the
overall mental health of the affected population. The tragedy is
particularly regrettable because iodine deficiency is entirely preventable (20). Iodine deficiency is the major cause of coinciding
maternal and fetal hypothyroidism, a combination that has the
greatest potential for exerting adverse effects on fetal nervous system development (21–23). Unfortunately, the affected populations have been virtually ignored as sources of prospective
information regarding in vivo brain morphological and metabolic
change in response to hypothyroidism. Yet, the so-called unaffected members of these groups may reveal much about subtle
functional effects of developmentally experienced hypothyroidism, effects that may be completely masked in overt cretinism.

By the same token, there are many patients in the iodine-
sufficient world with early-onset, relatively chronic, mild degrees

of learning impairment, social malfunction, or mood disorder. These individuals may be worthy of study with the aim of retrospectively identifying a source of transient or mild hypothyroidism (not necessarily related to iodine deficiency but occurring during perinatal life) as a cause for their functional debilities. Investigators considering such studies may be deterred by the fact that known examples of thyroid-related brain damage during development almost always reflect the results of severe disease, with gross abnormalities evident in the affected individuals. However, gradations of these severe effects are bound to occur. Efforts to unmask a thyroid-related etiology in minimally affected subjects may turn out to be a fruitful enterprise.

b. **Iodine excess**

A pulse of iodine, delivered in the form of skin antiseptics or iodine-containing drugs, not uncommonly precedes the appearance of hypo- or hyperthyroidism in individuals with diminished thyroid gland reserve, as in multinodular goiter, or in those with acquired defects of thyroid hormone biosynthesis, especially autoimmune thyroiditis (24). Similar responses are sometimes seen in patients with apparently normal glands (25). Iodine-induced thyroid dysfunction may persist long after the exogenous source of iodine has been removed.

Most healthy individuals show no functionally observable responses to excess iodine, although thyroid function may be inactivated temporarily by an iodine load (26). However, this, the so-called Wolff-Chaikoff phenomenon, is a short-lived process, and normal thyroid function is soon resumed. Exposure to excess iodine during late pregnancy may place the offspring at risk for goiter formation massive enough to interfere with initial respiratory efforts, causing secondary brain damage (27). Direct toxic effects of excess iodine are not infrequent, but these appear to be independent of changes in thyroid gland function.

c. **Naturally occurring goitrogens**

Thyroid gland function may be adversely affected by elements in the diet that inhibit peroxidase activity (28). The resulting de-

crease in iodothyronine biosynthetic potential may cause secondary TSH stimulation and goiter formation. These well-established
but often ignored sources of generally mild glandular malfunction
appear to produce only sporadic cases of identifiable disease, even
among seemingly uniform populations exposed to the same dietary goitrogens. However, the role of these dietary sources in individual patients may be significant even if occult. A thorough
search for the etiology of an obscure thyroid disorder should include consideration of these dietary sources of peroxidase inhibitors. As the full range of dietary inhibitors of peroxidase remains
to be identified, all dietary peculiarities, especially those occurring
during developmentally significant periods of life, should be carefully considered.

d. Life cycles and aging

Shifting requirements for thyroid hormones throughout life make
considerable demands on the thyroid gland. This is particularly
true for females, whose glandular activities vary with each phase
of the menstrual cycle, each pregnancy, and the ovarian involu-
tional period, as well as with the usual metabolic adjustments required during growth, development, illness, and psychological
stress (29). Structural features of the normal gland change as these
demands are experienced and responded to; histological areas of
hyperplasia and postinvolutional fibrosis accumulate. Such fairly
ubiquitous changes do not in themselves cause functional abnormalities, although they may lead to limitations of homeostatic vir-
tuosity. Because ovarian cyclicity and pregnancy are important
determinants of this type of structural-functional thyroid gland
reorganization, they may contribute to the high female-to-male
ratio (8:1) of patients with known thyroid disease. However, an
inherent X-linked predisposition probably more nearly explains
the selective sensitivity of females to these disorders; the strong
familial incidence of autoimmune thyroid disease also suggests
participation of genetic mechanisms. Underlying inborn abnormalities in B-cell functions (involved in cell-mediated immunity)
have been suggested as a common pathway leading to autoimmune susceptibility.

e. **Autoimmune thyroid disease**

In addition to the demands of life cycles and life situations, certain particular features of thyroid gland structural organization are thought to make this tissue especially vulnerable to autoimmune processes. In a manner characteristic of macrophages, but not of ordinary tissue cell types, thyroid follicular cells are capable of presenting antigen on their cell surfaces, allowing peroxidase, antigenically related microsomal proteins, thyroglobulin, and other follicular cell macromolecules to incite antibody production (30). Moreover, the structural similarities among elements in gastric mucosa and thyroid gland microsomes and thyroid peroxidase may encourage cross reactions among antibodies raised against these classes of protein (31,32). Therefore, thyroid gland autoimmunity should be suspected in patients manifesting parietal cell antibodies or frank pernicious anemia. Patients with the triad of insulin-dependent diabetes mellitus (type I), adrenal insufficiency, and Hashimoto's disease (thyroiditis) speak to the possibility of other shared antibody responses among different endocrine glands. Thus *disease in one endocrine system should signal interest in, and, under some circumstances, even full-fledged investigations of, all the others* (33).

Certain features of autoimmune thyroid disease deserve special mention. Hashimoto's disease is often occult and, therefore, frequently remains undiagnosed. It appears that, in some phases, dysregulation of hormone production may be subtle but associated changes in brain function may be unexpectedly prominent (34). Patients with autoimmune thyroiditis sometimes acquire defects in hormonogenesis that resemble those that are ordinarily inborn, such as failure of organification or coupling. These deficiencies may then be compensated for through overactivity of relatively intact functions of the gland. Because of the entrainment of compensatory mechanisms, gross abnormalities in peripheral thyroid function may not surface, but homeostatic responsiveness may be impaired and there may be unexpected untoward consequences. For example, even seemingly minimal thyroid lesions may lead to increased susceptibility to iodide-induced, overt hypo- or hyperthyroidism, emerging as superimpositions on the underlying thyroid disorder (24,25). These frank abnormalities may occur in settings that deflect attention away from the diagnosis of thyroid disease because they are often complicated by nonthyroidal medical or surgical illness.

Several researchers (35,36) have also observed an unusual concentration of symptomatic autoimmune disease occurring within the first few months after parturition. The cause is unknown, but a possible relationship to postpartum depression is intriguing.

Unfortunately, even when suspected, the diagnosis of autoimmune thyroid disease may be difficult to establish rigorously. The disease is notoriously subject to unaccountable remissions and exacerbations, so that, when looked for, the disease may be relatively quiescent. Although antiperoxidase, antimicrosomal, antithyroglobulin, and anti-TSH-receptor autoantibodies have been implicated in the genesis and progression of many cases of autoimmune thyroiditis, patients presenting with measurable antibody titers probably constitute only the tip of the iceberg. In cases where cell-mediated events predominate, humeral antibody production may be a secondary phenomenon and, as a result, circulating antibody titers may be low or late in appearance. Even tissue obtained at open biopsy may be difficult to classify; the difficulties are compounded if the tissue is obtained by needle biopsy. Because the diagnosis of autoimmune thyroid disease is so complex and sometimes so elusive, its identification as the cause of thyroid-related disorders of mental function is often delayed or even overlooked entirely. The reported high incidence of reduced cell-mediated immune function in patients with clinical depression makes the search for clarification even more relevant.

Autoimmune thyroid disease accounts for both Hashimoto's and Graves' disease, each generally but not necessarily accompanied by hypothyroidism and hyperthyroidism, respectively. It is always surprising to rediscover the diversity of antithyroid antibody effects: growth stimulating or inhibiting, function stimulating or inhibiting, alternately or even simultaneously affecting thyroid gland activity (30). Retrospectively obtained information in cases of current, easily diagnosed, overt Graves' disease–induced hyperthyroidism often reveals variable periods, sometimes extending over many years, replete with symptomatology in the physical and emotional realm, which might logically be attributed to thyroid abnormality. Moreover, Graves' disease may be preceded (months or years) by a well-substantiated period of hypothyroidism indistinguishable from the hypothyroidism of Hashimoto's thyroiditis. Careful histories from patients with full-blown syndromes of hyper- or hypothyroidism indicate that failure to diagnose individuals who are in the preovert phases of their disease must be common. These may be the most interesting cases to identify and study given the likely benefit to the patient, as well as the advancement of knowledge of the disorders.

Alternating periods of hyper- and hypofunction of the thyroid gland may also be seen in thyroiditis of the relapsing or lymphocytic type. Hyperthyroid phases are caused by thyroid cell death and massive release of stored hormone. These are followed by hypothyroid phases of variable duration in which recovery of the injured thyroid gland is delayed by TSH suppression due to a persistent leakage of hormone into the circulation (37,38). Patients with this condition could be in a particularly vulnerable state with regard to their mental functions. However, as indicated in the sections that follow, underlying problems in the brain appear to be a precondition for the development of significant mental disorders in response to altered thyroid gland function.

3.   THE BRAIN-PITUITARY-THYROID AXIS

Homeostatic control mechanisms normally maintain the euthyroid level of thyroid gland function. Tissue and whole body demands for shifting thyroid hormone supplies are perceived within and funneled through a brain pituitary unit linked to the thyroid gland through chemical and neural signals. New information regarding one brain component of this axis has recently come to the fore. The paraventricular nucleus (PVN) of the hypothalamus contains nerve cell bodies heavily committed to the synthesis of thyrotropin-releasing hormone (TRH). Rates of assembly of TRH precursor protein and subsequent release of TRH are modified through a number of different pathways, including noradrenergic and neuropeptide Y inputs to the PVN-TRH cells (39).

However, as presently understood (see Figure 1–3), the major influence on this process is derived from a negative feedback mechanism that detects deficiencies or excesses of thyroid hormone molecules reaching the PVN and brings about a corresponding increase or decrease in TRH synthesis and release. Not surprisingly, therefore, the PVN does not exhibit strong T_4-to-T_3 converting activity, in keeping with the suggestion that this brain nucleus is geared to react to hormone levels in blood as they are perceived by the brain (40–42). TRH, released in a pulsatile fashion from its synaptic terminals in the median eminence, enters the hypothalamic-pituitary portal circulation and reaches the pituitary thyrotrophs (43). To be active, TRH molecules must be amidated; in that state, they are subject to inactivation by peptidases and (de)amidases; these enzyme activities are themselves responsive to thyroid hormone levels in the median eminence and pituitary; the participation of all of these factors contributes to the final quantity of TRH available for receptor occupancy (44,45). In the absence of TRH, due to hypothalamic hypothyroidism for example, the molecular

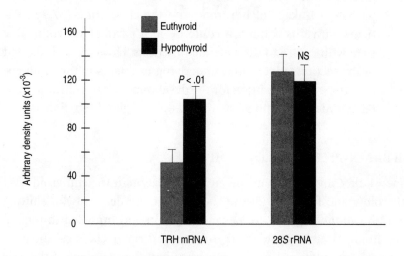

Figure 1–3. Comparison of quantitative Northern blot analysis of pro-thyrotropin-releasing hormone (TRH) mRNA from euthyroid and hypothyroid rat paraventricular nucleus (PVN) extracts. Density units (ordinate) determined by computer image analysis of Northern blots. Note selectivity of effect of hypothyroidism on TRH mRNA (i.e., no effect on 28S ribosomal RNA [rRNA]). *Source.* From Segerson TP, Kauer J, Wolfe HC, et al: "Thyroid Hormone Regulates TRH Biosynthesis in the Paraventricular Nucleus of the Rat Hypothalamus." *Science* 238:78–80, 1987. Copyright 1987 by AAAS. Used with permission.

form of TSH produced by thyrotropic cells exhibits defective biological activity even though it retains its ability to be detected in the immuno-assays for TSH (46,47).

TRH receptors decorating pituitary thyrotrophs transmit the constantly changing TRH message to the TSH-synthesizing apparatus via a calcium-phosphoinositol second messenger pathway, resulting in appropriate in-creases or decreases in TSH-subunit production rates and subsequent changes in TSH release rates (43). As a final consequence, circulating levels of TSH are modified. However, a negative feedback system operates inde-pendently at the level of the pituitary gland (48); high thyroid hormone concentrations perceived by the thyrotrophs will suppress TSH produc-tion and/or release even if TRH levels are markedly increased, as occurs during TRH testing in hyperthyroid patients. The strong influence of in-trapituitary thyroid hormones and thyroid hormone metabolism on TSH production and release rates accounts for many important aspects of the TRH stimulation test. Particular features and paradoxes about pituitary T_4 metabolism are discussed in subsequent sections of this chapter.

Although TRH and circulating levels of T_4 are the main coordinators of TSH synthesis and release rates, locally produced somatostatin and dopa-mine may also participate in this process (49,50). Both of these transmit-ters inhibit TSH release under circumstances that, although not yet fully defined, may turn out to be quite important. Inhibition of TSH release by dopamine is an issue frequently encountered in intensive care units in which patients with vascular collapse are sustained with infusions of large doses of the amine. Because dopamine has been implicated in the etiology of certain psychiatric disorders, participation of the transmitter in thyroid axis functions is of additional interest.

In common with many hormones of pituitary origin, a nighttime surge in TSH release occurs in healthy individuals (Figures 1–4 and 1–5). The TSH surge is apparently independent of changes in circulating hormones or known centrally acting substances (51,52). A normal sleep-wake cycle is required (53); the TSH surge is modified if the awake state is maintained for 24 hours. As noted in Figure 1–6, patients with nonthyroidal illness (NTI) or depression may also lose the nocturnal TSH surge (54–56).

TSH provides the directives that coordinate almost all aspects of thyroid gland function. It gives positive signals relative to glandular blood flow, iodine uptake rates and capacities, peroxidase activity, thyroglobulin iodination rates, iodotyrosyl coupling, and, eventually, release of hormone. When the TSH signal is perceived by thyroid hormone release mechanisms, endocytosis of some of the colloid across the follicular cell apical membrane brings colloid droplets into the follicle cell cytosol. There, in a process not unlike the digestion of proteins in the stomach, proteases in thyroid follicular cells, operating at an acid pH, release the constituent amino acids of thyroglobulin, including the iodoamino acids T_4, T_3 monoiodotyrosine (MIT), and diiodotyrosine (DIT). Absorption of iodothyronines into the venous capillaries occurs through the basal membrane of the thyroid follicular cell. Thus, all the activities of the thyroid gland illustrated in Figure 1–1, as well as those involved in iodothyronine release, are under the control of TSH.

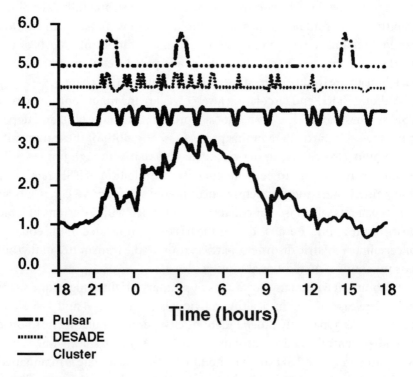

Figure 1–4. Twenty-four–hour thyroid-stimulating hormone secretion in a healthy male volunteer as analyzed by computer-assisted methods of analyzing pulsatile release (DESADE, Cluster, and Pulsar programs). Note surge occurring between 3 A.M. and 6 A.M. *Source.* From Brabant G, Prank K, Ranft U, et al: "Circadian and Pulsatile TSH Secretion Under Physiological and Pathophysiological Conditions." *Hormone and Metabolic Research* 23:12–17, 1990. Used with permission.

Although TSH is almost certainly the major factor directing the activity of the thyroid gland, it is far from the only factor. Epidermal growth factor is an essential mediator of thyroid gland growth (57), as are other growth factors including insulin (58), insulin-like growth factors (59), and others not necessarily known or understood. An array of these factors is involved in the normal growth, compensatory growth (following hemithyroidectomy, for example), or abnormal growth of the thyroid gland. In addition to humorally mediated controls, signals from the autonomic nervous system are also important. The superior cervical ganglia provide postganglionic noradrenergic fibers not only to submaxillary salivary and pineal glands but also to the thyroid gland. Both functional and structural properties of the gland are altered by changes in the activity of its sympathetic innervation (60). TSH effects, as well as growth responses of the gland, are influenced by transduction of noradrenergic message via α and β receptors

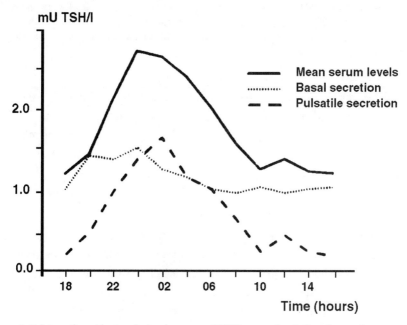

Figure 1–5. Mean thyroid-stimulating hormone (TSH) serum levels, basal secretion rate, and pulsatile secretion according to DESADE analysis. Data are shown as mean of 2-hour segments over 24 hours in 21 healthy male volunteers. *Source.* From Brabant G, Prank K, Ranft U, et al: "Circadian and Pulsatile TSH Secretion Under Physiological and Pathophysiological Conditions." *Hormone and Metabolic Research* 23:12–17, 1990. Used with permission.

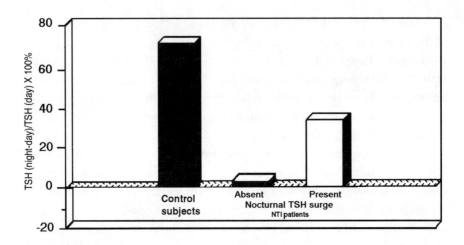

Figure 1–6. Decreased nocturnal thyroid-stimulating hormone (TSH) surge in nonthyroidal illness (NTI) patients. Nocturnal TSH surge (relative increase of nighttime TSH over daytime TSH) in control subjects and NTI patients without (*Absent*) and with (*Present*) nocturnal TSH surge. *Source.*   Adapted from Romijn JA, Wiersinga WM: "Decreased Nocturnal Surge of Thyrotropin in Nonthyroidal Illness." *Journal of Clinical Endocrinology and Metabolism* 70:35–42, 1990.

in blood vessel walls and plasma membranes of the thyroid follicular cells (61,62). Thus disorders originating in the brain in general, the PVN in particular, the pituitary thyrotrophs, and the peripheral autonomic nervous system may contribute to failure of homeostatic control of thyroid gland functioning.

4. SERUM BINDING PROTEINS

When iodothyronines enter the venous circulation they encounter a set of carrier proteins to which they bind with high, medium, or low affinity. As a result, a considerable store of hormone is held within the vascular system, serving as a supplement to the stores of hormone maintained within the colloid of thyroid follicles. However, hormone storage alone does not begin to describe the importance of the serum carrier proteins. Their interesting qualities stem from their diversity and their changing activities with alterations in physiological state (63).

During the time of their residence within serum, thyroid hormones, represented mainly by T_4, are presumably functionless. Only when they encounter cells and cellular enzymes and receptors are they able to mediate the cascade of effects associated with the euthyroid state. Serum iodothyronine-binding proteins are in an excellent position to influence those cellular encounters; their different strengths of hormone binding provide a mechanism for specifying selective hormone distribution to target tissue sites. At the same time, a number of different conditions prevailing at those sites may alter the strength of iodothyronine binding to circulating carrier proteins.

Unfortunately, the exact role of the serum binding proteins in these processes is not yet conceptualized in a generally accepted form, and the entire subject is riddled with controversy (64–66). Nevertheless, evolving features of the controversy are now seen to have direct implications for the actions of thyroid hormones in brain and are therefore relevant here.

Under ordinary circumstances, thyroxine-binding globulin (TBG) binds most of the T_4 in the circulation (about 70%). The rest is accounted for by a variety of hormone carriers including thyroxine-binding prealbumin (long known as *TBPA*; now called *transthyretin* or *TTR*), albumin, lipoproteins, apolipoprotein A-1, and a variety of unusual factors such as hepatitis B surface antigen and actinomycin D.

TBG is a low-capacity, high-affinity T_4-binding element; levels in the circulation are remarkably stable during all phases of healthy adult life. The molecular weight of TBG (92 kd) is reduced by half when stripped of its numerous oligosaccharide residues. As in the case of other glycoproteins, the carbohydrate residues appear to protect the protein from degradation by the liver. No doubt the conformational changes induced by the various degrees and forms of TBG glycosylation influence important interactive properties of the molecule.

The core protein of TBG contains the T_4-binding site, a single site on each TBG molecule. Despite its extensively glycosylated state, TBG is considered to be a rather fragile molecule, being readily disrupted by shaking, dilute acid, and other reagents commonly used in serum analytical procedures. Upon binding with T_4, the molecule becomes more compact and more stable. T_4-bound TBG communicates differential (biphasic) effects on TBG synthesis rates. The mature protein is highly analogous to antitrypsin and antichymotrypsin, both of which are serine antiproteinases (serpins). The relationship to serpins, shared with proteins that bind cortisol, has important implications for the selective delivery of their ligands to particular tissue sites. Pemberton et al. (67) have indicated a mechanism whereby the homology of TBG and cortisol-binding globulin (CBG) with serpins might affect the ability of the carrier proteins to mediate site-specific hormone release. The serpins are in the "stressed" configuration when susceptible to proteolytic cleavage, at which time they are heat labile; when cleaved, they assume the "relaxed" configuration and are heat stable. If TBG and CBG are exposed to elastase, an enzyme released from neutrophils at sites of inflammation, they are cleaved and become heat stable. Under these circumstances, CBG (but not TBG) releases its bound hormone. This change in capacity for cortisol binding by CBG suggests that cortisol (but not iodothyronine) release at inflammatory sites might be advantageous. However, under circumstances when site-directed release of thyroid hormones would be useful, cleavage of TBG by a different proteolytic agent might be effective in disrupting the binding site for iodothyronines.

A major physiological change in TBG levels is seen in pregnancy. Estrogen was thought to increase the synthesis of the protein (the gene for TBG is located on the X-chromosome), but increased TBG concentrations encountered in pregnancy may be due to the molecule's longer serum half-life associated with an increased extent of glycosylation. When estrogen is abruptly withdrawn after removal of the placenta, TBG levels fall rapidly; as this occurs, the large amounts of T_4, T_3, and rT_3 previously bound would become available for entry into tissues. The breast is one likely accommodation site for the excess hormone in that, with the onset of lactation, breast tissue deiodinase activity increases and large amounts of iodide are transported into the milk (68). Another possible recipient is the brain itself. The many CNS changes required for the onset of maternal behavior during the postpartum period could be mediated, in part, through thyroid hormone–related effects within the brain ensuing from the marked changes in peripheral thyroid hormone availability during that period. A possible relationship to postpartum depression, though obvious, is only speculative.

TTR (again, long known as thyroxine-binding prealbumin [TBPA]) is ranked second in importance to TBG because its binding activity relative to TBG is less, accounting for only about 15% of the total T_4 in serum. TTR is a 55-kd protein consisting of four identical subunits, which form a double-trumpet–shaped channel theoretically capable of carrying two T_4 molecules. However, only a single hormone molecule is bound at any one time due to a marked loss of T_4 affinity at the second site when the first is occupied.

A unique feature of TTR is its affinity for and active binding of one molecule of retinol-binding protein (RBP), which in turn binds retinol, the precursor of the tissue-active product, retinoic acid. No information is available regarding effects of RBP and TTR on the binding affinity of one or another of its ligands. Although TTR is far less active in binding T_4 than is TBG, its quantitative importance as a carrier increases when, for any reason, TBG binding is reduced. The importance of TTR is gaining ascendancy on several other grounds. Although primarily synthesized in the liver, TTR is also synthesized in choroid plexus epithelial cells and is concentrated in retina and pancreatic islets. Recently, receptors for TTR have been found on human astrocytoma cells (69). Because TTR is a repeating subunit constituent within amyloid precursor protein (63), the possibility that TTR may play a role in the development or expression of Alzheimer's disease is worth considering.

Albumin binding of T_3 and T_4 is of the nonspecific, high-capacity type; low-protein states, which may or may not lower TBG levels, will reduce its carrying capacity. Recently, serum albumin variants have been identified that exhibit marked increases in their thyroid hormone–binding affinities. In almost all instances, only T_4 carrier functions are increased, but, rarely, T_4 and rT_3 or T_4, T_3, and rT_3 binding may be affected. In some cases, even more rarely observed thus far, only T_3 carrier functions are expanded. All variants are accounted for by changes in the structure of the albumin molecule, due to alterations in gene structure, with resulting amino acid substitutions or deletions accounting for the change in iodothyronine-binding activity of the albumin molecule. Many genetic variations of TBG and TTR are also becoming known. These bring about positive or negative effects on their T_4-binding activity that are not necessarily quantified by changes in T_3 resin uptake tests. Therefore, in affected patients, radioimmunoassay measurements of the individual binding proteins or serum electrophoretic measurements of their relative iodothyronine-carrying capacity may be necessary for further elucidation of thyroid state.

Although the role of hormone carrier proteins in site-specific and function-specific delivery of hormone to tissues has been emphasized, these proteins also determine the size of the free-hormone pool in the circulation. The free-hormone hypothesis states that the metabolic clearance rate and the biological potency of protein-bound hormones are functions of the free-hormone concentration in the circulation as measured by equilibrium dialysis. This concept has held sway for decades and has persisted because, on the whole, it seemed to be clinically useful. Indeed, clinicians were essentially told that they did not particularly need to bother about changes in serum carrier properties as long as a "normal" free-hormone concentration was maintained. However, numerous troubling observations have been recorded that raise doubts about the hardness and fastness of this rule.

For example, the free-hormone hypothesis does not hold for TBG deficiency, even though TBG-deficient patients appear by all criteria to be euthyroid. In NTI, TBG affinity for T_4 and T_3 diminishes (70). Providing that the total T_4 level is no less than 2–3 μg/dl, free-hormone concentrations may remain normal because the dialyzable fraction is increased. Even so, the expected early disappearance of T_4 in NTI is not observed as in the case of TBG deficiency. Moreover, when T_4 falls to very low levels, the total free-hormone fraction also falls below the normal range. Nevertheless, TSH does not increase. Most telling is the fact that a few measurements of free-hormone fractions in selected tissue capillary networks indicate a variation from one site to another. In brain capillaries, the free-T_3 level is reported to be severalfold greater than that in the jugular vein (65).

In addition, new relationships and new implications of the relationships among different hormones are suggested by recently described carrier protein–ligand interactions. Thus, as previously noted, RBP and, therefore, retinol itself binds to TTR in serum; in turn TTR exists in high concentration in choroid plexus where its synthesis is controlled separately from that of serum TTR (71). Given new information about the unexpectedly close molecular ties between retinoic acid receptors and nuclear T_3 receptors (72,73) and between thyroid hormone and retinoic acid response elements in DNA (74) and evidence for nongenomic interactions of the two hormones at the plasma membrane (75), it seems reasonable that selected combinations of the hormones may be delivered to selected tissues by the diverse array of proteins, which, until recently, have been considered passive hormone carriers in the circulation. Another newly emphasized observation is that the extracellular segment of the transmembrane growth hormone receptor has been shown to be highly analogous to the serum carrier protein for growth hormone (76). This observation suggests that the function of hormone reception initiated by binding and the function of binding in the serum may both be mediated in selected cases by similarly derived proteins.

Derangements of thyroid hormone binding activities may not necessarily result in embarrassment to all tissues. However, it is not inconceivable that the brain might be especially vulnerable; it is likely that certain of its homeostatic control mechanisms may operate through localized interactions of binding proteins with brain barrier structures. In the special cases of choroid plexus and glial cell–localized TTR, mediation of highly regulated events seems likely. For these reasons, full consideration of potential sources of disturbed brain–thyroid hormone interactions would require attention not only to the free-hormone status, but also to the nature, capacity, and affinity of hormone carriers in serum.

5. SPECIAL FEATURES OF THYROID HORMONE PROCESSING IN PERIPHERAL TISSUES

5.1 Introduction

Events related to thyroid hormone actions in brain are perhaps best appreciated against the background of its actions in peripheral tissues. Although the brain is clearly unique, evidence suggests that individual somatic tissues also maintain unique requirements for thyroid hormones and use appropriate methods for satisfying those requirements.

In considering rates and routes of T_4 metabolism in any tissue, we have found it useful to think of iodothyronines as lately arrived aromatic amino acids evolved from tyrosine and, like tyrosine, participating as amino acid substrates in the synthesis of proteins and melanin and serving as precursor amino acids in a neurotransmitter pathway of metabolism (77). Whether these constructs describe mechanisms actually in use remains for future studies to elucidate. However, as a mode of approaching the issue of tissue utilization of thyroid hormones, the amino acid view of thyroid hormone action has been very useful. Thus as individuals grow, their requirements for iodothyronines increase, and during feeding, or even overfeeding, requirements for thyroid hormones increase proportionately. Similarly, during exercise, iodothyronine utilization and turnover, and therefore demand, increase as they do for other nutritional substrates (78). If exercise is so extreme that protein losses become significant, amino acid and thyroid hormone requirements may increase enormously. By contrast, in the fasting state the synthesis rate of T_3 is reduced. This is so for all other required amino acids because, in fasting, overall protein synthesis rates are low. It is noteworthy that when T_3 is administered during fasting it has no protein synthesis–promoting actions and, in fact, only appears to induce an amino acid imbalance in a previously balanced (if deficient) state. As in all cases of amino acid imbalance, protein catabolism is enhanced (79).

A normally functioning thyroid axis makes the appropriate adjustments to the changes in thyroid hormone requirements smoothly, whereas a malfunctioning unit may decompensate. In the combined exercise-fasting complex seen in some cases of anorexia nervosa, reduced requirements due to fasting are countered by an increase in requirements due to exercise. However, because metabolic demands are not the only ones in charge in this situation, the disorder is often accompanied by low serum levels of T_4 and T_3 (see Chapters 2 and 9).

Other features of the amino acid-like behavior of iodothyronines is seen in the body's response to primary deficiencies or excesses of the thyroid hormones themselves. As in the case of other essential amino acid deficiencies or excesses, the organism seeks to adapt to these conditions largely through changing to new rates and routes of T_4 metabolism. In amino acid deficiency states, the liver conserves the amino acids passing through its cellular apparatus, whereas, when the amino acids are oversupplied, the liver will dispose of them. In a similar fashion, the liver conserves what little T_4 is available in hypothyroidism, but it rapidly turns on the process of hormone disposal in hyperthyroidism. The behavior of the liver can thus be seen as adaptive, and this is particularly evident when the needs of the brain are taken into consideration. For, in hypothyroidism, as soon as the spared T_4 reaches the brain, it is quickly cannibalized for the purpose of maintaining near-normal levels of T_3 supplies in the CNS. Although this important example of responsivity to alterations in thyroid hormone availability on the part of liver and brain demonstrates that thyroid state is highly deterministic, the direction of the response is opposite in each of the two tissues, as illustrated in Figure 1–7. Considerably more attention is given to particulars of these responses in the following sections.

5.2 Role of Liver and Kidney

Evidence perceived on the evolutionary scale suggests that in early vertebrate species, when the anlage of the mammalian thyroid gland first appeared, thyroglobulin-like proteins present in superficial cells lining the pharynx of the primitive foregut exhibited the capacity to

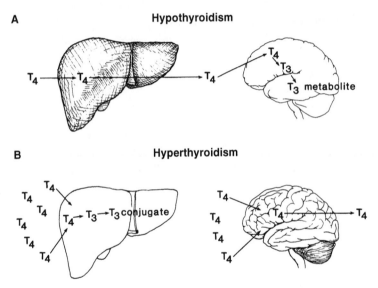

Figure 1–7. Coordinated responses in liver and brain help to maintain thyroid hormone homeostasis in the central nervous system. *Panel A:* In hypothyroidism, small amounts of thyroxine (T_4) remaining in the circulation pass through the liver unchanged, whereas, in the brain, T_4 is rapidly converted to triiodothyronine (T_3) and possibly other active metabolites. *Panel B:* In hyperthyroidism, excess T_4 entering the liver is subject to sulfation, rapidly converted to T_3, and excreted in urine and bile as inactive conjugates. Hepatic inactivation of T_4 and T_3 reduces overall T_3 availability. The brain further defends itself against hyperthyroidism by minimizing intracerebral T_3 formation and maintaining or increasing rates of T_4 disposal. *Source.* From Dratman MB, Crutchfield FL, Gordon JT: "Thyroid Hormones and Adrenergic Neurotransmitters," in *Catecholamines, Neuropharmacology and Central Nervous System: Theoretical Aspects.* Edited by Usdin E. New York, Alan R Liss, 1984, pp. 425–439. Used with permission.

trap iodine in tyrosyl residues and form T_4 (80). When sloughed into the gut lumen, the pharyngeal cells and their contents were digested, their free iodoamino acids were absorbed into the portal circulation, and the liver was their first port of call. Whatever survival value was imparted by the sequestration of the early thyroid gland anlage into a structure that delivered its products directly into the systemic circulation, it seems likely that the first-pass bypass of the liver was a contributory factor. Even so, the liver, performing its function as the body's metabolic monitor, eventually gets to scrutinize all compounds present in the circulation. The thyroid hormones are no exception; on dissociation from their carrier molecules in plasma, they make their way into hepatocytes. Like all moieties that enter the liver, iodothyronines encounter a branch point that leads either to activation or to disposal. A similar but less emphasized sorting process takes place in the kidney.

5.3 Tissue Thyroxine (T_4) Metabolizing Enzymes

In performing its thyroid hormone–promoting functions, the liver generates the more active form of the hormone, T_3, through the process of outer-ring monodeiodination (5'D) of T_4. Although it is premature to conclude that T_4 is a prohormone and T_3 always the active player in thyroid hormone–mediated events, it is useful to accept this view as a working hypothesis because it provides a rational explanation for otherwise obscure relationships and responses in the organism. The formation of T_3 from T_4 in liver is facilitated by prior conjugation of the phenolic hydroxyl group of T_4 with sulfate (81); the conjugate has a higher affinity for 5'D than for free T_4 itself. The process of liver and kidney cell T_4 sulfation may be particularly important in adaptation to the hyperthyroid state, in that it allows the fractional rate of T_3 formation to increase with increasing T_4 concentrations. Under such circumstances T_3 formed from T_4 sulfate represents a mechanism of disposal by liver; excretion of sulfate and glucuronide conjugates of T_3 into urine and bile becomes more and more active as more and more T_4 is presented to these tissues. By contrast, the behavior of the hepatic T_4 5'D in hypothyroidism is distinctly geared toward conservation of T_4 molecules. The different effects of thyroid state on tissue iodothyronine metabolism are addressed further in section 8 (on thyroid hormone homeostasis).

The fate of newly formed T_3 depends on homeostatic requirements, but, in the euthyroid state, a large proportion of hepatic 5'D-generated T_3 is released into the circulation. There it joins a pool, which may serve as the major source of T_3 for some tissues, notably heart. However, many tissues have an adequate supply of their own T_4 deiodinating enzymes. The T_4 molecules used in those tissues come from first-pass hormone or from unmetabolized T_4 that has entered and left the liver or kidney for further processing in extrahepatic tissues. T_3-forming enzymes in extrahepatic tissues are, for the most part, like the hepatic 5'D enzymes, the latter generally known as *type I* enzyme. (Note that the abbreviation *5'D* refers both to the process of outer-ring (or prime-ring) monodeiodination and to the enzymes mediating this process.)

The structure of the type I enzyme, an oxidoreductase, has recently been solved (82). It exhibits well-defined characteristics, including *1)* preferred localization in liver and kidney; *2)* specific kinetic features (e.g., a high apparent Michaelis constant [Km] and a high maximum capacity for T_4), and is therefore very active in hyperthyroidism; *3)* ping-pong kinetics; *4)* a requirement for thiols as cofactors; *5)* susceptibility to inhibition by propylthiouracil (PTU); and *6)* a covalently bound atom of selenium in its molecular structure in the form of the amino acid selenocysteine, which is incorporated in the enzyme's active site. (An important objection to the proposal that T_4 is an amino acid that is incorporated into protein is that it has not been found as a component of any protein molecule analyzed thus far. However, the rare amino acid selenocysteine has only been found in two eukaryote proteins, one of which is the 5'D. Selenocysteine is known to be incorporated into protein as such and not formed posttranslationally.) A role for selenium in T_4 metabolism was predicted by observations that dietary deficiency of this element resulted in marked reduction in T_3 production by liver and kidney (Table 1–1).

On the other hand, 5'D, type II, which also converts T_4 to T_3, exhibits catalytic properties quite different from those described for the type I isoform. First recognized in the pituitary (83) and soon thereafter in hypothyroid brain (84), the type II enzyme was subsequently identified in certain heavily adrenergically innervated tissues such as brown fat (85), pineal (86), harderian gland (87), and adrenal medulla (88). Type II enzyme is also thiol requiring, but otherwise differs from type I in that it *1)* is apparently much less abundant, even in those peripheral tissues in which it predominates; *2)* is of the low-Km and non-ping-pong variety in its kinetic behavior; *3)* is readily inhibited in vivo and in vitro by T_4 and rT_3, but highly active when iodothyronine concentrations are low, as in hypothyroidism; *4)* is not inhibited by PTU under physiological circumstances but, in vitro, can be inhibited by this agent if required thiols are in suboptimal concentration; and *5)* may have tissue-specific requirements for other cofactors (89).

The foregoing capsule description of type I and type II deiodinating enzymes should already indicate that in tissues that convert T_4 to T_3, the amount of T_4 that enters the tissue and the form of 5'D enzyme that is active in that tissue will determine the tissue's ability to obtain the quantity of T_3 required for its metabolic needs. However, the net amount of T_4 available to any tissue is also determined by the activity of another tissue-deiodinating enzyme, the type III (rT_3-forming) enzyme (90). The rate of T_4 catalysis by inner-ring deiodination has its own limitations, which are nevertheless in accord with what we presently consider to be the role of rT_3. The later iodothyronine has no agreed-upon function, although a (disputed) role for rT_3 as an in vivo 5'D inhibitor has been reported (91,92). Characteristic features of the three major tissue-monodeiodinating enzymes are listed in Table 1–2.

In vitro, rT_3 can readily inhibit 5'D activity. Although generally thought to be an inactive product of T_4 metabolism, rT_3 may never-

Table 1–1. Triiodothyronine (T_3) production (fmol/minute per mg of protein) in liver and kidney of selenium-deficient (Se-), selenium-replete (Se+), and selenium-replaced rats

| Organ | Se+ | Se- | Selenium replacement | |
			Low dose	High dose
Liver	5.02±1.33	1.88±1.30	0.95±0.95	3.76±0.63(NS)
Kidney	1.73±0.38	0.23±0.27	0.89±0.71	1.93±0.56(NS)

Note. Differences from Se+ significant unless otherwise noted (NS).
Source. From Beckett GJ, MacDougall DA, Nicol F, et al: "Inhibition of Type I and Type II Iodothyronine Deiodinase Activity in Rat Liver, Kidney and Brain Produced by Selenium Deficiency." *Biochemistry Journal* 259:887–892, 1989. Used with permission.

theless contribute importantly to homeostasis in that the rate of its formation will determine how much of the T_4 taken up into tissues is actually available for conversion to T_3. It would therefore seem teleologically sound that the rate of formation of this T_4 metabolite would increase in hyperthyroidism and decrease in hypothyroidism. And indeed, insofar as measurements of net serum and tissue rT_3 levels suggest, this is the case.

Despite the consonance of expectation and observation regarding the role of rT_3, an uneasiness on this issue seems to pervade many thoughtful presentations. Does the accumulation of rT_3 in NTI (of either somatic or nervous origin) mean something more than meets the eye? Since its discovery, investigators have considered the possibility that rT_3 may serve as a natural antagonist to T_3, whether independent of or deriving from its ability to inhibit the activities of T_4 5'D in various tissues. Another consideration that makes investigators hesitant to dismiss rT_3 as an entirely inactive iodothyronine is that it is by far the predominant iodothyronine in the fetal brain (where thyroid hormones are known to be absolutely essential for the progress of brain maturation) and may therefore play an active role in fetal brain development (93).

On the other hand, a plethora of papers shows an absolutely nil result of using or administering rT_3 to adults in proposed physiological or supraphysiological amounts (94). Unfortunately, both the pos-

Table 1–2.   Iodothyronine deiodinases in the rat central nervous system

Variable	Type I (5'D)	Type II (5'D)	Type III (5D)
Substrate preference	$rT_3>T_4>T_3$	$T_4>rT_3$	$T_3>T_4$
Km for T_4 (T_3)	1×10^{-6} M	1×10^{-9} M	6×10^{-9} M
Deiodination site	Outer ring	Outer ring	Inner ring
Effect of			
Iopanoic acid	Inhibited	Inhibited	Inhibited
Hypothyroidism	Inhibited	Stimulated	Inhibited
Hyperthyroidism	Stimulated[a]	Inhibited	Stimulated

Note. 5'D = outer-ring monodeiodinase; 5D = inner-ring monodeiodenase; rT_3 = reverse triiodothyronine; T_4 = thyroxine; T_3 = triiodothyronine; Km = Michaelis constant.
[a]Net effect.
Source. Adapted from Larsen PR: "Thyroid Hormone Metabolism in the Central Nervous System." *Acta Medica Austriaca* 15:5–10, 1988. Used with permission.

itive and the negative results with rT_3 suffer from the major and fairly obvious limitation that at present only the functional results of administering this product can be examined, and not the results of its formation in situ. Although progress toward measuring the steady state ratios of rT_3 to T_4 has been reported (95), uncertainty about the kinetics and functional implications of this metabolic step in tissues remains.

When administered, rT_3 is very rapidly destroyed by the very tissues that might conceivably use it as a T_3 antagonist (i.e., the T_3-forming tissues richly endowed with 5'D). Moreover, kidney and liver type I deiodinase enzymes have an even higher affinity for rT_3 than for T_4. Although the rate of rT_3 deiodination by tissues with type I enzyme is therefore potentially more rapid than that of T_4, the high capacity of the enzyme in the euthyroid and hyperthyroid states assures that all substrates will be accommodated. This is not the case in brain, however, where the situation is quite reversed. 5'D in brain prefers T_4, for which it has a very limited capacity. However, in hypothyroidism, the availability of T_3 is not normally jeopardized by T_4 depletion through rT_3 formation because the inner-ring deiodinating (5D) enzyme is suppressed in hormone-deficient states.

Nevertheless, in both hepatic and extrahepatic tissues, the fate of rT_3 formed in situ by 5D (type III) enzyme cannot be judged on the basis of the available evidence and may be quite different from that of rT_3 delivered through the circulation. The intracellular formation of rT_3 may take place in a compartment that positions the newly formed T_4 metabolite close to intracellular rT_3 receptors, or places it in contact with enzymes that convert it to a metabolically significant product (96).

The idea that tissue iodothyronine products may be differentially compartmentalized is not novel. For example, T_3 formed from T_4 as the 5'D liver product is directed toward the circulation and is not directly available for nuclear receptor binding in the hepatic cells in which it was made (97). In contrast, T_3 molecules formed in brain cells are retained and apparently engage with their T_3-binding nuclear receptor, without first entering the circulation.

Important insights into the role of rT_3 would be gained if a selective inhibitor of either the type II or the type III enzyme were known.

However, there are already signs on the horizon that even more direct evidence regarding these enzymes will soon become available. Thus, as previously noted, the structure of type I 5'D has been announced, following ingenious experiments in which RNA fractions transcribed from a rat liver cDNA library and injected into oocytes allowed expression of the gene coding for the enzyme (83). Despite the fact that selenium deficiency reduces the activity of both type I and type II enzymes (98), present evidence suggests that selenium is not incorporated into the type II enzyme molecule. The reduction of type II activity in the selenium-deficient animal is rationalized as follows: loss of type I enzyme in the otherwise thyroid-sufficient animal leads to an increase in unmetabolized T_4, a resultant increase in serum T_4, and a subsequent decrease in activity of low-Km type II enzymes, which are readily inhibited by excess T_4 (98a).

The varying specificities of T_4-metabolizing enzymes from one tissue type to another help to control the fate of T_4 transported into the tissue and ultimately the choice of the T_4-metabolic pathway to be followed there. They have another, possibly equally important, set of functions; they also determine the tissue half-life of the T_4 products. T_3, a very poor substrate for the enzymes responsible for its formation (5'D, type I and type II), is an excellent substrate for the rT_3-forming enzyme (5D), whereas rT_3 is an excellent substrate for 5'D, especially type I. In brains of hypothyroid individuals where 5D is low but 5'D is stimulated, the limited T_4 available is maximally utilized to enhance T_3 formation and limit T_3 deiodination. The spared T_3 molecules are then useful as ligands for nuclear or other putative T_3 receptors or as substrates for further T_3 activation. Thus protecting T_3 from deiodination might allow a higher rate of triiodothyroacetic acid (triac) formation from T_3.

The mention of triac is appropriate here because very similar questions arise about the importance of this molecule as have arisen about rT_3. It is well known that, in most instances, triac has a higher affinity for the T_3 nuclear receptor than any other naturally occurring iodocompound (99,100). Yet, when administered, triac is a weak T_3 agonist. Triac's poor showing as a thyroid hormone agonist has been evaluated in several laboratories and the agreed-on conclusion makes sense: the residence time of triac in bloodstream and tissues is so short that the opportunity for nuclear binding is minimal and the biological effect is weak. But what if the tissue residence time of triac formed in situ turned out to be quite different from that given exogenously? Or what if the site of triac formation turned out to be immediately proximate to the receptor and therefore optimally active under those circumstances? There are no straightforward answers to these questions. Like rT_3, triac given exogenously may not even get into the tissue parenchyma. But evidence that this molecule is present in a variety of tissues after labeled-T_4 and -T_3 administration suggests that the issue about triac and its role in mediating thyroid hormone effects has not yet been settled.

Most references to thyroid hormone metabolism imply deiodinative metabolism, especially the deiodination of T_4 to either T_3 or rT_3. Yet, as emphasized in Figure 1–8, a possible role for other T_3 metabolites as mediators of, at least, some aspects of thyroid hormone action has been perennially intriguing to investigators. (Note that triac is

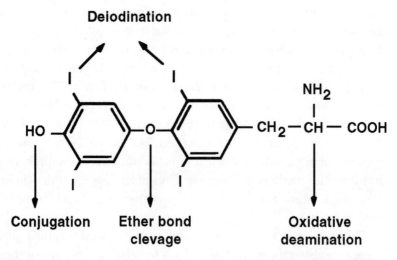

Figure 1–8. Common metabolic pathways for thyroxine. Schema shows potential for hydroxyl group conjugation, inner- and outer-ring monodeiodination, and side-chain alteration (the latter exemplified by production of the acetic acid derivative of the hormone through oxidative deamination). Ether bond cleavage yields diiodotyrosine. Sequential monodeiodination can produce the noniodinated metabolites of any of the above. *Source.* From Visser TJ, van Buuren JCJ, Rutgers M, et al: "The Role of Sulfation in Thyroid Hormone Metabolism." *Trends in Endocrinology and Metabolism* March/April:211–218, 1990. Used with permission.

only one of a number of possible side-chain–altered products of T_3.) For example, considerable interest has been focused on the (contested) claim that triiodothyronamine might be an in vivo–generated product of T_3 decarboxylation (101). Other modifications of the thyronine nucleus and/or side chain have been made synthetically and tested, without much success (102). Although still under investigation, and reasonable on theoretical grounds, no direct evidence has been mustered for the possibility that T_4 might enter a pathway of ring and side-chain metabolism in adrenergic nerve endings, which might lead to the formation of an iodothyronine-derived biogenic amine (77). Not investigated thus far is the possibility that amidation of the T_3 molecule might lead to expression of its latent peptide-like nature. Finally, given new attention paid to gases as neuroactive compounds (e.g., NO and CO), perhaps molecular iodine (I_2) deserves to be considered as well (102a).

5.4   Thyroxine (T_4) Metabolism in the Thyroid Axis

a.   Hypothalamus

As noted above, the PVN is a major (if not the major) hypothalamic thyroid axis structure in that, in response to circulating levels of T_3, it secretes amounts of TRH appropriate and necessary for modulating the production of TSH. A recent article (103) described a presumed disparity between elevations in hypothalamic mRNA levels for the TRH precursor protein and low levels of TRH during hypothyroidism. However, it is presumed that TRH would be actively transported out of the PVN and then secreted into the hypothalamic-hypophyseal portal circulation under those circumstances. Perhaps, therefore, low net levels of TRH should be expected. Because the PVN, as part of the hypothalamus, is a member of the circumventricular organ system, it may not be subject to the same blood-brain barrier (BBB) limitations as are other parts of the brain. Therefore, the PVN probably perceives the ratio of T_4 to T_3 that is actually present in the circulation. Such a direct relationship between PVN cells and the iodothyronine content of plasma is presumably necessary for driving the hypothalamic component of the feedback interaction, which accounts overall for the behavior of the thyroid axis. In that context, the participation of intra-PVN type II 5′D activity might not be appropriate (for the same reasons noted in the discussion below of pituitary 5′D) in that it might blunt the perception of lowered levels of T_3 in the circulation.

To engage this issue experimentally, deiodinase activity has been measured in the hypothalamus. It turns out that 5′D activity is low and 5D is high in homogenates prepared from whole hypothalami. However, that observation taken at face value is misleading; studies of 5′D activity based on punch-biopsy isolation of individual hypothalamic nuclei (Figure 1–9) reveal that some nuclei (but not the PVN) have as much as fourfold higher activity than that measured even in cortex or cerebellum, where the highest rates of regional deiodinase activity have been described (104). As can be inferred, it is difficult to gain functional biochemical information about one versus another brain nucleus because the level of investigation is ordinarily too gross for the problem at hand. In the case of the PVN, the anticipated result conforms with the experimental evidence: 5′D activity in the punch-biopsied PVN is indeed low.

b. **Pituitary gland**

Like the brain, the pituitary gland is a complex structure that houses the adenohypophysis and the neurohypophysis. Most of our knowledge about biochemical pathways of anterior pituitary iodocompounds and their kinetics is derived from studies performed in pituitary homogenates. All of the cell types responsible for the formation and secretion of the anterior pituitary hormones are mingled within the adenohypophysis and can only be identified with certainty through the use of differential immunohistochemical techniques. Although studies of pituitary homogenates have revealed some distinctive features of the gland as a whole that are important for understanding the operation of that tissue (83), we are still largely in the dark about thyroid hormone metabolism in individual adenohypophyseal cell types.

The predominant 5′D in the pituitary is of the type II variety; its fractional activity and rate of T_3 formation per unit weight of

tissue is among the highest measured in the body. As is characteristic of the type II isoform, hypothyroidism leads to enzyme induction and the maintenance of in situ–formed T_3 supplies at a
near-normal level. This response, if occurring in thyrotrophic
cells, would tend to soften their perception of reduced thyroid
hormone availability and delay or reduce the stimulus to TSH pro-

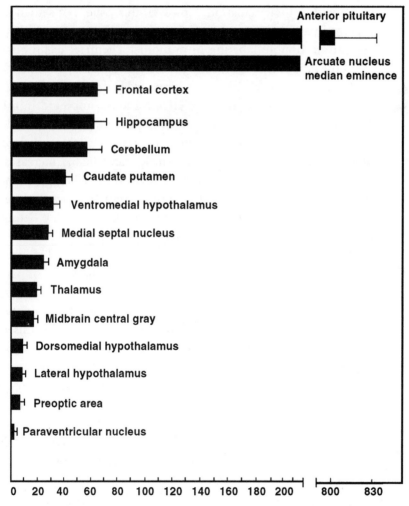

Figure 1–9. Regional distribution of 5′deiodinase type II activity measured as fmoles
iodide released per hour per mg protein ±SEM. *Source.* Adapted from Riskind PN,
Kolodny PN, Larsen PR: "The Regional Hypothalamic Distribution of Type II 5′-Mono-
deiodinase in Euthyroid and Hypothyroid Rats." *Brain Research* 420:194–198, 1987.

duction. It seems unlikely that such a result would be useful to the organism and, in fact, clinical and experimental observations indicate the contrary: TSH release increases promptly in response to even small reductions below normal in circulating thyroid hormone levels. Therefore it is possible that there is little 5'D activity within TSH-producing cells (thyrotrophs), and that the cells making the trophic hormone are responsive mainly to levels of hormone within the circulation. However, this issue, not settled at present, may be amenable to resolution with the use of high-resolution, double-labeling immunohistochemical techniques when the type II enzyme is fully characterized.

Whatever the mechanism, it appears likely that the nuclear receptor is involved and that the effective iodocompound in the TSH-forming cell is T_3. The issue is important because a single process, the TSH-forming process, is the most available indicator of intracellular thyroid hormone sufficiency. If TSH increases, hormone supplies (at least within the thyrotropic cellular apparatus) are inadequate, whereas, if TSH remains in the normal range, the needs of the thyrotropic cells are apparently satisfied. Whether this interpretation holds for patients with NTI, including illnesses in the psychiatric sphere, remains to be determined. The likelihood that TSH levels in serum reflect the thyroid status of particular tissues or individual brain nuclei is remote indeed. Thus, serum TSH levels, which serve as our best indicator of thyroid status, are no longer specific enough to answer the questions raised by our new level of appreciation that tissue T_4 diversity is complex, highly controlled, and therefore subject to local derangement.

Though not known to be part of the thyroid axis, the posterior pituitary has been separately examined for its 5'D activity (105). During hypothyroidism, type II activity was found, raising the possibility that the brain-derived neural lobe behaves like the brain with regard to thyroid hormone processing and requirements.

c. **Thyroid gland**

In all probability, no tissue is independent of the need for thyroid hormone, although not all tissues respond with an increase in oxygen consumption when given T_4 or T_3. The thyroid gland is a thyroid hormone–dependent structure and is reported to have a relatively rich supply of type II enzyme (106). In hypothyroidism, some level of positive control over iodothyronine biosynthesis is exerted by intrathyroidally released T_3 through an inductive effect on peroxidase activity (107). Thus the thyroid gland joins a growing list of tissues that mobilize a homeostatic response to hypothyroidism through the mechanisms inherent in 5'D activity.

5.5 Thyroxine (T_4) Metabolism in Selected Tissues With Rich Noradrenergic Innervation

In a series of important and ingenious studies, Leonard et al. (85) brought to light new aspects of interdependently acting noradrenergic and thyronergic events in brown fat. Greer and co-workers (86) have shown a similar interrelationship of the two systems in the pineal gland, as have others studying the harderian gland (87) and adrenal medulla (88). The processes involved have been investigated most exhaustively in brown fat (directed toward the maintenance of normal body temperatures during cold exposure). Formation of the uncoupling protein responsible for mitochondrial heat production in that tissue is the direct result of local sympathetic nervous system activity and the release of norepinephrine. However, the full transduction of the norepinephrine message requires T_4 and intact 5'D activity and therefore presumably T_3, not administered T_3 (except in industrial amounts), but T_3 formed in situ from T_4. The enzyme involved in this transformation is of the type II variety: resistant to the actions of PTU and induced by hypothyroidism.

Of great interest is the fact that the activity of 5'D in brown fat is, in turn, entirely dependent on the production of norepinephrine from its local sympathetic innervation (or on the addition of norepinephrine to preparations of chemically or surgically denervated brown fat). Thus for uncoupling protein to form and for heat production to proceed, both noradrenergic and thyronergic systems are required.

Pineal gland 5'D type II also shows a remarkable dependence on local noradrenergic processes. Because diurnal rhythms of amine production and release occur in response to diurnal light-dark cycles and because light-dark responsivity is an important feature of noradrenergic activity in the pineal gland, it was predicted that 5'D in that tissue would vary according to a similar cycle. This prediction was confirmed in a series of elegant experiments (Figure 1–10). Coordinated thyronoradrenergic activities in the pineal gland do not appear to be linked to melatonin production, and their exact role in pineal gland function is as yet unknown. However, the multisystem level of interaction between noradrenergic innervation and type II enzyme activity is probably not a coincidence. Whether this interaction is true for all type II–controlled deiodinative activities remains to be discovered. Another example of catecholamine–thyroid hormone deiodinase interaction was noted by Leonard (108), who demonstrated isoproterenol-stimulated T_4-to-T_3 converting activity (type II variety) in cultured rat brain astrocytes.

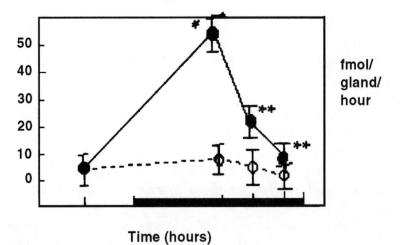

Time (hours)

Figure 1–10. Effects of diurnal light-dark cycle on 5'-deiodinase activity in the pineal gland. Pineal homogenates were incubated at 37° C for 60 minutes in the presence of 40 mM dithiothreitol and 2 nM iodine-125–labeled thyroxine. The dark bar indicates the daily dark period for the control group (*broken line* = no light-dark cycle; *solid line* = diurnal cycle). Deiodination rates are expressed as the mean ±SEM of values from eight animals. * = $P < .01$; ** = $P < .0001$ (versus controls). *Source.* From Guerrero JM, Puig-Domingo M, Reiter RJ: "Thyroxine 5'-Deiodinase Activity in Pineal Gland and Frontal Cortex: Nighttime Increase and the Effect of Either Continuous Light Exposure or Superior Cervical Ganglionectomy." *Endocrinology* 122:236–241, 1988. Used with permission.

SPECIAL FEATURES OF THYROID HORMONE PROCESSING IN ADULT BRAIN

6.1 Introduction

In the preceding sections, emphasis was placed on the many possibilities for the often subtle derangements of thyroid state encountered in clinical practice. In this section, considerable attention is given to the mechanisms that successfully maintain near-normal levels of thyroid hormones in brain and apparently near-normal levels of brain function despite full-blown abnormalities in thyroid gland function, readily measured chemically and fully expressed in somatic tissues.

Most patients with manifest thyroid disorders, although experiencing considerable discomfort in the mental sphere as they react to the dramatic changes in their bodies, manage their day-to-day lives fairly well and promptly dispense with most of their symptoms when rendered euthyroid. It is interesting that these patients, who may feel both anxious and depressed, generally do not show abnormal scores when tested by means of routine psychiatric diagnostic instruments.

However, a minority of patients develop serious mental problems as they experience changes in hormone status. Such patients include those who show major behavioral pathology early in the course of their disease or those who, having received definitive and enthusiastic pro- or antithyroid treatment with ensuing rapid changes in thyroid status, develop marked and sometimes lingering changes in mood, behavior, and/or cognition. These examples are relatively rare; most of the putative thyroid hormone–related psychopathological problems that come to clinical attention are found in individuals with relatively minor changes in thyroid function.

A reasonable explanation for this apparent paradox is available: an array of physiological mechanisms maintain thyroid hormone homeostasis in brain. These operate effectively in the vast majority of individuals, even those manifesting prolonged thyroid disease. However, seemingly fail-safe mechanisms can and do fail. In such cases, even mild fluctuations of hormone availability might produce serious consequences.

An underlying inability to maintain thyroid hormone homeostasis in the brain, coupled with peripheral conditions that produce nonphysiological fluctuations of tissue hormone distribution or availability, may provide the necessary and sufficient conditions for bringing about symptomatic, putatively thyroid-related changes in brain function. If such impaired individuals were to develop thyrotoxicosis, they could, according to this line of reasoning, become frankly psychotic. Or, depending on the brain site of vulnerability, they could develop other severe, uncommon (but not rare) brain-related symptoms (e.g., thyrotoxic chorea) (109).

On the other hand, troublesome mental symptoms associated with recurrent thyroid status change may manifest only transient or borderline changes in thyroid function profiles. Furthermore, in experimental animals it is possible to disrupt brain iodothyronine economy substantially, through the use of pharmacological or stressful challenges, without necessarily observing any noteworthy changes in serum hormone levels (Figure 1–11). Therefore, thyroid hormone–related abnormalities in brain may escape detection by present methods of diagnosis.

There is nothing necessarily exotic or covert about these relationships of thyroid and brain. Similar relationships are detectable in all bodily systems. For example, underlying (but possibly forever silent) heart disease may become a life-threatening condition when even mild hyperthyroidism prevails. Yet most patients with severe thyrotoxicosis show little more in the way of symptomatic cardiovascular effects than rapid pulses and hyperdynamic circulations. In most instances of so-called thyrotoxic heart disease, correction of the thyroid disease restores the patient to the accustomed state of cardiac function. However, it appears to be easier to correct peripheral tissue dysthyroidism than it is to make the proper corrections for the homeostatically impaired brain. Shifting the levels of hormones in the circulation may do little to bring the individual patient into a satisfactory state; satisfying thyroid hormone–related needs of particular brain networks may require adjustments in dose that disturb the body and/or the brain as a whole (110). Appropriately designed drugs that modify the access, metabolic processing, and intracellular actions of thyroid hormones may eventually provide some of the solutions. Already, thyroid hormone analogues have been developed that selectively influence some thyroid hormone–related phenomena without affecting others (111). Perhaps some will be appropriate for normalizing the brain.

Factors involved in determining thyroid hormone–processing rates in brain have been measured only under conditions in which central homeostasis prevails. Animal models representing central homeostatic failure may be available in, for example, the learned helplessness paradigm (112). However, brain–thyroid hormone kinetics have not yet been studied in these models. The discussion that follows may help to identify some of the sites where control mechanisms involved in brain-iodocompound processing may be vulnerable and therefore possibly instrumental in promoting pathophysiological changes in brain function.

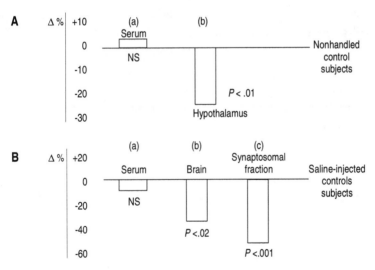

Figure 1–11. Changes in iodothyronine processing in brain produced by environmental or drug-induced events without concomitant changes in levels of serum thyroid hormones. *Panel A:* Decreased fractional thyroid hormone concentrations are noted in the hypothalamus of handled, as compared with nonhandled, controls (rats in isotopic equilibrium). *Panel B:* Levels of intravenously administered iodothyronines taken up into brain and synaptosomes are reduced by prior desipramine injection. Neither handling nor desipramine produced any significant change in fractional serum iodothyronine levels. *Source.* From Dratman MB, Crutchfield FL, Gordon JT: "Thyroid Hormones and Adrenergic Neurotransmitters," in *Catecholamines, Neuropharmacology and Central Nervous System: Theoretical Aspects.* Edited by Usdin E. New York, Alan R Liss, 1984, pp. 425–439. Used with permission.

6.2 Role of Brain Barriers

Among the many unresolved questions regarding thyroid hormone action in brain, the issue of access to sites involved in transduction of the hormone message is obviously important. Iodothyronines entering the brain from the cerebral circulation must first cross barriers at the blood-brain and choroid plexus–cerebrospinal fluid (CSF) interfaces. The route taken after entry through those barriers could bring about selective delivery of hormone to different regions of the brain, and those differences might be decisive in determining the ultimate functional effects of the hormone. Experiments performed to address this issue (113) demonstrated that hormone penetration into brain after crossing the choroid plexus–CSF barrier exhibited a markedly limited, essentially periventricular distribution. By contrast, hormone crossing the BBB was widely, though differentially, distributed. The functional implications of the differences in results produced by the two different routes of hormone entry are not known. However, ready access to circumventricular organs would appear to be favored by hormone crossing the choroid plexus–CSF barrier, whereas access to the panoply of nuclear T_3 receptors would be favored by hormone crossing the BBB. Therefore, unless information to the contrary becomes available, both routes of barrier transport should be taken into account in assessing the kinetics and actions of thyroid hormones in the brain.

Several new observations have bearing on this point. It appears that the BBB may provide the screen for rejecting the D isomers of thyroid hormones (114). If so, the fact that the nuclear T_3 receptor binds D-T_3 with affinity equal to that of L-T_3, even though the former enantiomer lacks thyromimetic activity, may (at least in brain) be irrelevant. Also, retinoic acid and T_3, each bound to its own receptor, can form a heterodimer capable of binding to thyroid response elements (TREs) (74). In view of the capacity of TTR to bind RBP, as well as T_4, coordinated retinol and thyroid hormone access to the brain may be a consequence of TTR localization in the choroid plexus and TTR secretion into the CSF by the choroid plexus. Of particular importance in this regard is that choroid plexus TTR is independently regulated and does not fluctuate with changes in serum TTR (115). It therefore appears that interactions at one versus another brain barrier, as well as the nature of those interactions, may have major physiological or pathological consequences for certain aspects of thyroid-related brain functions.

6.3 Disposition of Iodothyronines Crossing the Blood-Brain Barrier (BBB)

The morphological features of thyroid hormone distribution in brain have been determined on the basis of three separate methods of analysis: *1)* thaw-mount autoradiography, resolved at the film- and light-microscopic levels and prepared at short- and long-time intervals after intravenous (and in more limited experiments, after intrathecal) injection of labeled T_3, T_4, and rT_3 (113,116–118); *2)* in situ hybridization histochemistry showing the distribution of message for T_3 receptors of the α and β varieties and their subclasses, using film autoradiographic methods to demonstrate the labeled reaction products (119); and *3)* immunohistochemistry resolved at light- and electron-microscopic levels, using an antibody directed against the T_3 nuclear receptor and its variant forms (120). Each of these methods has its advantages and its limitations, and each makes contributions to understanding the morphological sites of binding and processing of the hormone in the brain.

a. Tracking of labeled hormones by autoradiography

    i. Brain distribution of intravenously administered iodine-125 (^{125}I)-labeled T_3 ($T_3{}^*$) Light-microscopic autoradiograms of serially sectioned brains revealed for the first time that intravenously delivered $T_3{}^*$ was saturably concentrated and retained in discrete neural systems (116). Wider brain surveys, more complete time course data, and information about the nature of the iodocompounds responsible for the labeling process were gained through use of the technically more accessible film autoradiographic method (Figure 1–12; *Panel A*), combined with parallel biochemical studies of brain homogenates (117,118).

    These investigations demonstrated that at all time intervals the label in the brain was mainly due to $T_3{}^*$ itself (>80%) or other iodothyronines* (about 15%) but probably not due to iodide* (about 3%), which is rapidly transported out of the brain. The reproducible labeling patterns seen in film autoradiograms indicated a widespread but selective localization of hormone. At early times after injections, label was saturably, nonuniformly, and prominently concentrated in selected regions of gray matter, in a pattern similar, but by no means identical, to those seen after administration of cerebral blood flow markers (indicating delivery, mainly, across the BBB). In competition studies with unlabeled T_3, decreased levels of radioactivity were noted in regions of specific binding, whereas in other regions radioactivity was noted to increase due to overflow of labeled hormone into nonspecific sites or saturation of deiodinative mechanisms of disposal.

Observations made at successively later time intervals after intravenous T_3* injection revealed evolving profiles of labeling (Figure 1–12; *Panel A*) best explained by movement of the hormone from original sites of incorporation in specific brain nuclei to terminal fields, through the mechanism of axonal transport. Because even at these late time intervals, inorganic iodide* levels were generally less than 5%, whereas T_3* (about 70%–80%) or other organic iodocompounds* (averaging 20%) clearly predominated, labeling patterns were considered relevant to the distribution of T_3* itself. Obviously, such attribution can be overturned by better methods of iodocompound analysis in localized brain regions. Note also that the persistence of T_3* as the predominant labeled iodocompound in brain after intravenous administration of the isotopically labeled hormone does not rule against the formation of important and functionally active T_3 metabolites in brain. The evidence only suggests that if there are such products they have shorter half-lives than T_3 itself.

ii. **Brain distribution of intravenously injected** [125]**I-labeled T_4** **(T_4*)**   Film autoradiograms prepared after intravenous injection of T_4* also showed a selective and saturable pattern of initial labeling (118). Although resolved more slowly over

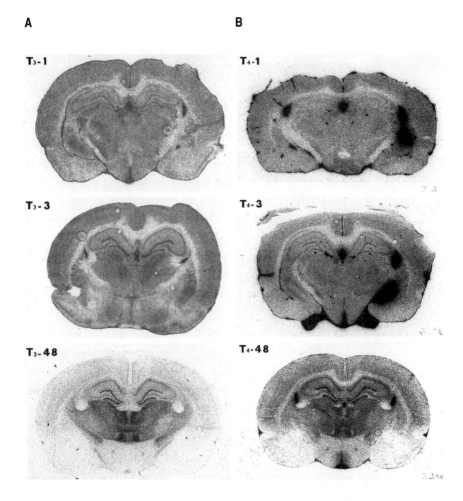

Figure 1–12. *Panel A:* Distribution of labeled triiodothyronine (T_3) in rat brain. Rats were decapitated at 1, 3, and 48 hours after intravenous iodine-125 (^{125}I)-labeled T_3 injection. Coronal brain sections at the level of the cortex, hippocampus, thalamus, and hypothalamus show change in distribution of radioactivity over time, accumulation in fornix at late time intervals, and selective distribution of radioactivity in thalamic nuclei. Label at all times due mainly (more than 80%) to T_3. Loss of radioactivity (especially in amygdala) is not due to artifact. (For more details and views of different brain levels, see Dratman et al. [117].) *Panel B:* Distribution of labeled thyroxine (T_4) in rat brain. Views of rat brain autoradiograms as in *Panel A* but obtained from rats injected with ^{125}I-labeled T_4. Note that changes in hormone distribution patterns over time are similar to those after ^{125}I-labeled T_3, but evolve more slowly. Autoradiographic reactions accounted for (more than 85%) by the sum of T_4 and T_3. (For a more complete discussion of biochemical and autoradiographic results in brains of rats receiving ^{125}I-labeled T_4, see Dratman and Crutchfield [118]).

time, the late distribution of radioactivity in terminal fields and fiber tracts was similar by all qualitative criteria to that seen after T_3^* administration. These relationships are exemplified by the autoradiograms shown in Figure 1–12 (compare *panel A* with *panel B*). Parallel biochemical studies of labeled brain homogenates revealed progressive replacement of T_4^* by T_3^*. Because the morphological characteristics of labeling patterns after T_4^* were completely disrupted by sodium ipodate, a powerful 5'D inhibitor, whereas labeling patterns after T_3^* were qualitatively unaffected by the drug, it was evident that patterns of brain labeling after T_4^* were due to in situ conversion and retention of T_3^* or T_3^* metabolites. Of further interest was the fact that treatment with PTU had no effect on labeling patterns after either T_3^* or T_4^* administration. Although this result supports well-accepted evidence that type II 5'D is resistant to PTU, interpretation of the lack of response in vivo is complicated by evidence suggesting that PTU cannot cross the BBB.

   Overall, the in vivo results following T_3^* and T_4^* administration were in keeping with the observations of thyroid hormone–deiodinase activity measured in dissected regions of rat brains. However, as already emphasized, the morphological and functional selectivity of brain–thyroid hormone interactions are hardly appreciated when regional dissections are the basis for comparing one unit of brain with another. These points are vividly appreciated on examining the detailed complexity of hormone distribution patterns in film autoradiograms and are further corroborated by evidence showing marked disparity between the results of measuring 5'D in whole hypothalamus and the results obtained from analyzing individual hypothalamic nuclei obtained by means of the punch-biopsy technique (104).

iii. Brain distribution of intravenously injected ^{125}I-labeled rT$_3$ (rT$_3^*$) Autoradiographic evidence obtained after administering rT$_3^*$ is in marked contrast with that seen after injecting T_3^* or T_4^* (118). The short half-life of rT$_3$ in serum is paralleled by a highly abbreviated residence time in brain. Early patterns of distribution resemble in every respect those seen after administering cerebral blood flow markers. Autoradiograms prepared at subsequent times fail to demonstrate any evidence of further differential distribution of the hormone. By the 3-hour interval, label coming from rT_3^* has entirely disappeared from the brain parenchyma. It therefore appears that administered rT_3 is not taken up into or, if taken up, is not retained by brain cells. Obviously, such studies give no information about the distribution and kinetics of rT_3 formed in situ.

b. **In situ hybridization histochemistry**

Autoradiography has been used to identify the distribution of mRNAs for T_3 nuclear receptors in brain using a labeled hybridizing probe (119). The rationale for these studies is described in greater detail in section 7.1 (on the c-*erb* A genes that code for the T_3 nuclear receptors). What is important at this point is that for each receptor subtype there were quite similar, but nevertheless distinctive, differences in profiles of regional localization of the message. Moreover, the studies confirm that the distribution of binding sites for T_3 seen at early times after intravenous administration of the labeled hormone is generally similar to the distribution of its T_3-binding receptors, although potentially interesting differences are evident.

c. **Immunohistochemical localization of Triiodothyronine (T_3) receptors in brain**

A detailed immunohistochemical study (120) has been reported recently describing use of any antibody directed against c-*erb* A gene products. Although not able to differentiate between T_3-binding and non-T_3-binding variant forms, this study showed a pattern of regional distribution generally similar to those previously described using other techniques. The antibody study included histological and electron-microscopic views of the immunocytochemical reaction products within cell nuclei, thereby achieving a new level of verification of T_3 nuclear receptor localization (120).

i. Cellular distribution All approaches taken to the study of
thyroid hormones in brain have led to the conclusion that a
large fraction of T_3 crossing the barrier systems and entering
the extracellular fluid space, as well as T_3 formed in situ from
T_4, is soon found bound in neurons (116). At the same time,
a number of studies have shown that T_4 is also taken up in glial
cells and that both nuclear receptors and 5'D activity are
found within astrocytes and oligodendroglia. Several techniques have been exploited in making these observations (e.g.,
gradient and/or differential centrifugations to separate neuronal and glial cells from mature brain [121,122], primary
cultures of glial cells from fetal brain [123], and separate neuronal and glial cell cultures obtained from tumor cell lines
[124,125]). The results demonstrated that by far the prepon-
derance of nuclear receptors are in neurons: in approximately
six- to eightfold greater concentration than in glial cells (Figure 1–13).

The mechanism of cellular uptake is not well defined because in vivo the uptake process cannot be separated from all
the other processes taking place simultaneously and no math-
ematical model for these events has yet been constructed.
When uptake of T_3 and T_4 into neurons was investigated
(using cultured neuroblastoma cells as the in vitro model), the
uptake process (see Figure 1–14) was found to be saturable,
sodium dependent, stereospecific, energy dependent, and
competitively inhibited by free L-system amino acids (124).
Transport into a glioma cell line was also demonstrated to be
mediated by a saturable, stereospecific, energy-dependent
process (125). However intriguing those observations may be
(suggesting an uptake mechanism for iodothyroamino acids
which is shared by other amino acids), they must be viewed
conservatively because they do not necessarily reflect the situation in adult brain cells in vivo.

ii. Subcellular distribution Use of differential centrifugation
and sucrose-gradient separation methods has allowed recovery of enriched subcellular fractions of brain homogenates

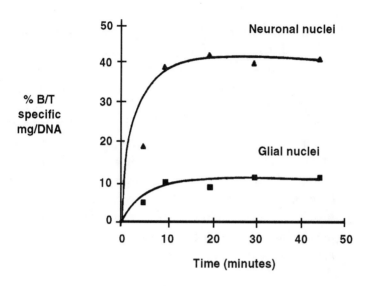

Figure 1–13. Time course of specific iodine-125 (^{125}I)-labeled triiodothyronine (T$_3$) binding in isolated neuronal and glial nuclei from brain of adult rats. Nuclei were incubated with ^{125}I-labeled T$_3$ (10^{-10} M) in binding buffer pH 7.4 at 37° C. Nonspecific binding, determined from parallel incubations with unlabeled T$_3$ (1 X 10^{-7} M), was subtracted from total ^{125}I-labeled T$_3$ and was 10%–15% of total binding. B/T = bound/total. *Source.* From Gullo D, Sinha AK, Woods R, et al: "Triiodothyronine Binding in Adult Rat Brain: Compartmentation of Receptor Populations in Purified Neuronal and Glial Nuclei." *Endocrinology* 120:325–331, 1987. Used with permission.

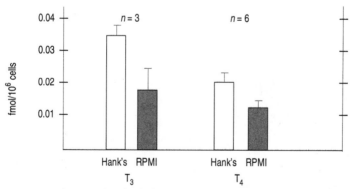

Figure 1–14. Nuclear uptake of triiodothyronine (T$_3$) or thyroxine (T$_4$) in neuroblasts incubated in cell culture medium or in Hank's solution plus HEPES containing no added amino acids. Note significant inhibition of both T$_4$ and T$_3$ uptake in presence of competing amino acids. *Source.* From Lakshmanan M, Goncalves E, Lessly G, et al: "The Transport of Thyroxine Into Mouse Neuroblastoma Cells, NB41A3: The Effect of L-System Amino Acids." *Endocrinology* 126:3245–3250, 1990. Used with permission.

(126). When these methods were used to investigate the subcellular distribution of intravenously delivered T_3* in brain,
the hormone was found to be differentially and reproductively
distributed among all the postnuclear subcellular organelles,
but to be most rapidly and selectively concentrated within the
synaptosomal fraction (127). The time course of these relationships is shown in Figure 1–15. A concentration gradient
of T_3 from brain cytosol to synaptosomes was already observed at 5 minutes after hormone injection (Figure 1–16); the
gradient increased linearly over the first hour and increased
further for at least 10 hours after receipt of the hormone. Approximately 85% of the synaptosomal radioactivity was released by osmotic disruption of the particles, providing

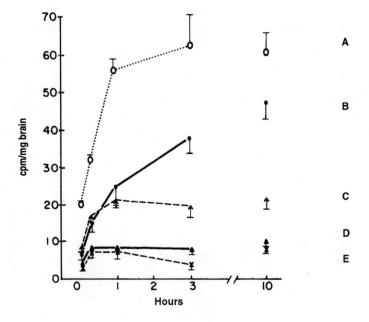

Figure 1–15. Radioactivity in subcellular particles of supranuclear fraction of rat brain
homogenate after intravenous iodine-125-labeled triiodothyronine. Data points show
mean counts per minute per mg brain ±SEM (ordinate) versus hours after intravenous
hormone injection (abscissa). A = synaptosomes; B = myelin; E = mitochondria; C and
D = intervening (unidentified) fractions in the gradient. *Source.*   From Dratman MB,
Crutchfield FL, Axelrod J, et al: "Localization of Triiodothyronine in Nerve Ending
Fractions of Rat Brain." *Proceedings of the National Academy of Sciences of the United
States of America* 73:941–944, 1976. Used with permission.

evidence that T_3 is taken up into nerve terminals and not merely bound to synaptosomal membranes. Radioactivity in other brain particles was entirely due to T_3^*, whereas, in synaptosomes, T_3^* was accompanied by a distinct peak of radioactivity amounting to 10% of the total, which was later identified as 3,3'-diiodothyronine (T_2). Thus, in vivo, T_3 is taken up, concentrated, and retained within nerve terminals.

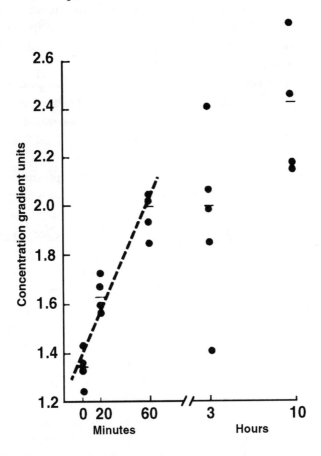

Figure 1–16. Ratios of labeled hormone in synaptosomes relative to brain cytosol after intravenous iodine-125-labeled triiodothyronine. The concentration gradient from cytosol to synaptosomes is linear through the first hour and shows a nonlinear increase thereafter. Each data point represents the ratio in an individual animal. *Source.* From Dratman MB, Crutchfield FL, Axelrod J, et al: "Localization of Triiodothyronine in Nerve Ending Fractions of Rat Brain." *Proceedings of the National Academy of Sciences of the United States of America* 73:941–944, 1976. Used with permission.

The presence of labeled T_2 suggested that type III deiodinase might be active in this brain fraction, a formulation that has since been confirmed by in vitro observations (128).

The kinetics of thyroid hormone uptake into synaptosomal preparations from rat brain have also been studied in vitro (129). These studies indicate that a saturable, sodium-requiring, and energy-dependent mechanism mediates the uptake process and show that the compartment of uptake is osmotically sensitive. The strict requirement for sodium favors an uptake mechanism similar to those mediating transport of amino acids.

The results, based on homogenization and gradient-separation methods after in vivo labeling of brain particles, are in keeping with autoradiographic evidence showing progressive accumulation of hormone in terminal fields of selected brain networks (117). Thus as represented in Figure 1–17, several lines of evidence now confirm that synaptosomal processing of T_3 is prominent and shares many features characteristic of aromatic amino acid processing in nerve terminals.

The capacity of synaptosomes to metabolize thyroid hormones in vivo was investigated further following intravenous $T_4{}^*$ administration (130). These experiments showed that radioactivity in synaptic particles was always greater than in any other particle separated per unit weight of brain and increased progressively relative to cytosol over the 15-hour period of observation. $T_3{}^*$, never identified as a separate peak in serum during those experiments, was observed in synaptosomes within 20 minutes and in brain cytosol within 1 hour after labeled-hormone administration; ratios of $T_3{}^*$ to $T_4{}^*$ were threefold greater in synaptosomes than in cytosol. The relationships of T_3-to-T_4 conversion ratios among various tissue components and brain fractions are illustrated in Figures 1–18 and 1–19.

Thus in vivo studies provided evidence for the presence of both 5D and 5'D enzymes in synaptosomes. Moreover, the rapid metabolism of T_4 and accumulation of T_3 suggested that the latter product or its triiodinated metabolites might act as mediators of the (proposed) synaptosomal mechanism of thyroid hormone action in the brain.

T_3 is not only taken up into synaptosomes through a well-defined, amino acid–related uptake mechanism, the hormone also binds to synaptosomal membranes (131). Studies of the binding process have revealed the presence of high-affinity synaptosomal membrane binding sites for T_3 that are non-uniformly distributed regionally and are therefore likely to be associated with discrete brain networks (132). The molecular characteristics and functional correlates of these binding elements have not yet been defined; some possibilities are illustrated in Figure 1–20.

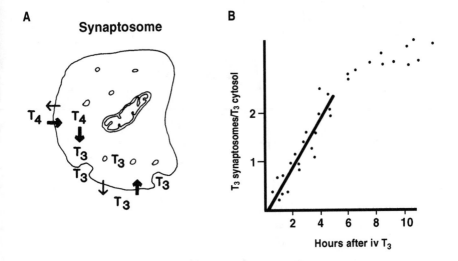

Figure 1–17. Mechanisms whereby high synaptosomal concentrations of triiodothyronine (T_3) might be favored. *Panel A:* Various sources of T_3 in synaptosomes: direct uptake from extracellular fluid (ECF), axonal transport from perikaryon, intra-synaptosomal conversion from thyroxine (T_4) after uptake of the latter from ECF, and detention at synaptosomal plasma membrane after binding to high-affinity sites. *Panel B:* Concentration gradient of T_3 from cytosol to synaptosomes over time after intravenous injection of hormone. Data were pooled from several separate experiments. *Source.* From Dratman MB, Crutchfield FL, Gordon JT: "Thyroid Hormones and Adrenergic Neurotransmitters," in *Catecholamines, Neuropharmacology and Central Nervous System: Theoretical Aspects.* Edited by Usdin E. New York, Alan R Liss, 1984, pp. 425–439. Used with permission.

7. THYROID HORMONE RECEPTORS IN BRAIN

According to present thinking, hormones are information-transmitting molecules that communicate their messages through a cascade of events initiated by their binding to high-affinity cellular receptors, the hormone fitting the receptor as a key fits a lock. Only the right key in the right lock

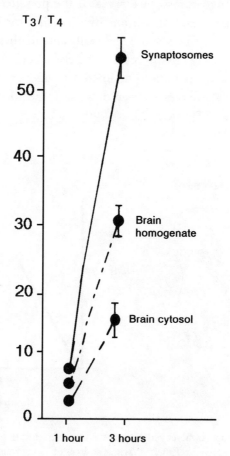

Figure 1–18. Fractional thyroxine (T_4) to triiodothyronine (T_3) conversion ratios in brain homogenates, cytosol, and synaptosomes. Rats were given an intravenous pulse of iodine-125–labeled T_4; brain homogenates and subcellular fractions of brain were extracted and iodothyronines were separated by high-performance liquid chromatography (HPLC). Data points show mean T_3/T_4 ±SD at 1 and 3 hours after isotope administration. *Source.* From Dratman MB, Crutchfield FL, Gordon JT: "Ontogeny of Thyroid Hormone-Processing Systems in Rat Brain," in *Iodine and the Brain.* Edited by DeLong GR, Robbins J, Condliffe PG. New York, Plenum, 1988, pp. 151–166. Used with permission.

will bring about the transduction of the hormone message, leading to the composite of structural and functional changes in cellular characteristics recognized as peculiar and specific to the actions of the hormone. However, despite the selectivity of receptors for their ligands, a large number of (seemingly) differently structured ligands can bind efficiently, even super-efficiently, to the receptor prototype and bring about all the actions of the ligand prototype.

7.1 Nuclear Receptors

The search for a thyroid hormone receptor extended over a period of many years and culminated in 1973 in the identification of nuclear binding sites for T_3 that fulfilled all of the then-required criteria of functional receptors (99). This discovery led to a font of new investigations, which in turn brought forth important information regarding the diverse effects of thyroid hormones on growth, development, and metabolic processes and established a rational connection (but

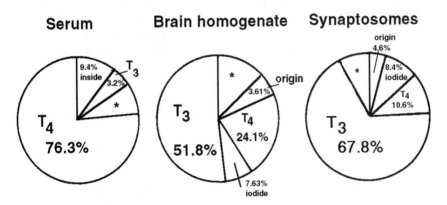

Figure 1–19. Concentration of endogenous iodocompounds in rat brain homogenates, synaptosomes, and serum. Pregnant Sprague-Dawley rats received Remington diet and iodine-125–labeled iodide in the drinking water from day 15 of gestation until weaning. Thereafter, offspring were continued on the low-iodine diet and labeled iodide until 40 days of age, at which stage iodocompound analyses were performed in brain homogenates and subcellular brain components. Note that the highest fractional concentrations of triiodothyronine (T_3) are in synaptosomes. T_4 = thyroxine; * = unidentified peaks and paper background. *Source.* From Dratman MB, Crutchfield FL: "Interactions of Adrenergic and Thyronergic Systems in the Development of Low T_3 Syndrome" (Serono Symposium No 40), in *The Low T_3 Syndrome.* Edited by Hesch RD. New York, Academic Press, 1981, pp. 115–126. Used with permission.

not a consistent cause-and-effect relationship) between T_3 nuclear receptor complex formation and the expression of many thyroid hormone effects in the organism.

In 1986, the T_3 nuclear receptor was identified as the product of the c-*erb* A proto-oncogene, the cellular homologue of a viral oncogene known as v-*erb* A (133). As represented in Figure 1–21, expression of the latter gene, together with a sister viral oncogene product (v-*erb* B), leads to the induction of an erythroid tumor in birds (avian erythroblastosis). However, the v-*erb* A gene product only collaborates with the v-*erb* B product to induce an oncogenetic effect; the latter gene is the prime mover in causing avian erythroblastosis (134). Although the cellular homologue c-*erb* A (the T_3 nuclear receptor gene) is referred to as a proto-oncogene, its claims to this role are somewhat in doubt. By contrast, c-*erb* B is a more nearly "true" proto-oncogene because its product, highly homologous to the epidermal growth factor (EGF) receptor, has autophosphorylating tyrosine kinase activity

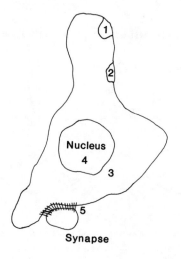

Receptor site: action

1. Plasma membrane: hormone uptake

2. Plasma membrane: T_3-stimulated transport of glucose, amino acids, ions, etc.

3. Cytosol: transport of T_3 to nucleus

4. Nucleus: altered gene transcription on formation of T_3-nuclear receptor complex

5. Synaptosomes: hormone transport? T_3-mediated information transfer?

Figure 1–20. Proposed triiodothyronine (T_3)-binding sites in neurons: plasma membrane receptors are described in cells of nonneuronal origin, but similar receptors are probably present in brain. High-affinity binding sites in cytosol, nuclei, and synaptosomes were characterized in brain fractions. Though looked for, mitochondrial receptors have not been found in brain (182). *Source.* From Dratman MB, Crutchfield FL, Gordon JT: "Thyroid Hormones and Adrenergic Neurotransmitters," in *Catecholamines, Neuropharmacology and Central Nervous System: Theoretical Aspects.* Edited by Usdin E. New York, Alan R Liss, 1984, pp. 425–439. Used with permission.

and entrains calcium-phosphoinositol second messenger pathways characteristic of the oncogenetic process (135,136).

Does the presence of these two genes in the same virus imply an original genetic linkage or a coordinated role in mammalian oncogenesis? This issue has not yet been settled (137,138). Retroviral oncogenes are considered to be transformed cellular genes that have been incorporated into the viral genome through the process of reverse transcription. The presence of *erb* A and *erb* B genes in the erythroblastosis-inducing virus might suggest that they are copies of linked cellular genes. However, they are separated in the virus by 12 base pairs and their presence on different chromosomes in the human but on the same chromosome in the mouse leaves the issue of their linkage still undetermined. Both of their cellular proto-oncogene products have normal growth effects in the organism and both cellular genes have, on some occasions, turned up in the same tumors. Moreover, as noted in the case of several different growth factors, the growth factor EGF and the growth promoter T_3 interact collaboratively (139,140).

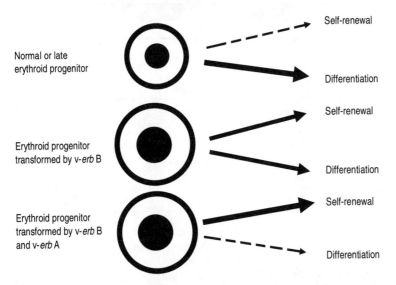

Figure 1–21. Action of viral genes involved in development of avian erythroblastosis. *Source.* Graf T, Beug H: "Role of the v-*erb* A and v-*erb* B Oncogenes of Avian Erythroblastosis Virus in Erythroid Cell Transformation." *Cell* 34:7–9, 1983

The c-*erb* A gene product, now equated with the T_3 nuclear receptor, is a so-called transacting DNA-binding protein with specific domains that determine its DNA- and ligand-binding activities (141). Variations in the size of these domains in different forms of the T_3 receptor are illustrated in Figure 1–22. The DNA site to which the receptor binds is the so-called thyroid response element (TRE), whereas the segment of the receptor that binds to the TRE is the DNA-binding domain. The TRE exhibits a defined, imperfect palindromic sequence of nucleic acids; the capacity of a gene to respond to T_3 requires that it have a TRE within its structure. The receptor generally binds to the TRE as a dimer (i.e., a complex of two receptors binding to a single TRE, each monomer binding to a half-palindrome). Within the 5′ end (ligand-binding domain) of the receptor is a helical stretch of amino acids that can be precisely aligned with a similar, complementary helix on a second receptor, forming a zipper-like structure that serves to hold the two receptors together as either a heterodimer or homodimer (142).

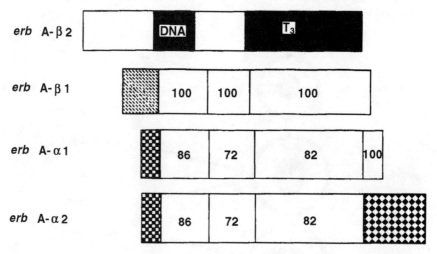

Figure 1–22. Suggested organization of rat nuclear receptors for triiodothyronine (T_3). The putative DNA- and T_3-binding domains are designated by analogy to the glucocorticoid receptor. Numbers within the boxes refer to percent nucleotide identity to *erb* A-β2. The *erb* A-α2 protein contains three more amino acids at its carboxyl terminus than do the proteins of *erb* A-α1. *Source.* Adapted from Hodin RA, Lazar MA: "Identification of a Thyroid Hormone Receptor That Is Pituitary-Specific." *Science* 244:76–79, 1989.

In theory, the following set of reactions occur in sequence: T_3 finds and binds to ligand-binding domain of the receptor protein and joins through hemizipper elements with another receptor; the resulting dimer in turn binds (as a transacting element) to the TRE. The binding of the new factors activate upstream DNA promoter elements, which act in a cis orientation to stimulate the polymerase reactions necessary for DNA transcription. The newly transcribed DNA is then copied into nuclear mRNA, which contains all of the constituents of the gene, both introns (untranslated DNA segments) and exons (usually translated or otherwise translationally involved segments). A subsequent edition (but not a new copy) of that mRNA involves a splicing step, which removes the introns and retains only exons. This process yields so-called mature mRNA, the mRNA that is now found in the cytosol and that determines the nature of the protein molecules to be synthesized by the ribosomes. This form of RNA is recognized in the in situ hybridization process. Because cytosolic mRNA is assembled in the sense direction, an antisense probe is required for hybridization, with a sense probe serving as a negative control. However (rarely, but nevertheless applicable to T_3 receptors), when the opposite DNA strand as well as the usual DNA strand is transcribed, both sense and antisense probes will hybridize.

The big news about c-*erb* A is that it has opened up a realm of possibilities for explaining the diverse biological roles of T_3. It turns out that while c-*erb* A codes for the T_3 receptor, other strongly homologous products of related genes (considered a gene superfamily) code for an entire family of receptors that includes the gonadal and adrenal steroids, the sterol hormone vitamin D, and the presumed morphogen, retinoic acid (143,144). The close structural relationships among all of these receptors raises issues about relationships among their ligands; the implications are only now beginning to unfold. One of the more interesting relationships thus far demonstrated, but not yet fully understood, is between T_3 and retinoic acid. The retinoic acid receptor (RAR) is capable of binding to a TRE, although a T_3 receptor cannot bind to a retinoic acid response element (RRE). An RAR and a T_3 receptor can dimerize, and the heterodimer can bind one of each ligand. The complex can, in turn, bind to a TRE. This result suggests that retinoic acid and T_3 may be coordinately involved in regulating gene expression (145). This result also suggests that the coordinated transport of both T_4 and retinol by TTR and the localization of TTR at selected sites (choroid plexus, retina, and pancreatic islets) may not be entirely coincidental and that it may instead have important implications for the mechanism of thyroid hormone action.

At least two main classes of the c-*erb* A genes have been recognized, yielding the so-called α and β forms of the receptors. These two receptor classes are now known to be coded for by two separate genes residing on two different chromosomes. Moreover, alternate splicing has led to their further classification into α1 and α2 and β1 and β2 subclasses (Figure 1–22). It turns out that these different classes of receptors have significantly different tissue distribution profiles (see Table 1–3), as well as different structural and binding characteristics: the α1, β1, and β2 receptors bind T_3, but the α2 receptor does not (146). The latter form has a truncated binding site, has no known ligand, has nevertheless retained its capacity to bind to a TRE, and exerts a so-called dominant negative effect through its occupation of a TRE (which is thereby no longer available for occupancy by a T_3-

Table 1–3. Relative abundance of thyroid hormone receptor subtypes (hTR) mRNAs per gram human tissues

Tissue	hTRβ	hTRα1 (3.2 kb)	hTRα1 (6.0 kb)	hTRα2
Kidney	1.0	1.0	1.0	1.0
Liver	0.2	0.1	0.2	0.2
Placenta	0.9	0.6	0.4	0.6
Tonsil	0.2	0.2	0.5	0.2
Spleen	1.2	1.2	1.6	1.5
Brain	UA	54.3	42.3	50.0
Prostate	UA	50.2	44.1	23.9
Thyroid	UA	135.6	60.6	87.5

Note. Relative amounts of TR mRNAs (per g tissue) in various human tissues. The relative amounts of mRNAs are expressed relative to the value for kidney normalized to 1.0. All values are the means of the following calculation in each experiment:

$$\frac{(mRNA\ abundance)/(mRNA\ abundance\ of\ kidney)}{(RNA\ recover)/(RNA\ recovery\ of\ kidney)}$$

UA = data unavailable. *Source.* From Sakurai A, Nakai A, DeGroot LJ: "Expression of Three Forms of Thyroid Hormone Receptor in Human Tissues." *Molecular Endocrinology* 3:392–399, 1989. Used with permission.

binding receptor) (147). The β2 receptor is also distinctive in that it is found mainly in the pituitary gland and is strongly downregulated by T₃. This form of the receptor may bind to the gene coding for the TSH subunits (148).

Customarily, DNA transcription occurs from a single one of the two DNA strands of a chromosome. However, sometimes the opposite strand is also transcribed. This duplicity has been noted in the case of transcription of c-*erb* Aα, yielding yet another receptor subtype that does not bind T₃. The transcript coming from the opposite strand is schematically represented in Figure 1–23; it is reversed in nucleic acid sequence, its mRNA is recognized by a sense probe, and it codes for still another dominant negative form (149).

Of considerable interest is the fact that c-*erb* A–encoded proteins are most heavily represented in the brain (146). It is possible that the strong presence of dominant negative types may allow a high degree of control, in that T₃ action might vary according to the active-counteractive receptor forms on hand. To a degree, T₃ also regulates the rate of its own receptor turnover, a function that varies according to the subtype and possibly to other parameters not yet fully defined. Thus the interplay of positive and negative elements, the presence of receptors of varying half-lives, the likelihood that at least some of the α2 and reverse forms bind to unknown ligands, and the preference for forming receptor dimers (of which some are of the heterologous

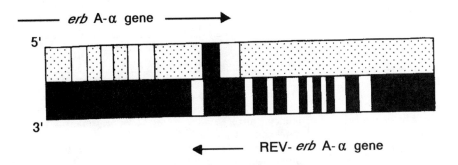

Figure 1–23. Overview of the organization of the *erb* A-α and REV-*erb* A-α genes (rat). *Source.* Adapted from Lazar MA, Hodin RA, Darling DS, et al: "A Novel Member of the Thyroid/Steroid Hormone Receptor Family Is Encoded by the Opposite Strand of the Rat c-erbAα Transcriptional Unit." *Molecular and Cellular Biology* 9:1128–1136, 1989.

type) all contribute to the potential for variability with which T_3, through its receptors, may influence gene expression in the brain.

Many negative results have been obtained in studies designed to demonstrate functional or biochemical effects of T_3 nuclear receptors in adult brain. However, recently Nikodem, Robbins, and their co-workers have characterized a TRE in the gene for myelin basic protein (MBP), which is active in both the developing and young adult rat brain. Notably, hypothyroidism initiated in the 5th and 6th week of life led to changes in expression of the MBP gene which were corrected by T_4 replacement. This represents the first demonstration of a TRE in a brain-specific gene and provides unequivocal evidence that thyroid hormones function in the adult CNS (149a).

One alternative model is based on evidence that a major change in the actions of many neuroactive compounds, particularly synaptically active compounds, comes about during the shift from one developmental phase to another (150). As noted in Table 1–4, many substances that regulate certain critical phases of neurogenesis and nerve cell specialization during brain development are better known and were originally identified for their important neuroregulatory or direct neurotransmitter roles in the differentiated, that is, adult, brain. Therefore, the early and important (but little emphasized) growth-promoting activities of biogenic amines, acetylcholine, γ-aminobutyric acid (GABA), and substance P are expressed well before the

Table 1–4. Role of neuroactive agents in the brain

Developing brain		Mature brain
Apparatus for neurotransmission		
Not yet in place	Forming or in place	In place
Mitogenic and differentiating effects on neuroblasts; control of morphogenetic cell movements	Pre- and transsynaptic actions as trophic agents inducing further developmental specializations (e.g., neurite elongation, myelinogenesis, and synaptogenesis)	Transsynaptic actions as neuromodulators or neurotransmitters

Source. Adapted from Dratman MB, Crutchfield FL, Gordon JT: "Ontogeny of Thyroid Hormone-Processing Systems in Rat Brain," in *Iodine and the Brain.* Edited by DeLong GR, Robbins J, Condliffe PG. New York, Plenum, 1988, pp. 151–166. Used with permission.

apparatus of neurotransmission has been set in place. Although receptors for these early activities are not known, they may be the same or different from those mediating the information transmitting synaptic activities of neuromodulators and neurotransmitters in the adult brain. After the apparatus of neurotransmission is fully in place, these originally growth- and maturation-inducing substances become heavily involved in synaptic functions. Although remnants of their original activities are reflected in their continued involvement in neurite growth and plasticity, the neurotransmitters are mainly responsible, in adult brain, for regulating, modulating, or directly transmitting information across synapses.

Developmentally determined major changes in the actions of known neurotransmitters set a pattern for neuroactive compounds in general and raise the possibility that thyroid hormones may also pursue their roles in the brain through a series of different, developmentally determined mechanisms. Early effects of T_3 on neuroblast proliferation and differentiation occur before the apparatus for neurotransmission has developed, and the likelihood that these effects are mediated through the nuclear receptor seems highly convincing although not yet directly demonstrated. Later (noted in the first weeks of postnatal life of the rat), a T_3-processing synaptosomal apparatus emerges (details of this process discussed below). This phase of nerve cell specialization and neurite elongation may also involve nuclear receptors, but affirmative evidence of this involement is thus far not available.

In the differentiated brain, a thyroid hormone–dependent mechanism for maintaining plasticity is suggested by evidence that, in adult-onset hypothyroidism, the density of dendritic spines of cortical pyramidal cells is significantly reduced and susceptible to at least some degree of repair by institution of thyroid hormone treatment (151). At the same time, evidence that thyroid hormones may modify or mediate intercellular communication is indicated by 1) biochemical evidence of a high degree of intraneuronal thyroid hormone metabolizing and synaptosomal concentrating activity, particularly in hypothyroidism; 2) morphological evidence of active axonal transport with resulting high concentration of hormone in terminal fields; 3) presence of high-affinity synaptosomal membrane binding sites for

T_3; and *4)* earlier heart rate response of hypothyroid animals to intrathecal than to intravenous injection of thyroid hormone. Proposed molecular mechanisms for transynaptic neuroregulatory functions of T_3 or T_3 metabolites are described below.

7.2 Plasma Membrane Receptors

Receptors for thyroid hormones were originally assumed to be in the plasma membrane and were sought there for many years. Thus far, at least three separate T_3 membrane binding entities mediating several separate cellular functions have been identified. A membrane receptor studied in detail by Segal (152) and Segal and Ingbar (153) binds T_3 with high affinity and is associated with immediate changes in cellular glucose, calcium, and amino acid transport functions; these responses are modified in the presence of norepinephrine. Recently, Segal (154) has provided further evidence that transduction of the biochemical information communicated by the interaction of the membrane receptor with T_3 involves calcium uptake. However intriguing the possibility that these events might reflect universal T_3-dependent cellular phenomena, there is no direct information available that might link the membrane receptor identified in somatic cells with any parallel receptors in brain cells.

Another category of thyroid hormone plasma membrane receptors has been extensively studied by Cheng et al. (155). These receptors mediate the endocytosis of T_3 into fibroblasts through a mechanism reminiscent of that described for the uptake of low-density lipoprotein (LDL). Like LDL, T_3 is taken up into coated pits and travels to the lysosomes within vesicles. Further studies have revealed that T_4 entry into LDL-competent fibroblasts is enhanced by LDL (156). In addition, the membrane receptors involved in transport of the aromatic amino acid, T_3, into erythrocytes are reported to be closely linked to the transport of other aromatic amino acids into these cells (157).

Still another form of plasma membrane receptor for thyroid hormones has been studied in depth by Davis et al. (158). These receptors are linked to the calcium ATPase family of transmembrane proteins and are stimulated by the binding of T_4 and T_4 analogues. As in the case of other plasma membrane receptors for thyroid hormones, no direct information is available regarding their presence in brain cells.

7.3 Mitochondrial Receptors

The rate of total body energy transformation is one of the major and obvious consequences of thyroid hormone action. Although several lines of evidence have suggested that effects of iodothyronines on metabolic rates and oxygen and glucose consumption are correlates of their primary effects on protein synthesis, a direct effect of the hormones on mitochondrial activity mediated through a mitochondrial receptor seems reasonable. Evidence for the possibility that the ADP-ATP translocase functions as such a receptor has been assembled by Sterling and colleagues (159), but the issue remains unsettled. No evidence has been offered to suggest that mitochondrial binding sites in the CNS account for the actions of the hormone in brain.

7.4 Synaptosomal Receptors

The demonstration several years ago that a high-affinity membrane binding site for T_3 is found in enriched synaptosomal preparations from rat brain raises the possibility that a nerve terminal–associated receptor for T_3 mediates some of the actions of the hormone in brain (131,132). These binding sites have an affinity for T_3 similar to that of T_3 for the nuclear receptor. Found in low concentrations during fetal life, synaptosomal binding sites begin to increase shortly after birth, suggesting their possible participation in T_3-dependent nerve cell specialization, neurite elongation, and synaptogenesis. Synaptosomal T_3-binding sites reach their maximum concentration in the adult. They are also heterogeneously distributed regionally, indicating a likely association with selected neural networks. No experimental information is available about any functional implications of T_3 synaptosomal binding. However, these in vitro observations conform with those made in vivo following intravenous injection of labeled T_3 in adult rats, as well as with observations made in developing rats in the course of isotope equilibrium experiments.

8. THYROID HORMONE HOMEOSTASIS IN BRAIN

Only a few observations speak directly to the issue of thyroid hormone action in adult brain. Among the most impressive are those demonstrating that in hypothyroidism the disposition of available thyroid hormone molecules highly favors the brain (160). After thyroidectomy, the liver desists from converting T_4 to T_3 or otherwise metabolizing the hormone (as it does in the case of other scarce, limited, but important, substrates), allowing more of what is available to be used by other tissues with 5'D capability. If we accept the premise that T_3, rather than T_4, is the active thyroid hormone molecule, this action would serve to make the hypothyroid rat liver, as well as tissues dependent on it for their source of T_3, even more hypothyroid. However, the biological rationale for this action of the liver is appreciated when the response of the brain is taken into account. In that context, it is apparent that the brain is prepared to take maximal advantage of the sparing action of liver by markedly increasing its own fractional rate of T_3 production from T_4. These mechanisms make the brain among the most active of all T_3-forming (and presumably T_3-utilizing) tissues during hypothyroidism. Some of these relationships are illustrated in Figure 1–7.

As a result of these coordinated efforts, total levels of T_4 and T_3 in brain are reduced relatively little in hypothyroidism. Because diverting T_4 for use by the brain requires both somatic and CNS tissue responses, it appears that this homeostatic adjustment provides some advantage to the entire hypothyroid organism. Endogenous levels of T_3 and T_4 in serum, liver, and brain during different thyroid states are shown in Figure 1–24.

The brain, in collaboration with the liver, also makes homeostatic adjustments in hyperthyroidism. Although, as derived from calculating initial reaction rate kinetics, T_4 and T_3 uptake and turnover in somatic tissues are markedly increased in this condition, T_3 levels and T_3 turnover in brain are not noted to be significantly different in the hypo-, eu-, and hyperthyroid states.

Most studies describe a decrease in T_3 turnover in hypothyroid rat brain (161). However, these conclusions reflect measurements made at equilibrium. The difference in results derived from different methods of kinetic analysis may indicate that there is more than one phase of T_3 turnover (e.g., an initial [early] phase and an equilibrium [later] phase). Further studies of brain T_3 turnover in altered thyroid states are clearly indicated because, if in hypothyroidism a phase of maintained T_3 turnover is validated, the possibility of a T_3-derived active metabolite would be favored.

Issues related to thyroid hormone homeostasis arise when treatment with thyroid hormone is contemplated. In particular, uncertainties emerge in situations in which the degree of peripheral thyroid function is only mildly abnormal but evidence of altered CNS function argues for prompt and appropriate clinical intervention. The evidence overall favors treatment with T_4 rather than T_3, but if the clinical evidence suggests that failure of thyroid hormone homeostasis is the problem (as proposed in previous sections of this chapter) and if dysregulation is at the level of central T_4 5′ deiodination, perhaps T_3 would be the best choice. Despite speculations to the contrary, hard autoradiographic and biochemical evidence developed in both thyroidectomized and intact animals clearly indicates that T_3 enters the brain from the bloodstream, engages with nuclear receptors, and migrates through axons to reach terminal fields (117). Therefore, there is no reason why administered T_3 should not be effective if diminished 5′D activity were the limiting problem. On the other hand, as one treats with T_3, thyroid gland activity and, particularly, T_4 production rates fall. Is it possible to support the brain entirely with exogenously ad-

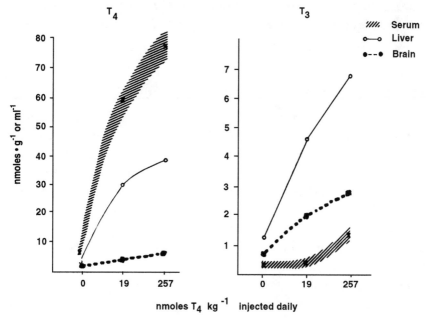

Figure 1–24. Endogenous concentrations of thyroxine (T_4) and triiodothyronine (T_3) in rat liver, brain, and serum during altered states of thyroid function. Tissue homogenates were extracted with chloroform-methanol; iodothyronines in extracts and serum were measured by radioimmunoassay. Values are arithmetic means ±SD. *Source.* From Dratman MB, Crutchfield FL, Gordon JT, et al: "Iodothyronine Homeostasis in Rat Brain During Hypo- and Hyperthyroidism." *American Journal of Physiology* 245:E185–E193, 1983. Used with permission.

ministered T_3? The evidence suggests that T_4 is necessary because, despite the use of even large doses of T_3, which effectively suppress T_4 production by the thyroid, the brain manages to maintain a close-to-normal level of both hormones. Nevertheless, brain T_3-to-T_4 ratios are significantly increased under those conditions (M. B. Schoenhoff, M. B. Dratman, unpublished observations, March 1988).

If for some reason the clinical decision is to press for maximally tolerated doses of T_4, continued intracerebral production of T_3 in the brain would, under normal circumstances, be inhibited. But again, if the presumed dysregulation lies at the level of the T_3-forming enzymes, inhibition may not occur (i.e., the deiodinase may be nonsuppressible). In the face of these dilemmas, it is not possible to pontificate. What is badly needed is some method for measuring brain–thyroid hormone processing in vivo. Brain glucose metabolism can be measured in vivo using labeled 2-deoxyglucose and positron-emission tomography (PET) scanning (162). An in vivo technique involving use of an appropriate T_3 analogue would be welcome.

9. THYROID HORMONE ACTIONS IN ADULT BRAIN

Efficient homeostatic responses that protect the brain during adult-onset hypothyroidism and hyperthyroidism speak strongly for lifelong requirements by the CNS for thyroid hormones. Several other reports speak to this issue as well. However, before mentioning them, a caveat must be introduced. Long-standing changes in thyroid function lead to considerable changes in dynamics of the cerebral circulation (163), and these, rather than direct effects of the hormone in brain, may be responsible for symptoms of brain dysfunction. Although many changes in adult brain function have been described, only a few well-controlled sets of observations appears to provide direct information about thyroid hormone action in the brain. The first observations came from experiments in which heart rate responses were compared in conscious hypothyroid rats given T_3 intrathecally or intravenously (164). As noted in Figure 1–25, a significant increase in heart rate occurred within 18 hours after 1.5 nmol T_3/100 g body weight was delivered intrathecally through a cannula previously placed in the lateral cerebral ventricle. Injection of the same T_3 dose intravenously through an indwelling jugular catheter, injection of vehicle only by either route, and injection of T_4 and rT_3 intrathecally produced no significant increase in heart rate during the 48-hour postinjection period of observation. The effects of intrathecal T_3 administration on heart rate emerged even though integrated serum T_3 concentrations were significantly lower after intrathecal versus after intravenous T_3 injection. Results indicating that thyroid hormone effects on heart rate are exerted within the brain, as well as within the heart, point to a correlation between peripheral and central noradrenergic and thyronergic mechanisms.

Some recent in vitro observations deserve thoughtful consideration.

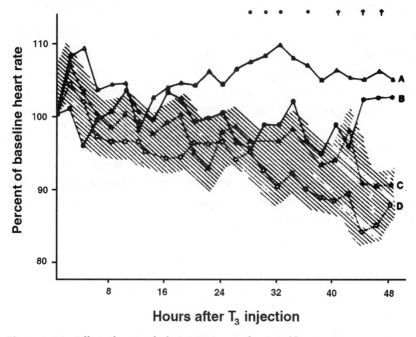

Hours after T_3 injection

Figure 1–25. Effect of route of administration on fractional heart rate response to triiodothyronine (T_3). Pairs of rats receiving T_3 1 μg/100 g body weight or NaOH by intravenous or intrathecal injection were observed simultaneously. Mean fractional changes from baseline are shown in 2-hourly intervals after intrathecal T_3 (A), intravenous T_3 (B), intrathecal NaOH (C), or intravenous NaOH (D). Shaded area shows composite range of standard deviation for NaOH-treated groups, which were not significantly different from each other. Fractional heart rate responses in intrathecally T_3-treated rats were significantly greater than in those given intravenous T_3 ($P< .04$) or in NaOH-treated groups. *Source.* From Dratman MB, Crutchfield FL, Gordon JT: "Ontogeny of Thyroid Hormone-Processing Systems in Rat Brain," in *Iodine and the Brain.* Edited by DeLong GR, Robbins J, Condliffe PG. New York, Plenum, 1988, pp. 151–166. Used with permission.

Mason, Prange, and co-workers have investigated effects of thyroid hormones on GABA release by synaptosomes with results that further the idea that interrelationships between thyroid hormones and other neurotransmitters are by no means limited to tyrosine-derived systems (165). More recently, their studies of changes in calcium processing by synaptosomes have suggested that in the synaptosomal systems in which it is concentrated, T_3 may play a part in modulating uptake and/or release of a number of neurotransmitters (166).

10. THYROID HORMONE ACTIONS IN THE DEVELOPING BRAIN

Brain maturation in human subjects is dependent on the orderly execution of a developmental program that is based on inherent mechanisms and is generally quite resistant to external influences. For example, balanced nutritional deprivation must be extreme before changes in structure and function of the developing brain become evident. Nevertheless imbalance relevant to even one ingredient such as phenylalanine or iodothyronines during fetal and early postnatal life causes marked derangement in the execution of the normal developmental program. The result is widespread but heterogeneous, which in the case of hypothyroidism causes regional abnormalities in growth of nerve-cell processes and impaired synaptogenesis (167). Most striking from the clinical standpoint is the irreversible nature of the resulting brain damage. All too many individuals with cretinism have this preventable form of stunted brain development. When the mental function of hypothyroid children remains uncorrected, or is corrected too late, the difference in outcome is dramatic compared with that of children receiving early thyroid hormone treatment (168).

It is suspected, but not yet proven, that thyroid hormone effects on the brain start well before delivery. However, the hypothyroid fetus may be protected somewhat by placental hormones if the mother has normal thyroid function and iodine deficiency is not the limiting problem. After delivery, the effects of hypothyroidism, unbuffered except by small quantities of hormone transported in the milk, proceed apace. Therefore, the worst ravages of perinatal hypothyroidism may be avoided by immediate correction after neonatal hypothyroidism has been diagnosed. As a result of these clinical observations and the basic investigations that have followed, thyroid hormones are now considered to be a major regulator, possibly the most important single regulator, of normal brain maturation.

Descriptions of the evolution of thyroid-deficient newborns treated with hormones shortly after birth indicate that "cretinism" is not an all-or-none entity. As noted above, certain individuals with early-appearing and persistent disorders of mood, behavior, and/or cognition may be expressing the results of partial thyroid hormone–related damage to the developing brain.

The big issue has always been: By what mechanism(s) is the thyroid hormone acting as it brings the brain into a normal state of maturation?

Some informed speculations on this issue are now available, based on several lines of experimental evidence: 1) investigations of nuclear receptor occupancy during the period of neuroblast proliferation, 2) studies of the ontogeny of c-*erb* A subclasses during development, 3) studies of the effects of the hormone on gene expression during the so-called critical period of brain maturation, and 4) observations of the ontogeny of regional and subcellular iodocompound distribution and processing during the same period of brain maturation (169,170). Conclusions derived from these different lines of evidence, and especially those provided by studies of early fetal brain development, generally support the view (without yet establishing cause and effect) that, during the period of neuroblast proliferation and differentiation, thyroid hormone–dependent fetal brain growth and development are largely due to exquisitely timed interactions of T_3 receptors with TREs in DNA, with the resultant orderly sequences of changes in gene expression that are required for the earliest phase of brain-cell differentiation.

Efforts to determine the ontogeny of the nuclear receptor during the critical period have not yet provided any definitive information linking changes in *erb* A receptor subtype abundance with ontogenetic features of brain development. However, the observations made in families with the syndrome of generalized hormone resistance (171) have suggested that such changes may be found when studies are carried out in more evolved animal models than those offered by rodents.

Because of the widespread nature of thyroid hormone effects in the developing brain, a formulation offered by Nunez and colleagues (144)— that T_3 deficiencies may prevent normal development of the cytoskeleton through a deficiency of microtubule-associated proteins—was received with great enthusiasm. Moreover, the evidence supporting this idea is impressive and convincing. Nevertheless, efforts to link T₃ actions in the developing brain to expression of genes for microtubule-associated proteins and other potentially important CNS targets, have so far not been supported by Northern (mRNA) analyses of brains examined at various stages of development (172).

Finally, experiments tracking the disposition of endogenous iodothyronines in developing brain have provided evidence that the perinatal rat brain may be sensitive to hypothyroidism because the iodothyronines may serve as essential substrates for the CNS during the time that its apparatus for neurotransmission is being completed (5,169). Details of the ontogeny of such systems were obtained in rat pups who were nurtured on ¹²⁵I-iodide-containing milk from dams receiving daily supplements of ¹²⁵I-iodide in their drinking water. This regimen (i.e., producing isotopic equilibrium throughout the pup body) allowed iodocompounds present in the developing rat brain to be measured and localized throughout the early postnatal phase of rat brain development. The results showed that significant differences in distribution of iodocompounds in different brain regions were already evident on day 1 of life and that developmental progress was associated with significantly different rates of accumulation of the hormones (Figure 1–26). Early in the postnatal period, most of the hormones were in brain cytosol. By the time of weaning, they were predominantly localized in brain particles, particularly in synaptosomes (in the osmotically sensitive compartment, as well as bound to synaptosomal membranes) (Figures 1–27 and 1–28). Through this process, the stage may be set for a series of developmental events pertaining to neurite growth and synapse formation in the particular neural systems that process iodothyronines, wherein arborizing nerve terminals containing more and more T₃ may be recognized by postsynaptic elements endowed with increasing numbers of T₃ recognition sites (postsynaptic membrane and nuclear receptors) (5).

Eventually, processes characteristic of the developing brain merge with those supporting the differentiated brain. Such mergers are usefully explained if the hormones of the thyroid gland are conceptualized as amino acids involved in protein synthesis during early phases of brain development (an involvement probably orchestrated by nuclear receptors for T₃). After establishment of the apparatus of neurotransmission the hormones may function as neuroactive amino acids (or as amino acid precursors of neuroactive compounds), which modify information transmission at synapses. A scheme is shown in Figure 1–29 whereby various molecular alterations or additions to T$_3$ might allow it to serve in this capacity.

11. CONCLUDING REMARKS

It is anticipated that when a new volume discussing possible thyroid hormone–related aspects of brain dysfunctions is published for psychiatrists 5 years from now, its message will be dramatically different from that delivered in this volume. We are on the cusp of making fundamental discov-

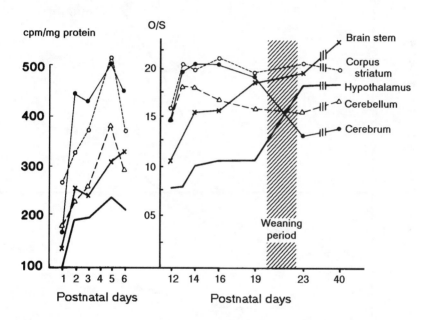

Figure 1–26. Regional distribution of endogenous brain iodocompounds during development. Iodocompound measurements made from postnatal day 1 through 40 showed that, relative to brain stem (where levels increased progressively during the period of observation), levels in corpus striatum were maintained at a generally high level; in cerebellum, levels were maintained at an intermediate level; in hypothalamus, there was a slow rise with marked increase during weaning; and in cerebrum, levels were initially high and then had a significant decrease with weaning. Little further regional change was noted from day 23 to 40, at which time all values were significantly different from each other ($P < .05$). CPM = counts per minute; O/S = ratio of brain to serum iodocompounds expressed as cpm/ml. *Source.* From Dratman MB, Crutchfield FL, Gordon JT: "Ontogeny of Thyroid Hormone-Processing Systems in Rat Brain," in *Iodine and the Brain.* Edited by DeLong GR, Robbins J, Condliffe PG. New York, Plenum, 1988, pp. 151–166. Used with permission.

eries about the mechanisms of thyroid hormone action in the brain and its implications for abnormalities of brain function. To use the information as it emerges will require a broad understanding of many of the issues touched on in this chapter: mechanisms of thyroid axis functions and their

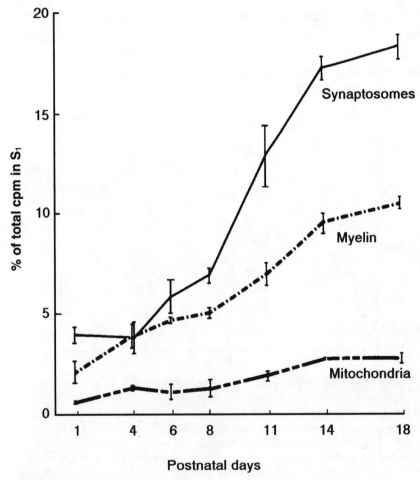

Figure 1–27. Endogenous iodocompounds in rat brain during development: localization in supranuclear (S_1) subcellular particles. Data show mean percentage of total iodocompounds in synaptosomes, myelin, and mitochondria; differences among the different particles are significant ($P < .001$) both as to amounts and rates of change. *Source.* From Dratman MB, Crutchfield FL, Gordon JT: "Ontogeny of Thyroid Hormone-Processing Systems in Rat Brain," in *Iodine and the Brain.* Edited by DeLong GR, Robbins J, Condliffe PG. New York, Plenum, 1988, pp. 151–166. Used with permission.

vicissitudes, peripheral pathways of processing the hormones and transducing their messages, particulars of hormone delivery systems from thyroid to brain, nature and extent of collaborative functions among thyroid hormones and other neuroactive moieties, and finally the peripheral, as well as intracerebral, regulatory mechanisms and dysregulations that determine the difference between thyroid hormone–dependent brain health and disease.

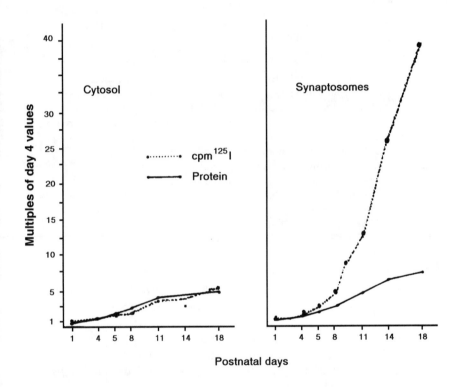

Figure 1–28. Developmental changes in iodocompound binding sites in synaptosomes and cytosol. Rat pup brains were analyzed at intervals during the nursing period. Individual data points represent mean levels in cytosol and synaptosomes per brain ($n \geq$ 10), expressed as a multiple of the mean day 4 value. Note that after day 4, ratios of protein to iodocompound content were constant for cytosol but changed significantly for synaptosomes ($P < .001$); differences between cytosol and synaptosomal iodocompounds per mg protein were significant ($P < .001$). CPM = counts per minute. *Source.* From Dratman MB, Crutchfield FL, Gordon JT: "Ontogeny of Thyroid Hormone-Processing Systems in Rat Brain," in *Iodine and the Brain.* Edited by DeLong GR, Robbins J, Condliffe PG. New York, Plenum, 1988, pp. 151–166. Used with permission.

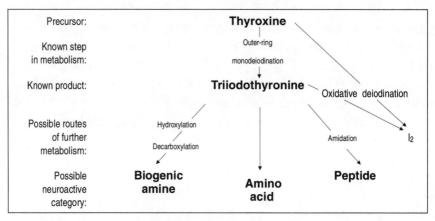

Figure 1–29. Proposed thyroxine-derived neuromodulators: possible routes of formation. Thyroxine, after outer-ring monodeiodination, may enter into a "false" transmitter pathway of metabolism leading to the formation of thyronine-derived catecholamine analogues; the outer-ring monodeiodination product, triiodothyronine, may itself serve as an amino acid neuromodulator; iodothyronines, may be viewed as dipeptides (i.e., derived from the condensation of two tyrosyl residues), which if amidated or otherwise modified may serve as peptidergic neuromodulators; deiodinations mediated by peroxidases or other oxidative enzymes may lead to the formation of a gaseous neuroactive molecule in the form of I_2. *Source.* From Dratman MB: "Early Ontogeny of Iodocompound-Processing Neural Systems in Rat Brain." *Discussions in Neurosciences* 1:73–76, 1984. Used with permission.

REFERENCES

1. Lissitzky S, Torresani J, Carayon P, et al.: Physiology of the thyroid, in Endocrinology. Edited by DeGroot LJ. Philadelphia, PA, WB Saunders, 1989, pp 512–540
2. Halmi NS: Thyroidal iodide transport. Vitam Horm 19:133–163, 1961
3. Taurog A: Hormone synthesis: thyroid iodine metabolism, in The Thyroid, 5th Edition. Edited by Ingbar SH, Braverman LE. Philadelphia, PA, JB Lippincott, 1986, pp 53–97
4. Ekholm R, Wollman SH: Site of iodination in the rat thyroid gland deduced from electron microscopic autoradiographs. Endocrinology 97:1432–1444, 1975
5. Dratman MB: Early ontogeny of iodocompound-processing neural systems in rat brain. Discussions in Neurosciences 1:73–76, 1984
6. Wollman SH, Lowenstein JE: Rates of colloid droplet and apical vessicle production and membrane turnover during thyroglobulin secretion and resorption. Endocrinology 93:248–252, 1973
7. Dunn AD, Dunn JT: Thyroglobulin degradation by thyroidal proteases: action of purified cathepsin D. Endocrinology 111:280–289, 1982

8. Melander A, Ericson ME, Sundler F, et al: Sympathetic innervation of the mouse thyroid and its significance in thyroid hormone secretion. Endocrinology 94:959–966, 1974

9. Oppenheimer JH, Surks MI: Quantitative aspects of hormone production, distribution, metabolism, and activity, in Handbook of Physiology, Vol 3. Edited by Greep RO, Astwood EB, Greer MA, et al. Washington, DC, American Physiological Society, 1974, pp 197–214

10. Hennenmann G (ed): Thyroid Hormone Metabolism. New York, Marcel Dekker, 1986

11. Gavin LA, Moeller M, McMahon FA, et al: Carbohydrate feeding increases total body and specific tissue 3,5,3'-triiodothyronine neogenesis in the rat. Endocrinology 123:1075–1081, 1988

12. O'Connell M, Robbins DC, Horton ES, et al: Changes in serum concentrations of 3,3,5'-triiodothyronine and 3,5,3'-triiodothyronine during prolonged moderate exercise. J Clin Endocrinol Metab 49:242–246, 1979

13. Baumgartner A, Meinhold H: Sleep deprivation and thyroid hormone concentrations. Psychiatry Res 19:241–242, 1986

14. Fregley MJ: Activity of the hypothalamic pituitary-thyroid axis during exposure to cold. Pharmacol Ther 41:85–142, 1989

15. Reed HL, Silverman ED, Shakir KMM, et al: Changes in serum triiodothyronine (T_3) kinetics after prolonged antarctic residence: the polar T_3 syndrome. J Clin Endocrinol Metab 70:965–974, 1990

16. Puig-Domingo M, Guerrero J-M, Vaughan MK, et al: Activation of cerebrocortical type II 5'-deiodinase activity in Syrian hamsters kept under short photoperiod and reduced ambient temperature. Brain Res Bull 22:975–979, 1989

17. Oppenheimer JH, Surks MI: Quantitative aspects of hormone production, distribution, metabolism, and activity, in Handbook of Physiology, Vol 3. Edited by Greep RO, Astwood EB, Greer MA, et al. Washington, DC, American Physiological Society, 1974, pp 197–214

18. Delange F: Regional variations of iodine nutrition and thyroid function during the neonatal period in Europe. Biol Neonate 49:322–330, 1986

19. Hetzel BS: An overview of the prevention and control of iodine deficiency disorders, in The Prevention and Control of Iodine Deficiency Disorders. Edited by Hetzel BS, Dunn JT, Stanbury JB. Amsterdam, Elsevier, 1987, pp 7–31

20. Hetzel BS: The chances of success, in The Story of Iodine Deficiency. Edited by Hetzel BS. New York, Oxford University Press, 1989, pp 228–230

21. Hetzel BS: A global review of endemic cretinsm, in The Story of Iodine Deficiency. Edited by Hetzel BS. New York, Oxford University Press, 1989, pp 36–51

22. Escobar del Rey F, Ruiz de Ona C, Bernal J, et al: Generalized deficiency of 3,5,3'-triiodo-L-thyronine (T_3) in tissues from rats on a low iodine intake, despite normal circulating T_3 levels. Acta Endocrinol (Copenh) 120:490–496, 1989

23. Escobar de Rey F, Mallol J, Pastor R, et al: Effects of maternal iodine deficiency on thyroid hormone economy of lactating dams and pups: maintenance of normal cerebral 3,5,3'-triiodo-L-thyronine concentrations in pups during major phases of brain development. Endocrinology 121:803–811, 1987

24. Braverman LE, Ingbar SH, Vagenakis AH, et al: Enhanced susceptibility to iodide myxedema in patients with Hashimoto's disease. J Clin Endocrinol Metab 32:515–521, 1971

25. Savoie JC, Massin JP, Thomopoulos P, et al: Iodine-induced thyrotoxicosis in apparently normal thyroid glands. J Clin Endocrinol Metab 41:685–691, 1975

26. Hashizume K, Akasu F, Takazawa K, et al: The inhibitory effect of acute administration of excess iodide on the formation of adenosine 3',5'-monophosphate induced by thyrotropin in mouse thyroid lobes. Endocrinology 99:1463–1468, 1976

27. Bernhard WG, Gubin H, Schiller G: Congenital goiter: report of a fatal case with postmortem findings. Archives of Pathology 60:635–368, 1955

28. Greer MA: The natural occurrence of goitrogenic agents. Recent Prog Horm Res 18:187–219, 1962

29. Dratman MB, Eskin BA: Human thyroid: ovarian relationships, I: influence of serum from various phases of ovarian cycle on goitrogenesis. Am J Obstet Gynecol 89:646–650, 1964

30. Burman KD, Baker JR Jr: Immune mechanisms in Graves' disease. Endocr Rev 6:183–232, 1985

31. McLachlan SM, Rapoport B: Evidence for a potential common T-cell epitope between human thyroid peroxidase and human thyroglobulin with implications for the pathogenesis of autoimmune thyroid disease. Autoimmunity 5:101–106, 1989

32. Mariotti S, Aneli S, Rut J, et al: Comparison of serum thyroid microsomal and thyroid peroxidase antibodies in thyroid disease. Journal of Clinical Endocrinology 65:987–993, 1987

33. Blizzard RM, Chee D, Davis W: The incidence of parathyroid and other antibodies in the serum of patients with idiopathic hypoparathyroidism. Clin Exper Immunol 1:119–128, 1966

34. Haggerty JJ Jr, Evans DL, Golden RN, et al: The presence of antithyroid antibodies in patients with affective and nonaffective psychiatric disorders. Biol Psychiatry 27:51–60, 1990

35. Amino N, Mori H, Iwatani Y, et al: High prevalence of transient postpartum thyrotoxicosis and hypothyroidism. N Engl J Med 306:849–852, 1982

36. Jansson R, Bernander S, Karlsson A, et al: Autoimmune thyroid dysfunction in the postpartum period. J Clin Endocrinol Metab 58:681–687, 1984

37. Maagoe H, Reintoft I, Christensen HE, et al: Lymphocytic thyroiditis, II: the course of the disease in relation to morphologic, immunologic and clinical findings at the time of biopsy. Acta Medica Scandinavica 202:469–473, 1977

38. Hayashi Y, Tamai H, Fukata S, et al: A long term clinical, immunological and histological follow-up study of patients with goitrous chronic lymphocytic thyroiditis. J Clin Endocrinol Metab 61:1172–1178, 1985
39. Toni R, Jackson IMD, Lechan RM: Neuropeptide-Y-immunoreactive innervation of thyrotropin-releasing hormone-synthesizing neurons in the rat hypothalamic paraventricular nucleus. Endocrinology 26:2444–2453, 1990
40. Segerson TP, Kauer J, Wolfe HC, et al: Thyroid hormone regulates TRH biosynthesis in the paraventricular nucleus of the rat hypothalamus. Science 238:78–80, 1987
41. Yamada M, Wilber JF: Reciprocal regulation of preprothyrotropin-releasing hormone (TRH) mRNA in the rat anterior hypothalamus by thyroid hormone: dissociation from TRH concentrations during hypothyroidism. Neuropeptides 15:49–53, 1990
42. Taylor T, Wondisford FE, Blaine T, et al: The paraventricular nucleus of the hypothalamus has a major role in thyroid hormone feedback regulation of thyrotropin synthesis and secretion. Endocrinology 126:317–324, 1990
43. Gershengorn MC: Thyrotropin releasing hormone: a review of the mechanisms of acute stimulation of pituitary hormone release. Mol Cell Biochem 45:163–179, 1982
44. Ponce G, Charli J-L, Pasten JA, et al: Tissue specific regulation of pyroglutamate aminopeptidase II activity by thyroid hormones. Neuroendocrinology 48:211–213, 1988
45. Suen C-S, Wilk S: Regulation of thyrotropin releasing hormone degrading enzymes in rat brain and pituitary by L-3,5,3'-triiodothyronine. J Neurochem 52:884–888, 1989
46. Amr SM, Kubota K, Tramontano D, et al: The carbohydrate moiety of bovine thyrotropin is essential for full bioactivity but not for receptor recognition. Endocrinology 120:345–352, 1982
47. Beck-Peccoz P, Amr S, Menezes-Ferreira MM, et al: Decreased receptor binding of biologically inactive thyrotropin in central hypothyroidism: effect of treatment with thyrotropin-releasing hormone. N Engl J Med 312:1085–1090, 1985
48. Saberi M, Utiger RD: Augmentation of thyrotropin responses to thyrotropin-releasing hormone following small decreases in serum thyroid hormone concentrations. J Clin Endocrinol Metab 40:435–441, 1975
49. Weeke J, Christensen SE, Hansen AP, et al: Somatostatin and the 24 h levels of serum TSH, T3, T4 and reverse T3 in normals, diabetics, and patients treated for myxedema. Acta Endocrinol 94:30–37, 1980
50. Sowers JR, Catania RA, Hershman JM: Evidence for dopaminergic control of circadian variation in thyrotropin secretion. J Clin Endocrinol Metab 54:673–675, 1982
51. Vanhaelst L, Van Cauter E, Degaute JP, et al: Circadian variations of serum thyrotropin levels in man. J Clin Endocrinol Metab 35:479–482, 1972

52. Brabant G, Prank K, Ranft U, et al: Circadian and pulsatile TSH secretion under physiological and pathophysiological conditions. Horm Metab Res 23:12–17, 1990
53. Parker DC, Pekary AE, Hershman JM: Effect of normal and reversed sleep-wake cycles upon nyctohemeral rhythmicity of plasma thyrotropin: evidence suggestive of an inhibitory influence in sleep. J Clin Endocrinol Metab 43:318–329, 1976
54. Romijn JA, Wiersinga WM: Decreased nocturnal surge of thyrotropin in nonthyroidal illness. J Clin Endocrinol Metab 70:35–42, 1990
55. Souetre E, Salvati E, Wehr TA, et al: Twenty-four-hour profiles of body temperature and plasma TSH in bipolar patients during depression and during remission and in normal control subjects. Am J Psychiatry 145:1133–1137, 1988
56. Bartalena L, Placidi GF, Martino E, et al: Nocturnal serum thyrotropin (TSH) surge and the TSH response to TSH-releasing hormone: dissociated behavior in untreated depressives. J Clin Endocrinol Metab 71:650–655, 1990
57. Westermark K, Westermark B, Karlsson FA, et al: Location of epidermal growth factor receptors on porcine thyroid follicle cells and receptor regulation by thyrotropin. Endocrinology 118:1040–1046, 1986
58. Sho K, Knodo Y: Insulin modulates thyrotropin-induced follicle reconstruction and iodine metabolism in hog thyroid cells cultured in a chemically defined medium. Biochem Biophys Res Commun 118:385–391, 1984
59. Roger PP, Dumont JE: Factors controlling proliferation and differentiation of canine thyroid cells cultured in reduced serum conditions: effect of thyrotropin, cyclic AMP and growth factors. Mol Cell Endocrinol 36:79–93, 1984
60. Forster VT, Peschke E, Peschke D: Karyometrical and histological investigations of the nucleus paraventricularis after ganglionectomy and exposure to cold under consideration of the thyroid circuit and the pineal gland. Anat Anz 169:203–211, 1989
61. Melander A, Sundler F: Interaction between catecholamines, 5-hydroxytryptamine and TSH on secretion of thyroid hormone. Endocrinology 90:88–193, 1972
62. Maayan ML, Debons AF, Krimsky I, et al: Inhibition of thyrotropin and dibutyryl cyclic AMP-induced secretion of thyroxine and triiodothyronine by catecholamines. Endocrinology 101:289–291, 1977
63. Bartalena L: Recent achievements in studies on thyroid hormone-binding proteins. Endocr Rev 11:47–64, 1990
64. Pardridge WM: Transport of thyroid hormones in tissues in vivo, in Thyroid Hormone Metabolism. Edited by Wu S-Y, Hershman JH. Oxford, England, Blackwell Scientific, 1990, pp 123–143

65. Ekins RP, Edwards PR, Pardridge WM, et al: Plasma protein-mediated transport of steroid and thyroid hormones: a critique: further comments (letter). Am J Physiol 255:403–409, 1988

66. Ekins RP, Edwards PR, Pardridge WM, et al: Plasma protein-mediated transport of steroid and thyroid hormones: further comment (letter). Am J Physiol 258:394–396, 1990

67. Pemberton PA, Stein PE, Pepys MB, et al: Hormone binding globulins undergo serpin conformational change in inflammation. Nature 336:257–258, 1988

68. Etling N, Gehin-Fouque F: Iodinated compounds and thyroxine binding to albumin in human breast milk. Pediatr Res 18:901–903, 1984

69. Divino CM, Schussler GC: Transthyretin receptors on human astrocytoma cells. J Clin Endocrinol Metab 71:1265–1268, 1990

70. Nicoloff JT: Thyroid function in non-thyroidal disease, in Endocrinology. Edited by DeGroot LJ. Philadelphia, PA, WB Saunders, 1989

71. Schreiber G, Aldred AR, Jaworowski A, et al: Thyroxine transport from blood to brain via transthyretin synthesis in choroid plexus. Am J Physiol 258:R338–R345, 1990

72. Petkovich M, Brand NJ, Krust A, et al: A human retinoic acid receptor which belongs to the family of nuclear receptors. Nature 330:444–450, 1987

73. Evans RM: The steroid and thyroid hormone receptor superfamily. Science 240:889–895, 1988

74. Umesono K, Giguere V, Glass CK, et al: Retinoic acid and thyroid hormone induce gene expression through a common responsive element. Nature 336:262–265, 1988

75. Smith TJ, Davis FB, Davis PJ: Retinoic acid is a modulator of thyroid hormone activation of Ca2+-ATPase in the human erythrocyte membrane. J Biol Chem 264:687–689, 1989

76. Smith WC, Kuniyoski J, Talamantes F: Mouse serum growth hormone binding protein has GH receptor extracellular and substituted transmembrane domains. Mol Endocrinol 3:984–990, 1989

77. Dratman MB: On the mechanism of action of thyroxin, an amino acid analog of tyrosine. J Theor Biol 46:255–270, 1974

78. Katzeff HL, Bovbjerg D, Mark DA: Exercise regulation of triiodothyronine metabolism. Am J Physiol 255:E824–E828, 1988

79. Harper AE: Balance and imbalance of amino acids. Annals of the New York Academy of Medicine 69:1025–1041, 1958

80. Barrington EJW: Some endocrinological aspects of the protochordata, in Comparative Endocrinology. Edited by Gorbman A. New York, Wiley, 1959, p 250–256

81. Visser TJ, van Buuren JCJ, Rutgers M, et al: The role of sulfation in thyroid hormone metabolism. Trends in Endocrinology and Metabolism March/April:211–218, 1990

82. Berry MJ, Banu L, Larsen PR: Type I iodothyronine deiodinase is a seleno-cysteine-containing enzyme. Nature 349:438–440, 1991

83. Cheron RG, Kaplan MM, Larsen PR: Physiological and pharmacological influences on thyroxine to 3,5,3'-triiodothyronine conversion and nuclear 3,5,3'-triiodothyronine binding in rat anterior pituitary. J Clin Invest 64:1402–1414, 1979

84. Kaplan MM, Yaskoski KA: Phenolic and tyrosyl ring deiodination of iodothyronines in rat brain homogenates. J Clin Invest 66:551–562, 1980

85. Leonard JL, Mellen SA, Larsen PR: Thyroxine 5'-deiodinase activity in brown adipose tissue. Endocrinology 112:1153, 1982

86. Tanaka K, Murakami M, Greer MA: Type-II thyroxine 5'-deiodinase is present in the rat pineal gland. Biochem Biophys Res Commun 137:863–868, 1986

87. Hoffman RA, Habeeb P, Buzzell GR: Further studies on the regulation of the Harderian glands of golden hamsters by the thyroid gland. J Compr Physiol 160:269–275, 1990

88. Anguiano B, Aceves C, Navarro L, et al: Neuroendocrine regulation of adrenal 5'-monodeiodination during acute cold exposure in the rat, I: effects of hypophysectomy. Endocrinology 128:504–508, 1991

89. Visser TJ, Leonard JL, Kaplan MM, et al: Kinetic evidence suggesting two mechanisms for iodothyronine 5'-deiodination in rat cerebral cortex. Proc Natl Acad Sci U S A 79:5080–5084, 1982

90. Kaplan MM, Visser TJ, Yaskoski KA, et al: Characteristics of iodothyronine tyrosyl ring deiodination by rat cerebral cortical microsomes. Endocrinology 112:35–42, 1983

91. Obregon M-J, Larsen PR, Silva JE: The role of 3,3',5'-triiodothyronine in the regulation of Type II iodothyronine 5'-deiodinase in the rat cerebral cortex. Endocrinology 119:2186–2192, 1986

92. Kaiser CA, Goumaz MO, Berger AG: In vivo inhibition of the 5'-deiodinase Type II in brain cortex and pituitary by reverse triiodothyronine. Endocrinology 119:762–770, 1986

93. Kobayashi A, Shimazaki M, Hamada N, et al: Reverse triiodothyronine nuclear binding in rat brain. Osaka City Med J 36:29–35, 1990

94. Shulkin BL, Utiger RD: Reverse triiodothyronine does not alter pituitary-thyroid function in normal subjects. J Clin Endocrinol Metab 58:1184–1187, 1984

95. Goumaz MO, Kaiser CA, Burger AG: Brain cortex reverse triiodothyronine (rT3) and triiodothyronine concentrations under steady state infusions of thyroxine and rT3. Endocrinology 120:1590–1596, 1987

96. Goswame A, Rosenberg IN: Regulation of iodothyronine 5'-deiodinases: effects of thiol blockers and altered substrate levels in vivo and in vitro. Endocrinology 126:2597–2606, 1990

97. Silva JE, Dick TE, Larsen PR: The contribution of local tissue thyroxine monodeiodination to the nuclear 3,5,3'-triiodothyronine in pituitary, liver, and kidney of euthyroid rats. Endocrinology 103:1196–1207, 1978
98. Beckett GJ, MacDougall DA, Nicol F, et al: Inhibition of Type I and Type II iodothyronine deiodinase activity in rat liver, kidney and brain produced by selenium deficiency. Biochem J 259:887–892, 1989
98a. Berry MJ, Larsen P: The role of selenium in thyroid hormone action. Endocr Rev 13:207–219, 1992
99. Oppenheimer JH, Schwartz HL, Surks MI: Effect of iodothyronines and iodotyrosines on the displacement of (125)I-T3 form hepatic and heart nuclei in vivo: structural requirements for nuclear binding and possible relationship to hormonal activity. Biochem Biophys Res Commun 55:544–550, 1973
100. Schueler PA, Schwartz HL, Strait KA, et al: Binding of 3,5,3'-triiodothyronine (T3) and its analogs to the in vitro translational products of C-erbA protooncogenes: differences in the affinity of the α- and β-forms for the acetic acid analog and failure of the human testis and kidney α-2 products to bind T3. Mol Endocrinol 4:227–234, 1990
101. Meyer T, Hesch RD: Triiodothyronine: a beta-adrenergic metabolite of triiodothyronine? Horm Metab Res 15:602–606, 1983
102. Thibault O: Recherches sur la nature de la thyroxine active: renforcement par la thyroamine synthetique. Annals of Endocrinology 13:949–957, 1952
102a. Lowenstein CJ, Snyder SH: Nitric oxide: a novel biologic messenger. Cell 70:705–707, 1992
103. Yamada M, Wilber JF: Reciprocal regulation of preprothyrotropin-releasing hormone (TRH) mRNA in the rat anterior hypothalamus by thyroid hormone: dissociation from TRH concentrations during hypothyroidism. Neuropeptides 15:49–53, 1990
104. Riskind PN, Kolodny PN, Larsen PR: The regional hypothalamic distribution of type II 5'-monodeiodinase in euthyroid and hypothyroid rats. Brain Res 420:194–198, 1987
105. Tanaka K, Murakami M, Greer MA: Thyoxine 5'-deiodinase and thyroid hormone metabolism in intermediate and neural lobes of rat posterior pituitary. Neuroendocrinology 46:494–498, 1987
106. Erikson VJ, Cavalieri RR, Rosenberg LL: Phenolic and non-phenolic ring iodothyronine deiodinases from rat thyroid gland. Endocrinology 108:1257–1264, 1981
107. Nakamura M, Yamazaki I, Ohtaki S: Iodothyronine-induced catalytic activity of thyroid peroxidase. J Biochem 108:804–810, 1990
108. Leonard J: Dibutyryl cAMP induction of type II 5'deiodinase activity in rat brain astrocytes in culture. Biochem Biophys Res Commun 151:1164–1172, 1988
109. Ahronheim JC: Hyperthyroid chorea in an elderly woman associated with sole elevation of T3. J Am Geriatr Soc 36:242–244, 1988

110. Bauer MS, Whybrow PC: Rapid cycling bipolar affective disorder. Arch Gen Psychiatry 47:435–440, 1990
111. Underwood AH, Emmett JC, Ellis D, et al: A thyromimetic that decreases plasma cholesterol levels without increasing cardiac activity. Nature 324:425–429, 1986
112. Martin P, Brochet D, Soubrie P, et al: Triiodothyronine-induced reversal of learned helplessness in rats. Biol Psychiatry 20:1023–1025, 1985
113. Dratman MB, Crutchfield FL, Schoenhoff MB: Transport of iodothyronines from bloodstream to brain: contributions by blood-brain and choroid plexus: cerebrospinal fluid barriers. Brain Res 554:229–236, 1991
114. Terasaki T, Pardridge WM: Stereospecificity of triiodothyronine transport into brain, liver, and salivary gland: role of carrier- and plasma protein-mediated transport. Endocrinology 121:1185–1191, 1987
115. Dickson PW, Aldred AR, Marley PD, et al: Rat choroid plexus specializes in the synthesis and the secretion of transthyretin (prealbumin): regulation of transthyretin synthesis in choroid plexus is independent from that in liver. J Biol Chem 261:3475–3478, 1986
116. Dratman MB, Futaesaku Y, Crutchfield FL, et al: Iodine-125-labeled triiodothyronine in rat brain: evidence for localization in discrete neural systems. Science 215:309–312, 1982
117. Dratman MB, Crutchfield FL, Futaesaku Y, et al: (125-I) Triiodothyronine in the rat brain: evidence for neural localization and axonal transport derived from thaw-mount film autoradiography. Journal of Comprehensive Neurology 260:392–408, 1987
118. Dratman MB, Crutchfield FL: Thyroxine, triiodothyronine, and reverse triiodothyronine processing in the cerebellum: autoradiographic studies in adult rats. Endocrinology 125:1723–1733, 1989
119. Bradley DJ, Young WS III, Weinberger C: Differential expression of alpha and beta thyroid hormone receptor genes in rat brain and pituitary. Neurobiology 86:7250–7254, 1989
120. Puymirat J, Miehe M, Marchand R, et al: Immunocytochemical localization of thyroid hormone receptors in the adult rat brain. Thyroid 1:173–184, 1991
121. Yokota T, Nakamura H, Akamizu T, et al: Thyroid hormone receptors in neuronal and glial nuclei from mature rat brain. Endocrinology 118:1770–1776, 1986
122. Gullo D, Sinha AK, Woods R, et al: Triiodothyronine binding in adult rat brain: compartmentation of receptor populations in purified neuronal and glial nuclei. Endocrinology 120:325–331, 1987
123. Courtin F, Chantoux F, Francon J: Thyroid hormone metabolism by glial cells in primary culture. Mol Cell Endocrinol 48:167–178
124. Lakshmanan M, Goncalves E, Lessly G, et al: The transport of thyroxine into mouse neuroblastoma cells, NB41A3: the effect of L-system amino acids. Endocrinology 126:3245–3250, 1990

125. Goncalves E, Lakshmanan M, Pontecorvi A, et al: Thyroid hormone transport in a human glioma cell line. Mol Cell Endocrinol 69:157–165, 1990
126. Whittaker VP: The separation of subcellular structures from brain tissue. Biochemical Society Symposium Transactions 23:109–126, 1963
127. Dratman MB, Crutchfield FL, Axelrod J, et al: Localization of triiodothyronine in nerve ending fractions of rat brain. Proc Natl Acad Sci U S A 73:941–944, 1976
128. Tanaka K, Inada M: Inner ring monodeiodination of thyroxine and 3,5,3'-L-triiodothyronine in rat brain. Endocrinology 109:1619–1624, 1981
129. Kastellakis A, Valcana T: Characterization of thyroid hormone transport in synaptosomes from rat brain. Mol Cell Endocrinol 67:231–241, 1989
130. Dratman MB, Crutchfield FL: Synaptosomal 125-I triiodothyronine after intravenous 125-I thyroxine. Am J Physiol 235:E638–E647, 1978
131. Mashio Y, Inada M, Tanaka K, et al: High affinity 3,5,3'-L-triiodothyronine binding to synaptosomes in rat cerebral cortex. Endocrinology 110:1257–1261, 1982
132. Mashio Y, Inada M, Tanaka K, et al: Synaptosomal T_3 binding sites in rat brain: their localization on synaptic membrane and regional distribution. Acta Endocrinol (Copenh) 104:134–138, 1983
133. Weinberger C, Thompson CC, Org ES, et al: The c-erbA gene encodes a thyroid hormone receptor. Nature 324:641–646, 1986
134. Debuire B, Henry C: Sequencing the erb A gene of avian erythroblastosis virus reveals a new type of oncogene. Science 224:1456–1459, 1984
135. Druker BJ, Mamon HJ, Roberts TM: Oncogenes, growth factors, and signal transduction. N Engl J Med 321:1383–1391, 1989
136. Graf T, Beug H: Role of the v-erb A and v-erb B oncogenes of avian erythroblastosis virus in erythroid cell transformation. Cell 34:7–9, 1983
137. Zabel BU, Fourner REK, Lalley PA, et al: Cellular homologs of the avian erythroblastosis virus erb-A and erb-B genes are syntenic in mouse but asyntenic in man. Proc Natl Acad Sci U S A 81:4874–4878, 1984
138. Spurr NK, Solomon E: Chromosomal localization of the human homologues to the oncogenes erb A and B. EMBO J 3:159–163, 1984
139. Walker P, Weischel ME Jr, Eveleth D, et al: Ontogenesis of NGF and EGF in submaxillary gland and NGF in brain of immature male mice: correlations with ontogenesis of serum levels of thyroid hormones. Pediatric Journal 16:520–524, 1982
140. Salido EC, Lakshmanan J, Koy S, et al: Effect of thyroxine administration on the expression of epidermal growth factor in the kidney and submandibular gland of neonatal mice: an immunocytochemical and in situ hybridization study. Endocrinology 127:2263–2269, 1990
141. Mitsuhashi T, Tennyson GE, Nikodem VM: Alternative splicing generates messages encoding rat c-erb A proteins that do not bind thyroid hormone. Proc Natl Acad Sci U S A 85:5804–5808, 1988

142. Forman BM, Samuels HH: Minireview: interactions among a subfamily of nuclear hormone receptors: the regulatory zipper model. Mol Endocrinol 4:1293–1300, 1990

143. Goldberg Y, Glineur C, Bosselut R, et al: Thyroid hormone action and the erbA oncogene family. Biochimie 71:279–291, 1989

144. Nunez EA: The erb-A family receptors for thyroid hormones, steroids, vitamin D and retinoic acid: characteristics and modulation. Current Opinions on Cell Biology 1:177–185, 1989

145. Glass CK, Lipkin SM, Devary OV, et al: Positive and negative regulation of gene transcription by a retinoic acid-thyroid hormone receptor heterodimer. Cell 59:697–708, 1989

146. Sakurai A, Nakai A, DeGroot LJ: Expression of three forms of thyroid hormone receptor in human tissues. Mol Endocrinol 3:392–399, 1989

147. Koenig RJ, Lazar MA: Inhibition of thyroid hormone action by a non-hormone binding c-erbA protein generated by alternative mRNA splicing. Nature 337:659–661, 1989

148. Hodin RA, Lazar MA: Identification of a thyroid hormone receptor that is pituitary-specific. Science 244:76–79, 1989

149. Lazar MA, Hodin RA, Darling DS, et al: A novel member of the thyroid/ steroid hormone receptor family is encoded by the opposite strand of the rat c-erbAx transcriptional unit. Mol Cell Biol 9:1128–1136, 1989

149a. Farsetti A, Mitsuhashi T, Desvergne B, et al: Molecular basis of thyroid hormone regulation of myelin basic protein gene expression in rodent brain. J Biol Chem 266:23226–23232, 1991

150. Lauder JM: Hormonal and humoral influences on brain development. Psychoneuroendocrinology 8:121, 1983

151. Ruiz-Marcos A, Sanchez-Toscano F, Escobar del Rey F, et al: Reversible morphological alterations of cortical neurons in juvenile and adult hypothyroidism in the rat. Brain Res 185:91–102, 1980

152. Segal J: Acute effect of thyroid hormone on the heart: an extranuclear increase in sugar uptake. J Mol Cell Cardiol 21:323, 1989

153. Segal J, Ingbar SH: Stimulation of 2-deoxy-D-glucose uptake in rat thymocytes in vitro by physiological concentrations of triiodothyronine, insulin, or epinephrine. Endocrinology 107:1354, 1980

154. Segal J: Calcium is the first messenger for the action of thyroid hormone at the level of the plasma membrane: first evidence for an acute effect of thyroid hormone on calcium uptake in the heart. Endocrinology 126:2693–2702, 1990

155. Cheng S-Y, Maxfield FR, Robbins J, et al: Receptor-mediated uptake of 3,3′,5-triiodo-L-thyronine by cultured fibroblasts. Cell Biology 77:3425–3429, 1980

156. Benvenga S, Robbins J: Enhancement of thyroxine entry into low density lipoprotein (LDL) receptor-competent fibroblasts by LDL: an additional mode of entry of thyroxine into cells. Endocrinology 126:933–941, 1990

157. Zhou Y, Samson M, Osty J, et al: Evidence for a close link between the thyroid hormone transport system and the aromatic amino acid transport system T in erythrocytes. J Biol Chem 265:17000–17004, 1990

158. Davis FB, Cody V, Davis PJ, et al: Stimulation by thyroid hormone analogues of red blood cell Ca2+-ATPase activity in vitro: correlations between hormone structure and biological activity in a human cell system. J Biol Chem 258:12373–12377, 1983

159. Sterling F: Thyroid hormone action: identification of the mitochondrial thyroid receptor as adenine nucleotide translocase. Thyroid 1:167–171, 1991

160. Dratman MB, Crutchfield FL, Gordon JT, et al: Iodothyronine homeostasis in rat brain during hypo- and hyperthyroidism. Am J Physiol 245:E185–E193, 1983

161. Larsen PR: Thyroid hormone metabolism in the central nervous system. Acta Med Austriaca 15:5–10, 1988

162. Reivich AJ, Kuhl D, Wolf A, et al: The (18F) fluoro-deoxyglucose method for the measurement of local cerebral glucose in man. Circ Res 44:127–137, 1979

163. Kety SS, Schmidt CF: The nitrous oxide method for the quantitative determination of cerebral blood flow in man. J Clin Invest 27:476–483, 1948

164. Goldman M, Dratman MB, Crutchfield FL, et al: Intrathecal triiodothyronine administration causes greater heart rate stimulation in hypothyroid rats than intravenously delivered hormone: evidence for a central nervous system site of thyroid hormone action. J Clin Invest 76:1622–1625, 1985

165. Mason GA, Walker CH, Prange AJ Jr: Modulation of gamma-aminobutyric acid uptake of rat brain synaptosomes by thyroid hormones. Neuropsychopharmacology 1:63–70, 1987

166. Mason GA, Walker CH, Prange AJ Jr: Depolarization-dependent 45Ca uptake by synaptosomes of rat cerebral cortex is enhanced by L-triiodothyronine. Neuropsychopharmacology 3:291–295, 1990

167. Eayrs JT: Thyroid hypofunction and the development of the central nervous system. Nature 172:403–405, 1953

168. Dussault JH, Glorieux J: Screening for congenital hypothyroidism: beneficial effects on neuropsychological development, in Iodine and the Brain. Edited by DeLong GR, Robbins J, Condliffe PG. New York, Plenum, 1988, pp 203–208

169. Crutchfield FL, Dratman MB: Early ontogeny of iodocompound-processing neural systems in rat brain. Pediatr Res 17:8–14, 1983

170. Dratman MB, Crutchfield FL, Gordon JT: Ontogeny of thyroid hormone-processing systems in rat brain, in Iodine and the Brain. Edited by DeLong GR, Robbins J, Condliffe PG. New York, Plenum, 1988, pp 151–166

171. Usala SJ, Bale AE, Gesundheit N, et al: Tight linkage between the syndrome of generalized thyroid hormone resistance and the human c-erbAB gene. Mol Endocrinol 2:1217–1220, 1988

172. Munoz A, Rodriguez-Pena A, Perez-Castillo A, et al: Effects of neonatal hypothyroidism on rat brain gene expression. Mol Endocrinol 5:273–280, 1991
173. Guerrero JM, Puig-Domingo M, Reiter RJ: Thyroxine 5'-deiodinase activity in pineal gland and frontal cortex: nighttime increase and the effect of either continuous light exposure or superior cervical ganglionectomy. Endocrinology 122:236–241, 1988
174. Dratman MB, Crutchfield FL, Gordon JT: Thyroid hormones and adrenergic neurotransmitters, in Catecholamines, Neuropharmacology and Central Nervous System: Theoretical Aspects. Edited by Usdin E. New York, Alan R Liss, 1984, pp 425–439
175. Dratman MB, Crutchfield FL: Interactions of adrenergic and thyronergic systems in the development of low T3 syndrome (Serono Symposium No 40: The Low T3 Syndrome). Edited by Hesch RD. New York, Academic Press, 1981, pp 115–126

Chapter 2

Nutrition, Energy Metabolism, and Thyroid Hormones

Anthony J. Levitt, M.D.
Russell T. Joffe, M.D.

CONTENTS

4. Mechanisms of Thermogenesis
   4.1 Cellular Heat Production
   4.2 Thyroid-Induced Thermogenesis
       a. Sodium potassium transport
       b. Calcium
       c. Substrate cycling
       d. Mitochondria
       e. Muscle
5. Nutritional Effects of Thyroid Hormones and Psychiatric Illness
   5.1 Depression
   5.2 Eating Disorders
   5.3 Other
6. Conclusions

___

1. INTRODUCTION

Thyroid function is profoundly influenced by nutritional changes at virtually every level of the thyroid axis. The hypothalamic-pituitary axis, the
thyroid gland itself, and the peripheral metabolism of thyroid hormones
are highly sensitive to changes in both nutritional intake and energy metabolism. In this chapter, we review evidence for the impact of nutritional
intake on thyroid hormone physiology and action and then outline the
complex association between energy metabolism and thyroid function. We
also review the possible mechanisms by which thyroid hormones influence
energy metabolism. Finally, we discuss the possible relevance of nutrition
and energy metabolism to the measurement of thyroid function in psychiatric disorders.

2. NUTRITIONAL INTAKE AND THYROID FUNCTION

2.1 Thyroid Axis

Under normal conditions, a reduction in circulating levels of triiodothyronine (T_3) leads to an increase in the secretion of thyroid-stimulating hormone (TSH). Therefore, it may be expected that the decline
in circulating T_3 that occurs with fasting will be associated with a rise

in TSH or an augmented TSH response to thyrotropin-releasing hormone (TRH). However, several studies (1–21) have reported either a decreased or unchanged basal TSH and a blunted or unchanged TSH response to TRH during starvation. In addition, overnutrition results in an increase in T_3 concentration and production but does not lead to the expected blunting of the TSH response to TRH (22,23). The reasons for these apparently paradoxical responses of TSH are not yet known. However, several explanations have been put forward.

Some investigators (6,24) have suggested that under- and overnutrition affect the sensitivity of hypothalamic-pituitary feedback to T_3. Burger et al. (6) demonstrated only a 20% inhibition of TSH response to TRH in fasting subjects with the addition of 15 μg T_3, 2 hours before testing. In contrast, Burman et al. (15) proposed that the intrapituitary sensitivity to T_3 is normal in the fasting state. They reported that the addition of iopanoic acid, which has been shown, in vitro, to block intrapituitary conversion of thyroxine (T_4) to T_3, abolishes the decline in TSH that occurs in the fasted state. The addition of T_3 alone or with iopanoic acid led to appropriate suppression of TSH. These findings imply that the T_3-feedback mechanisms are intact in fasting (i.e., there is no decreased sensitivity of the thyrotroph). Burman and others (5,6) have therefore advanced the hypothesis that the apparent lack of responsiveness in TSH to lower peripheral levels of T_3 during fasting may be explained by an enhanced intrapituitary conversion of T_4 to T_3.

Although TSH secretion is primarily regulated by TRH, the TSH response during starvation or overnutrition may be regulated by several other mechanisms. Evidence for this was presented by Spencer et al. (11) who compared basal and TRH-stimulated TSH and TRH levels in mildly obese fasting female subjects given either saline or continuous TRH infusion. The sequence of changes in thyroid hormones and the decline in TSH on the second day of fasting were the same in both groups. Furthermore, the normal circadian fluctuation in TSH was observed in both groups. The investigators concluded that the transient fall in TSH with fasting is not necessarily TRH mediated.

Several other neuroendocrine systems have been examined to determine other possible influences on TSH response in altered nutrition. Although dopamine has a potent effect on TSH, it is unlikely to play a role in the nutritional influence on TSH. Rojdmark (25) has shown that metoclopramide, a dopamine agonist, does not reverse the suppression of TSH that occurs with starvation. Similarly, glucocorticoids, which also play a role in regulating TSH secretion in normal physiological conditions, are unlikely to be involved. There is, however, evidence that somatostatin may be involved in the regulation of TSH response (26–28). Decreased blood glucose that results from undernutrition has been shown to lead to an increase in secretion of growth hormone, which in turn leads to increase in somatostatin. Increased somatostatin secretion may result in a lowered TSH secretion. Support for this mechanism comes from several sources (24,29). Nonetheless, the discrete role of somatostatin remains speculative and unknown. Other factors, such as the α-adrenergic and serotonergic systems and insulin, have been implicated in the regulation of TSH (29), but it is beyond the scope of this review to elaborate in detail on each of these hypotheses. Nevertheless, the mechanisms for alterations in the TSH levels and the response to TRH with altered nutrition probably result from a complicated interplay of these neuroendocrine factors and cannot be explained simply by changes in TRH secretion or peripheral thyroid hormones dynamics alone.

2.2 Thyroid Gland

Several components of the diet influence the production of thyroid hormones in the thyroid gland.

a. Iodide

The thyroid gland is the only organ in the body requiring iodide for normal functioning, although other tissues, such as salivary glands, gastric mucosa, and choroid plexus, can secrete iodide against a gradient. Iodide is transported from plasma to thyroidal cells mostly under the influence of TSH and, then, through the process of deiodination, is recycled. An adequate daily intake of iodide is approximately 150 µg (30). In some areas of the world where iodide content in the diet is low, goiter is endemic; for this reason many countries encourage the use of iodinated salts. If there is an abrupt increase in iodide in the diet, hyperthyroidism may result.

b. Trace elements

Heavy metals have been shown to influence thyroid function at several levels of the hypothalamic-pituitary-thyroid axis. In addition, thyroid hormones may influence the metabolism of heavy metals. Red blood cell zinc concentrations may be reduced in patients with hyperthyroidism (31), and an inverse relationship between T_4 concentrations and red blood cell zinc has been reported. Recently, Yoshida et al. (31) demonstrated an inverse relationship between both T_3 and T_4 levels and red blood cell zinc concentration in hyperthyroid patients at baseline. They also showed that, as T_3 and T_4 fall into the euthyroid range with treatment, red blood cell zinc rises. There is, however, a lag of approximately 8 weeks in the rise in zinc, and the authors suggested that red blood cell zinc may be an integrated index of thyroid hormone levels.

Wada and King (32) demonstrated that both T_4 levels and resting metabolic rate declined during the course of a low-zinc diet and both returned toward normal when subjects were refed a diet containing higher amounts of zinc. These changes could not be explained by alteration in dietary carbohydrates because there was no fall in T_3, as would be expected. Plasma magnesium concentrations have also been reported to be reduced in hyperthyroid patients and increased in hypothyroid patients (33). Furthermore, Shibutani et al.(34) demonstrated an inverse relationship between both plasma and red cell magnesium and thyroid hormone levels. Also rats fed a magnesium-deficient diet demonstrated reduced T_4 levels and an enlargement of the thyroid gland (35). Therefore, dietary intake of metals such as zinc and magnesium may potentially influence thyroid function. However, because most studies have been with hyper- and hypothyroid patients, extension of these findings to subjects with normal thyroid function may be unwarranted.

Although lithium is present in extremely small concentrations in red blood cells in healthy individuals and, therefore, probably has little effect on thyroid function, in patients treated with lithium (e.g., for bipolar affective disorder) there may be an effect on thyroid function (36). (For a more detailed discussion of the effect of lithium on the thyroid gland, see Chapter 6.)

c. Sympathetic nervous system

The thyroid gland is densely innervated by the autonomic nervous system with an increase in secretion of hormones resulting from either β or α stimulation. Furthermore, β blockade tends to suppress thyroid function. There is growing evidence that dietary carbohydrates may influence thyroid hormones through the action of the sympathetic nervous system on the thyroid gland (37).

2.3 Peripheral Metabolism

In this section we first describe the peripheral metabolism of thyroid hormones, focusing on deiodination. Second, we examine the effects of dietary components, particularly carbohydrates, on peripheral metabolism. Finally, we characterize the effects of nutrition on thyroid-binding globulins (TBGs).

a. Deiodination

The production and deiodination of thyroid hormones is demonstrated in Figures 2–1 and 2–2. Twenty percent of T_3 comes directly from the thyroid gland and 80% from the peripheral deiodination of T_4. Between 2.5% and 6% of reverse triiodothyronine (rT_3) comes directly from the thyroid gland, and 94%–97.5% comes from the deiodination of T_4 (38). Approximately 41% of T_4 is deiodinated to T_3 and 38% to rT_3 (39). T_4 may be deiodinated by either inner-ring or outer-ring deiodinases (Figure 2–2).

It is now established that there are three separate types of deiodinases (40). Type I deiodinase is nonselective and deiodinates both rings. There are two subtypes of this enzyme: one is found in large quantities in the liver and kidneys and is insensitive to TSH; the other is found in the thyroid gland and is sensitive to TSH (41–43). Type II deiodinase is a true 5′ deiodinase; it only deiodinates the outer (or phenolic) ring. It is found in the brain, in the pituitary gland, and in muscle and is also insensitive to TSH. It has been recently proposed that the major proportion of circulating T_3 comes from both type II and type I deiodination. Type III deiodinase acts exclusively on the inner-ring (or tyrosyl ring) and is responsible for the production of the major proportion of rT_3, although type I deiodinase also plays a role in inner-ring deiodination. Peripheral thyroid hormone levels represent the dynamic balance between production rate and degradation of these hormones, and this is to a large part dependent on the activity of these three enzymes. Therefore, measurement of the kinetics of thyroid hormones, and/or the activity of these enzymes, may be of more value than static plasma levels in understanding the changes in thyroid activity that accompany changes in nutrition. In the following discussion, we focus on changes in thyroid hormones and kinetics with various dietary alterations, with specific reference to

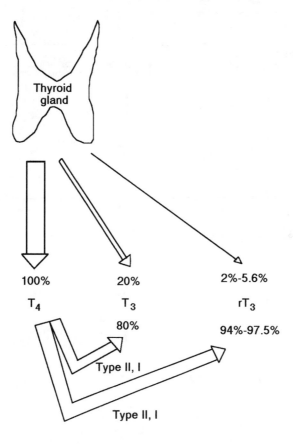

Figure 2–1. Production of thyroid hormones from the thyroid gland and peripheral thyroxine (T_4) deiodination. T_3 = triiodothyronine; rT_3 = reverse triiodothyronine. Deiodinase enzymes: type I = nonselective, deiodinates both rings; type II = true 5′ deiodinase, deiodinates only the outer (or phenolic) ring; type III = deiodinates only the inner (or tyrosyl) ring.

deiodination. Thyroid hormones may also be metabolized by
other mechanisms. For example, Engler and Burger (39) have reported that only 56% of T_3 degradation and 28% of rT_3 degradation is by monodeiodination alone. Nonetheless, the process most
relevant to the discussion of the effects of nutrition on thyroid
function is deiodination.

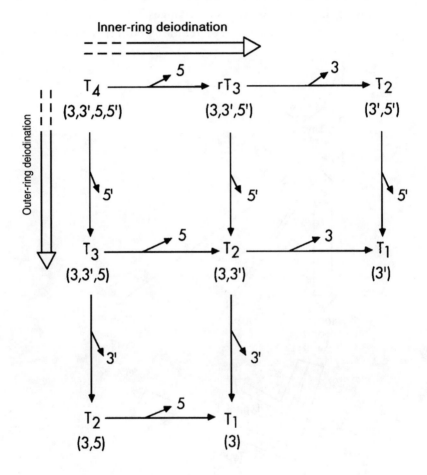

Figure 2–2. Monodeiodination of thyroid hormones. Numbers refer to position of
iodine on tyrosyl or inner ring (3,5) and phenolic or outer ring (3′,5′). Deiodinase types
II and I are responsible for outer-ring deiodination. Types III and I are responsible for
inner-ring deiodination. T_1 = monoiodotyrosine; T_2 = diiodotyrosine; T_3 =
triiodothyronine; rT_3 = reverse triiodothyronine; T_4 = thyroxine.

b. Diet composition

i. Thyroxine (T₄) Plasma levels of T_4 change little during fasting or carbohydrate restriction (1,7–10,13–21,44–53) or overfeeding (23). In some cases it has been shown that free T_4 increases transiently (11) and then returns to normal levels (19). This phenomenon is likely due to displacement of T_4 from TBG and thyroid-binding prealbumin (TBPA) (or transthyretin [TTR]) by free fatty acids. However, during a prolonged fast, due to a general decrease in nutrient intake, there is a progressive decline in both TBG and iodide resulting in changes in T_4 levels (10,19).

ii. Triiodothyronine (T₃) and reverse triiodothyronine (rT₃) In contrast to T_4, changes in T_3 and rT_3 are determined by several factors, including the caloric content, the composition of the diet, and the length of starvation. Overfeeding results in increased T_3 production and clearance and decreased rT_3 (23, 54). In contrast, the concentration of T_3 decreases and rT_3 increases with fasting and caloric restrictions (1,4,5,7–16,18–22, 47,50–53,55–65). The decrease in T_3 is usually noted within the first 24 hours, and nonthyroidal production of T_3 may be reduced up to 69% with fasting (66). After this point in time there is a gradual increase in levels, but T_3 rarely returns to prefasting levels during the course of the fast. Concentrations of rT_3 and free rT_3 increase with fasting and then return to normal or slightly higher than normal by the second week of fasting.

These changes in T_3 and rT_3 have been suggested to be the result of the same mechanism. The decrease in T_3 concentration is likely due to a decrease in T_3 production (39,50,54,67) as a result of lowered activity of type I deiodinase. Because rT_3 degradation also depends on type I deiodinase, fasting will result in a reduced clearance of rT_3 and will lead to an increase in plasma concentration. However, the changes in production and clearance of thyroid hormones with altered nutrition cannot simply be explained by this one mechanism.

In a recent study that extensively evaluated the kinetics of thyroid hormones in fasting, LoPresti et al. (67) reported that 13 days of fasting in five euthyroid obese men resulted in increased serum rT_3 levels and decreased serum T_3. Fasting resulted in decreased rT_3 clearance, but did not affect rT_3 production. The decreased clearance of rT_3 in fasting was most likely due almost entirely to changes in type I deiodinase activity. The decreased activity of the type I deiodinase may have also reduced the conversion of T_4 to T_3 and explains, in part, the lowered T_3 during fasting. However, the time course and relative magnitude of changes in rT_3 clearance and T_3 production were different. Therefore, an alteration in a single enzyme is unlikely to explain the changes in both rT_3 and T_3. Type II deiodinase is also involved in the clearance of T_3, and alternate pathways of disposal for both T_3 and T_4 may be increased in starvation (39,54). In a second phase of this study, subjects were refed. This did not restore rT_3 clearance, but did result in decreased rT_3 production, which explained the observed fall in serum rT_3. These findings suggest that regulation of thyroid hormone metabolism during fasting and refeeding is complex. Furthermore, it appears that type III deiodinase, unlike type I, is not particularly sensitive to changes in starvation, as rT_3 production did not change during fasting. It may, however, be affected during refeeding, as rT_3 production was depressed on the fourth day of refeeding.

Further evidence for the central role of alteration in type I deiodinase activity in fasting was presented by Katzeff et al. (53). They reported that caloric restriction inhibits T_3 production in the periphery but not the pituitary, whereas iopanoic acid inhibits production in both the periphery and the pituitary. They concluded that caloric restriction may only inhibit type I and may spare intrapituitary type II deiodinase activity. This would appear highly adaptive, as it would allow for the maintenance of normal brain function and reduced peripheral oxygen consumption during starvation.

As previously mentioned, almost all studies examining changes that occur in thyroid function with caloric restriction have reported a decrease in T_3 levels and an increase in rT_3

levels. However, several lines of evidence suggest that this effect may be modulated by the presence or absence of carbohydrates. First, the addition of small amounts of carbohydrate to a low-calorie diet has been shown to prevent the normal rise in rT_3 associated with caloric restriction. Second, diets high in calories result in a shift to outer-ring deiodination of rT_3, a result of either increased type I activity or increased alternative pathways of degradation (54). Third, complete carbohydrate restriction can, in fact, mimic the effects of starvation on thyroid function (48). Finally, a critical amount of carbohydrate may need to be present in the diet before the effects of total calories on thyroid hormone metabolism are noted. Pasquali et al. (68) found that T_3 levels were only sensitive to carbohydrate levels of 120 g/day or less, although dietary caloric intake varied between 360 and 1,200 calories/day. These investigators suggested that a "permissive" amount of carbohydrate must be present, after which total calories in the diet may modulate thyroid hormone metabolism.

Although the evidence above supports a somewhat specific effect of carbohydrates on thyroid hormone metabolism, there is evidence to suggest the contrary. For example, Danforth (69) suggested that the effect of carbohydrate may occur only at higher levels of caloric intake. Davidson and Chopra (70) studied six normal-weight subjects fed five separate diets, three isocaloric diets, and two hypercaloric diets with differing levels of carbohydrates. T_3 levels were most highly correlated with total calories and not with carbohydrate levels. Furthermore, Bogardus et al. (cited in 24) found that adding 75 g/day carbohydrate to a 830-kcal/day diet containing no carbohydrate failed to avert a decrease in T_3. However, because these studies involved different levels of starvation and different replacement of carbohydrate, firm conclusions are difficult to make.

In summary, peripheral thyroid hormone metabolism is highly sensitive to changes in nutrition, particularly to caloric intake. The sensitivity is mediated in part through the change in activity of the deiodinase enzymes, which may be affected by carbohydrate content in the diet. Of note, it appears that type III deiodinase is not affected by brief undernutrition because the production rate of rT_3 is not affected. The increase in rT_3 with fasting is in fact due to decreased clearance of rT_3, not to an increased production from T_4. Type II deiodinase, on the other hand, is modulated by nutritional factors, although there may be differential effects on the central versus the peripheral enzyme activity. Type I deiodinase is probably the most sensitive to reduced caloric intake, with activity decreasing by more than 50% during starvation (53). As a result of the sensitivity of type I deiodinase, some investigators have suggested that rT_3 levels may be a sensitive index of type I deiodinase activity.

iii. Thyroid-binding globulins (TBGs) Not all changes in thyroid hormones can be attributed to alterations in metabolism or degradation. During periods of over- or undernutrition, there are also changes in the transport proteins TBG and TBPA. With regard to overfeeding, excess dietary carbohydrate results in increases in both TBG and TBPA (71). With regard to undernutrition, Unger (10) demonstrated that there was a decrease in TBG in subjects after a 4-day fast. There was a significant positive correlation ($P < .05$) between TBG levels and both TSH and T_3 levels. In this study, TSH declined with fasting, and, as TBG is also under influence of TSH, the author suggested that the decrease in TBG and T_3 are both the result of decreased TSH.

There is some conjecture as to what extent carbohydrates influence these proteins. Stokholm (18) demonstrated that TBPA decreases in subjects given a low-calorie diet, regardless of whether carbohydrate was added. Bogardus et al. (cited in 24) added either 75 g carbohydrate or isocaloric amounts of fat to a 830-kcal/day diet. TBPA decreased in both states, but TBG decreased, in concert with total T_3, only when there was no carbohydrate added. Therefore, some of the changes in total T_3 that occur during a low-calorie diet may be due to decreases in TBG. In contrast, Kelleher et al. (12) reported that

TBPA is modulated by carbohydrate intake independent of caloric intake. Taken together, these studies suggest that thyroid-binding proteins appear to be affected to some extent by both caloric intake and dietary composition. Indeed, a general reduction in nutrient intake during starvation may result in decreased protein intake and consequent reduction in transport proteins. These findings amplify the importance of measuring free thyroid hormone and transport proteins in the assessment of changes in thyroid function in altered nutrition.

2.4 Summary

Undernutrition is associated with relatively predictable changes in thyroid physiology from the hypothalamus to the peripheral metabolism of thyroid hormones. Fasting may be associated with altered sensitivity of the hypothalamus and/or pituitary gland to normal feedback mechanisms. Alternatively, there may be an alteration in the intrapituitary conversion of T_4 to T_3. The role of other neuroendocrine systems in the regulation of thyroid function during changes in nutrition is probable, but there are insufficient data to make firm conclusions.

Furthermore, undernutrition is associated with altered nutrient delivery to the thyroid gland and a decrease in activity of some of the peripheral enzymes responsible for the metabolism of thyroid hormones. Changes in transport proteins also affect the levels of thyroid hormones, and all these influences are probably amplified if carbohydrate is specifically restricted. These multilevel and complex changes in thyroid metabolism appear essential for maintaining homeostasis, specifically the energy economy of the body. However, thyroid hormones are not only responsive to a decreased energy intake; they also modify and are influenced by changes in energy expenditure. For example, type I deiodinase may be more sensitive to the balance between caloric intake and expenditure than to either one of those factors alone. Therefore, it is essential to understand the association between thyroid hormones and both components of energy balance, namely caloric intake and energy expenditure. In the next section, we deal with this issue.

3. ENERGY BALANCE AND THYROID HORMONES

3.1 Introduction

Energy balance is determined by the difference between caloric intake and energy expenditure and can be summarized by the equation

Energy balance (EB) = Caloric intake (CI) − Energy expenditure (EE)

Energy expenditure is comprised of several heat-producing–energy-consuming processes outlined in Figure 2–3 and below.

● **Resting metabolic rate (RMR):** The largest component of thermogenesis is basal metabolic rate, or the rate of oxygen consumption at rest in the postabsorptive state at thermoneutral temperatures. Because this basal state is sometimes difficult to achieve, RMR is the usual measure of this component of energy expenditure. RMR

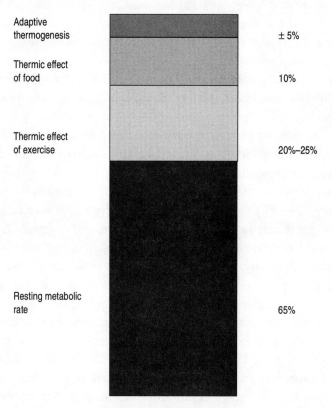

Figure 2-3. Components of energy expenditure.

is always slightly higher than basal metabolic rate because of mental activity and muscle tone present at rest and represents 60%–75% of total daily energy expenditure (72). RMR is related to the rate of energy turnover in the cell. Because 95% of heat-consuming cellular processes require oxygen, oxygen consumption can be used to estimate metabolic rate (72,73).

- **Thermic effect of exercise (TEE):** TEE is the energy expended during voluntary muscle activity. Of all the components of energy expenditure, this is the most variable. In standard conditions, TEE represents approximately 30% of energy expenditure, but the rate of expenditure during heavy exercise can be as high as 10–15 times the RMR (72,74).
- **Thermic effect of food (TEF) or diet-induced thermogenesis:** TEF refers to the rise in energy expenditure after the ingestion of food. It reflects an obligatory component that is probably due to the absorption, transport, metabolism, and storage of ingested food (72,75). In addition, there is an adaptive component that responds to over- or undereating, as well as to the specific substances in the diet. In a standard diet, TEF represents approximately 10% of total daily energy expenditure (75).
- **Adaptive thermogenesis (AT):** AT is thought to represent heat production that yields no useful work but that appears to serve adaptive or homeostatic needs (72,75).

Thyroid hormones are involved primarily in the regulation of RMR and have little influence on TEF or TEE (76). It has been long known that hypothyroid patients have an abnormally low RMR and that hyperthyroid patients have increased RMR as compared with healthy subjects. The thermogenic effect of thyroid hormone is observed about 12–24 hours after administration (77). T_4 has very little effect on thermogenesis in vitro, whereas all tissues, with the exception of brain, spleen, and gonad, respond with increased thermogenesis when T_3 is added (77).

3.2 Energy Expenditure

The association between energy expenditure and thyroid function in humans is complex. In the first section below, we review studies that have manipulated thyroid hormones levels by either adding exogenous thyroid hormone or altering the peripheral metabolism of thyroid hormone and evaluated the effects of these manipulations on energy expenditure. In the second section, we examine studies that have altered one or both components of energy balance and evaluated the effects of altered energy balance on thyroid hormones.

a. Manipulation of thyroid hormones

   i. *Exogenous thyroid hormones* The induction of mild thyrotoxicosis by the administration of oral or intravenous thyroid hormones has relatively consistent effects on energy expenditure. For example, Abraham et al. (78) reported on changes in metabolic rate in 14 obese patients treated with T_3 for 7–62 days as part of a weight-loss program. There was a mean increase in RMR of 6% in the entire group, with 10 out of 14 showing increased RMR. Rozen et al. (61) treated 20 obese subjects with a low-calorie diet, with the addition of either placebo or T_3. Placebo treatment and diet led to a reduction in T_3 and oxygen consumption. When patients were treated with T_3, which resulted in normalization of their T_3 levels, there was no such drop in RMR. This study suggests that addition of T_3 may blunt the expected decline in both RMR and T_3 that occurs with caloric restriction. Nair et al. (79), in a group of 3 obese subjects who had fasted for 1 week, reported that T_3 declined by 53% and RMR by 11.7%. Five other patients received T_3 in addition to the fast; both plasma T_3 and RMR increased, although not to prefast levels.

   The thermogenic effect of exogenous thyroid hormones does not appear to result from an interaction with the sympathetic nervous system. Gelfand et al. (80) demonstrated that 1 week of 150 µg/day T_3 resulted in a 20% increase in RMR. Infusion of a β-blocker had no impact on T_3-induced changes in RMR. However, the thermogenic effect of epinephrine was augmented by T_3. The investigators concluded that the sympathetic nervous system is not responsible for the increased RMR resulting from administration of T_3, although T_3 does augment the thermogenic effect of epinephrine. Others have suggested that the thermogenic effects of thyroid hormones may, in fact, involve an interaction between the sympathetic nervous system and insulin (81,82). Recently, Piolino et al. (81) studied eight healthy control subjects who were rendered euinsulinemic and euglycemic. In keeping with the findings of Gelfand et al. (80), they found that the addition of T_4 in these patients increased RMR and enhanced the thermogenic response to epinephrine. However, in the hypoinsulinemic state, the effect of thyrotoxicosis on the epinephrine-induced thermogenesis disappeared, suggesting an interaction between T_4, insulin, and epinephrine in the regulation of RMR. Although the hypoinsulinemic state affected epinephrine-induced thermogenesis, the direct thermogenic effect of thyroid hormones does not seem to be affected in the hypoinsulinemic state (82).

In summary, with few exceptions (e.g., Moore et al. [83]) studies confirm that exogenous administration of thyroid hormones leads to predictable changes in RMR and that the changes in RMR are probably not mediated directly by the sympathetic nervous system.

ii. Iopanoic acid   Iopanoic acid blocks conversion of T_4 to T_3 and is not itself thermogenic. Therefore, the administration of iopanoic acid provides an opportunity to investigate the effects of lowering circulating and intrapituitary levels of T_3 on energy expenditure. There are few data available on the effects of iopanoic acid on energy expenditure. Acheson and Burger (84) noted that in healthy control subjects on a low-calorie diet, T_3 fell in concert with metabolic rate. However, the addition of iopanoic acid to a normal diet resulted in a decline in T_3, but prevented the expected decline in RMR. The investigators concluded that the decline in T_3 with fasting may be of little significance to the decline in RMR. Of note, there was an increase in T_4 during the administration of iopanoic acid, but it is unlikely that there was a potent direct effect of T_4 on RMR.

In contrast, in a study of eight obese men on a low-calorie diet, Katzeff et al. (53) concluded that caloric restriction inhibited T_3 production peripherally and not centrally, but that iopanoic acid inhibited T_3 production both in the periphery and the pituitary. The authors hypothesized that fasting will result in decreased type I deiodinase activity. Because type I deiodinase is found predominantly in the liver and kidney and these two organs are responsible for approximately 40% of thermogenesis at rest, fasting will result in a decline in RMR. However, RMR was not measured, and it remains possible that the decline in T_3 associated with fasting may not be entirely responsible for changes in RMR.

b. Altered energy balance

In this section, we review the relationship between thyroid hormones and RMR, as well as other components of energy expenditure, in conditions of altered nutrition. Results from studies evaluating the relationship between thyroid hormones and energy expenditure at various levels of caloric intake are inconsistent. Although both T_3 and RMR decrease with fasting (19,20,49,52,57, 61,79,85), few authors report modest correlations between the decline in T_3 and the decline in RMR (50,57,59,79), whereas the majority report no significant relationship (19,20,49,52,58,85). One such positive study is that by Serog et al. (57), who studied 14 healthy subjects on a low-carbohydrate intake and found a reduced oxygen consumption and reduced plasma T_3 levels. When patients were then stabilized at a low intake, both oxygen consumption and T_3 increased, but not to prefast levels. In contrast, Davies et al. (58) treated 2 groups of 8 obese subjects, one with a 330-calories/day diet and the other with a 780-calories/day diet. Despite a fall in both T_3 and RMR there was no significant correlation in the changes in both. Clearly, factors other than thyroid hormones play a more significant role in the decrease in RMR associated with fasting.

Thyroid hormones play little role in thermogenic events such as TEF that occur over the short term. However, because the sympathetic nervous system is strongly implicated in TEF (86) and T_3 may enhance epinephrine-induced thermogenesis, it remains possible that thyroid hormones play a permissive role in TEF (86). Poehlman et al. (85) compared 12 vegetarians and 11 nonvegetarians and found that both TEF and T_3 were lower in the vegetarians. The investigators concluded, perhaps prematurely, that prolonged low-calorie intake results in depressed T_3 and lower TEF. Further evaluation of this potential relationship is warranted. Thyroid hormones appear to play little role in TEE. The possible function of thyroid hormones in the regulation of AT in humans is, of course, unknown.

Several investigators have examined the effects of refeeding or overfeeding on thyroid hormones and energy expenditure. Barrows and Snook (52) followed 15 obese persons on a 420-kcal diet for 4–6 months, followed by realimentation. The diet alone produced a decrease whereas realimentation increased both T_3 and RMR. Neither T_3 nor RMR were restored to their original baseline levels during the refeeding period. Little information is available on the effects of overfeeding on both thyroid hormones and RMR. Acheson et al. (87) mimicked the effects of overfeeding on T_3 by adding small amounts of T_3 to subjects already taking T_4. The increase in T_3 was associated with increase in RMR, but not with changes in TEF or TEE. Woo et al. (cited in 24) found that overfed patients had a rise in both T_3 and RMR. Despite the relative consistency of these findings, a causative relationship between changes in T_3 and RMR during overfeeding cannot be inferred from these studies.

Woo et al. (cited in 24), found a relationship between RMR and T_3 during overfeeding. In that study, overfeeding plus exercise did not affect T_3, but did lead to an increase in RMR. The authors concluded that there was no linear relationship between changes in T_3 and RMR, in all conditions. Notably, when the energy balance was altered, by increasing energy expenditure, the relationship between thyroid hormones and RMR was affected. This raises the important issue of whether the relationship between thyroid hormones and RMR is influenced by the level of caloric intake or by the relative excess or deficit of calories or by both. We address this issue below.

Woo et al. (cited in 24) induced a negative energy balance at a high-caloric intake and found a dissociation of the relationship between T_3 and RMR. Phinney et al. (88), on the other hand, in-

duced a negative energy balance at a low-calorie intake. They studied two groups of obese patients on a calorie-restricted diet, one
with added exercise to increase the energy deficit. Both free T_3 and
RMR decreased in the diet-only group and both fell significantly
more in the diet-and-exercise group.

Garrell et al. (89) attempted to further evaluate this issue by
creating a negative energy balance at high-, low-, and normal-
caloric intake in the same individuals. They evaluated 6 healthy
control subjects who were in "energy balance" at three different
levels of caloric intake. The subjects then increased their energy
expenditure by exercising to induce negative energy balance at the
same three levels of caloric intake. There was a significant increase
in the ratio of T_4 to T_3 ($P < .01$) during periods of negative energy
balance as compared with "zero" energy balance (Figure 2–4). The
increased ratio suggests that a negative energy balance is associated with reduced conversion of T_4 to T_3. The type I deiodinase
responsible for this conversion in the periphery is known to be
affected by reduced caloric intake. This finding raises the possibility that the enzyme is sensitive to the relative and not absolute
caloric deficit. However, several studies do not support such a hypothesis. Mathieson et al. (49) treated 12 obese patients with a
high-carbohydrate or a low-carbohydrate diet. The high-carbohydrate group also exercised. T_3 declined to a greater degree in the
low-carbohydrate group, but the fall in RMR was equivalent between the two groups.

The reasons for the differences in result are hard to reconcile
because the methods, subjects, diets, and energy balance differ
between studies. In addition, the nature of the calories ingested
may influence thyroid hormones and RMR. To test this possibility, McCargar et al. (90) fed high-carbohydrate or high-fat diets
to six healthy male subjects in basal conditions and at 75% of
original energy balance (i.e., 25% energy deficit). During energy
deficit in both diets, there was a decline in mean T_3 (carbohydrate
12%, fat 12%) and mean RMR (carbohydrate 2.5%, fat 3.2%) regardless of the type of diet. However, mean RMR, but not T_3, was
lower in the subject group fed high-fat diets in both the energy-
balance and the energy-deficit state, suggesting that both diet

composition and energy balance impact on RMR.

Taken together these findings might suggest that thyroid hormone levels may be influenced, in certain subjects, by energy balance rather than by either energy expenditure or caloric intake alone. Furthermore, there may also be some sensitivity to the type of calories ingested (i.e., fat or carbohydrate). It is of interest to note that primary changes in energy balance produce somewhat inconsistent secondary changes in thyroid hormones, whereas exogenous administration of thyroid hormones produce predictable secondary changes in RMR. Therefore, although thyroid hor-

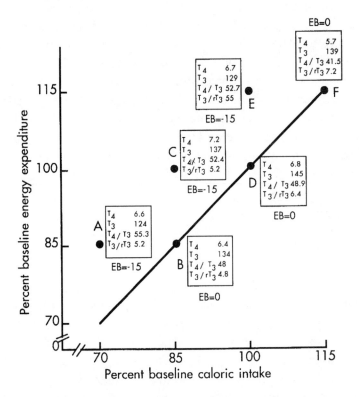

Figure 2–4. The effect of negative energy balance (EB) on thyroid hormones (T_3 = triiodothyronine; rT_3 = reverse triiodothyronine; T_4 = thyroxine). All values represent means. Mean T_4/T_3 for all points of negative energy balance (A, C, and E) is significantly greater ($P < .01$) than points at energy balance (B, D, and F). Mean T_3/rT_3 at point B is significantly lower ($P < .05$) than at point F. *Source.* Adapted from Garrell DR, Todd KS, Pugeat MM et al: "Hormonal Changes in Normal Men Under Marginally Negative Energy Balance." *American Journal of Clinical Nutrition* 39:930–936, 1984.

mones appear to have a direct effect on RMR when delivered exogenously, other regulatory mechanisms must act to influence RMR when thyroid hormone levels change as the result of altered nutrition and energy balance.

In summary, most, but not all, studies support the view that thyroid hormones are involved in the regulation of energy expenditure, particularly RMR. However, it is unlikely that changes in thyroid hormones levels alone can explain changes in RMR during under- or overnutrition. There appears to be a complex interplay between feedback mechanisms, deiodinase enzyme activity, the sympathetic nervous system, and insulin during under- and overnutrition, and these have complex effects on thyroid hormone levels and RMR. Further work is required to elucidate the nature of this relationship. In addition, changes in thyroid hormones may be more closely associated with alterations in energy balance than with changes in caloric intake or energy expenditure alone. However, the direct effect on thermogenesis of thyroid hormones either in vitro or when administered exogenously to humans appears consistent. In the next section, we describe the potential cellular mechanisms by which thyroid hormones may exert this influence on thermogenesis.

4. MECHANISMS OF THERMOGENESIS

4.1 Cellular Heat Production

The mitochondrion is responsible for the generation of heat within the cell. It is here that oxidation provides the majority of the energy required for physiological functioning of the cell. For the most part, energy is stored in the phosphate ester bond in adenosine triphosphate (ATP). The cellular processes that hydrolyze ATP for energy include ion transport; synthesis of proteins, carbohydrates, lipids, and so on; muscle contraction; secretory, absorptive, and storage processes; and various other degradation processes. These metabolic processes regulate thermogenesis only if oxidation is highly coupled with phosphorylation. However, as described below, there is also the possibility that some thermogenesis is not tightly coupled.

4.2 Thyroid-Induced Thermogenesis

a. Sodium potassium transport

Early researchers hypothesized that thyroid hormones uncoupled mitochondrial oxidative phosphorylation (77). However, Ismail-Beigi and Edelman (91,92) presented evidence to suggest that thyroid hormones increase the active transmembrane transport of Na^+. Because active Na^+ transport occurs in all target cells for thyroid hormone action and active Na^+ transport is estimated to contribute up to 85% of cellular oxygen consumption, this process is the most likely candidate for the effects of thyroid hormone on thermogenesis. Na^+ transport–dependent respiration or thermogenesis has been shown to be responsive to thyroid hormone in rat liver, kidney, muscle, and jejunal mucosa, but not brain or the gonads (92).

The relationship between T_3 and oxygen consumption in vitro is linear with a 12-hour lag effect and a plateau at 48 hours (77). The most likely mechanism for this increase in activity is either the activation of preexisting Na^+ pumps or an increase in the number of pumps or both (77). T_3 increases the biosynthesis of the Na^+/K^+ ATPase enzymes in various tissues. The possible mechanism for the induction of synthesis is the action of thyroid hormones at the nucleus of the cell to regulate RNA production and protein synthesis (93).

b. Calcium

Although there exists sufficient evidence to suggest that thyroid hormone is important in intracellular calcium homeostasis, calcium cycling is thought to contribute only approximately 7% to the increase in metabolic rate that results from the administration of thyroid hormone (94). It is beyond the scope of this chapter to review the current evidence for the role of calcium in thermogenesis.

c. Substrate cycling

Substrate cycling refers to the simultaneous function of two opposing and energy-requiring pathways of metabolism (24,94,95). This action produces energy or heat without useful work. For example, when glycolysis and gluconeogenesis occur at the same time there is a recycling of glucose using 3-carbon precursors, such as lactate. This type of recycling may occur in healthy subjects, and the degree to which this occurs probably depends on glycogen stores, energy balance, and diet composition. The role of thyroid hormone in substrate cycling is as yet undetermined. However, it has been suggested that hyperthyroidism is associated with increased cycling of glucose up to 15%–30% (95). Another metabolic pathway that may be involved in substrate cycling is that of fatty acid, with simultaneous oxidation and synthesis of free fatty acids. Again, evidence for the involvement of the thyroid in this pathway is suggested by the observation that increased oxidation of free fatty acids may occur in patients with hyperthyroidism (96).

An additional potential source of wasteful energy-consuming mechanisms in hyperthyroid patients are the so-called futile cycles. These cycles are created when single reversible steps in metabolism proceed simultaneously (95). Although some evidence exists for the contribution of these mechanisms to the increased thermogenesis in hyperthyroid rats (97), the role in humans is less well defined. Furthermore, the role of any of the mechanisms of wasteful energy production within the normal range of thyroid function is still unclear.

d. Mitochondria

Thyroid hormones appear to have both an acute and chronic effect on the mitochondria. Some investigators have suggested that T_3 may exert its influence via the regulation of adenosine nucleotide transcriptase (ANT), which transports ATP to the cytosol for essential metabolic functions (98). However, the balance of more recent data suggest T_3 neither affects gene expression nor binds to the molecule of ANT. Hoppner et al. (98) concluded that the effect of thyroid hormones on the mitochondria in the short term may be due to binding of T_3 to either mitochondrial or cell membrane proteins or through an increase in nuclear activity. Long-term changes in thermogenesis are likely due to changes in the size in number or the active respiratory units (i.e., mitochondria).

Of particular note, Horst et al. (99) have proposed a different scheme for thyroid hormone control of mitochondrial activity. Using isolated perfused liver cells from hypothyroid rats, they demonstrated that T_3, T_4, and 3,5 diiodothyronine (T_2) in low concentrations significantly increased oxygen consumption within 90 minutes of administration. T_2 resulted in the most rapid increase. Furthermore, when deiodination of T_4 to T_3 and T_3 to T_2 was blocked with propylthiouracil, only T_2, when added to the cells, retained its stimulatory effect. The investigators suggested that T_2 acts directly and rapidly via the mitochondrial pathway, whereas T_3 has its long-term effect by the induction of enzymes. This fascinating work requires replication and further evaluation.

e. Muscle

Thyroid hormone increases energy turnover during muscular contractions by several putative mechanisms: 1) proliferation of sarcoplasmic reticulum, 2) change in the excitation-contraction coupling process, 3) calcium cycling, 4) changes in the properties of the contractile elements themselves, and 5) alteration of Na^+ homeostasis, which may further influence calcium exchange (94). Although thyroid hormones may increase energy turnover in muscle through these mechanisms and may only have a permissive effect in the thermogenesis of shivering, there is little clinical evidence that thyroid hormones are involved in the regulation of the thermic effect of exercise (72,73,75).

In summary, thyroid hormones influence thermogenesis by several mechanisms, the most important being their regulation of Na^+/K^+ ATPase. The role of short-term direct effects on the mitochondria remain controversial.

5. NUTRITIONAL EFFECTS OF THYROID HORMONES AND PSYCHIATRIC ILLNESS

Several major psychiatric disorders are frequently associated with significant changes in body weight and nutritional status (100). Furthermore, there is a large body of evidence suggesting that these same psychiatric disorders are also associated with changes in thyroid function. Although a direct relationship has not been extensively investigated, it is possible that either primary changes in thyroid hormone are responsible for some of the nutritional-metabolic changes or nutritional-metabolic changes result in the alterations of thyroid function observed (101). In the following section, we briefly outline some of the possible relationships that occur in selected psychiatric disorders.

5.1 Depression

Major depression is often associated with changes in body weight (102, 103). In the short term, provided that body composition remains reasonably stable, changes in body weight that may occur in depression are as a result of alteration in the energy balance between caloric intake and energy expenditure. The most frequent manifestation of depression is weight loss, which may be a result of either a deficient caloric intake or excessive energy expenditure. As yet, no study has examined all the components of energy balance simultaneously in depressed patients either during the depressed phase or in recovery.

With regard to caloric intake, most studies show that the majority of depressed patients lose their appetite during the depressive phase of the illness (104,105). Though appetite is not physiologically equivalent to caloric intake, the likelihood is that these patients also have a reduced caloric intake. Furthermore, depression may be associated with altered food preference (106). No study to date of which we are aware, however, has systematically evaluated caloric intake in depressed subjects, although Tayek et al. (107) have evaluated caloric intake in six profoundly marasmic adults with depression before and after electroconvulsive therapy.

There is also recent evidence to suggest that depression is associated with increased energy expenditure. Gaist et al. (108) reported that patients with winter depression have a higher baseline RMR compared with healthy control subjects. Fernstrom et al. have shown that most antidepressant agents result in a reduction in RMR (109), although fluvoxamine, a serotonin reuptake blocker, resulted in increased RMR (110). The studies from this group are complicated by the fact that small numbers were involved and only patients who responded to treatment were evaluated.

Our group (A. J. Levitt, R. T. Joffe, J. Allard, unpublished data, April 1990) examined RMR in four depressed female patients before and after treatment with either imipramine or desipramine. Of these patients two responded and two did not respond to treatment, yet all four had reductions in RMR, with insignificant changes in TEF (Figure 2–5).

However, few data exist to make conclusions regarding the effects of antidepressants on overall energy expenditure. Depression may be a state of increased RMR and decreased caloric intake and, therefore, a state of negative energy balance. This might lead to the commonly observed weight loss that occurs with depressive illness. Furthermore, treatment with standard antidepressant agents such as tricyclic antidepressants and monoamine oxidase inhibitors may result in a decrease in RMR and an increase in caloric intake and, therefore, a relative positive energy balance, hence, weight gain. The effects of

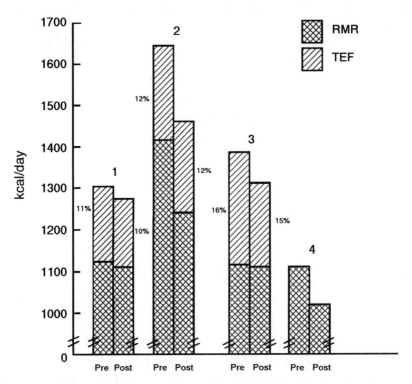

Figure 2–5. Change in resting metabolic rate (RMR) and thermic effect of food (TEF) in two patients who did not respond (*1* and *2*) and two patients who responded (*3* and *4*) to tricyclic antidepressants. TEF values not available for patient 4. There was a trend to lower RMR in all four patients following treatment.

these and other antidepressants depend on the initial energy balance, response to treatment, and specific pharmacological properties of the medications. As yet, the possible role of thyroid hormones in these changes in energy balance has not been systematically investigated. Studies to date have not evaluated caloric intake nor the specific content of the diet, both of which may have influenced thyroid function. Nor has measure of all components of energy expenditure been completed in depressed subjects before and after treatment.

The other major regulator of energy expenditure is the sympathetic nervous system (86). Changes in sympathetic nervous system function have been consistently reported in patients who have major depression. These include increased norepinephrine turnover (111); reduced 24-hour output of urinary sulfatoxymelatonin (112); increased levels of norepinephrine and its metabolites in cerebrospinal fluid, plasma, and urine (113); and alterations in all these parameters with treatment for depression. However, there have been no systematic studies of the relationship between changes in measures of the sympathetic nervous system function and changes in nutrition and energy balance in depression. One could hypothesize that because there is a general trend to increased noradrenergic activity in depression that this may be a contributing factor to increased energy expenditure in depressed patients. Furthermore, the decline in noradrenergic function that occurs with antidepressant agents may also be associated with the reduction in energy expenditure that occurs with treatment with standard antidepressants. Finally, because the sympathetic nervous system has a significant interaction with thyroid function, these two main regulators of energy balance need to be examined together with energy balance both in depression and during treatment.

Major depression itself is known to be associated with alteration in thyroid function. Blunting of the TSH response to TRH has been reported in 30%–40% of depressed subjects (see Chapter 6). However, several studies have reported that this finding may simply reflect change in body weight (or energy balance) that accompanies depression (114). One of the most consistent findings during the depressed phase is an increase in T_4 production (115). Although T_4 is less metabolically active than is T_3, this would be in keeping with the increased

RMR that has been observed. Treatment for depression with a variety of antidepressant agents and with electroconvulsive therapy is associated with a decline in both T_4 and T_3 (115).

Interestingly, depressed patients who respond to antidepressant treatment have been shown to have a greater decline in thyroid function than those who do not respond (115). Again, this is in keeping with the suggestion that patients who respond to antidepressant treatment tend to have a reduction in RMR, whereas those who do not have either no change or an increase. To date there have been no studies that directly evaluate energy balance and thyroid function in the same individuals before and after treatment. It has yet to be determined which physiological event is primary (i.e., does the reduction in thyroid hormone as a result of central changes affect the changes in energy balance, or do changes in energy balance influence the regulation of thyroid hormone production or clearance). Although it is difficult to untangle this question, the study of the relationship between thyroid hormone and energy balance in depression may be essential to help understand the changes in thyroid function observed in depression (101).

5.2 Eating Disorders

Anorexia nervosa is associated with starvation and changes in both thyroid hormone levels and energy balance. It is interesting to note that the changes are not as substantial in anorexia nervosa as they are in acute starvation (see Chapter 9). It has been hypothesized that this may be due to a relative adaptation by the body in anorexia nervosa due to the more chronic nature of the starvation. It is also important to note that in healthy starved subjects and in patients with anorexia nervosa who are refed, the T_3 and the RMR do not necessarily increase to prestarvation levels. This continued suppression of RMR in anorexia nervosa may be a risk factor for more accelerated weight gain during recovery. This has obvious implications for patients who are preoccupied with thinness.

In addition, although little direct evidence is available, this process may also apply to patients with bulimia nervosa. Recent data suggest that obese subjects who have dramatic fluctuations in their weight may have an alteration in the "set point" of their RMR (116, R. M. Black, S. H. Kennedy, A. S. Kaplan, A. J. Levitt, J. S. Allard, G. H. Anderson, unpublished data, March, 1991). If patients with bulimia nervosa, who are often premorbidly obese, lose large amounts of weight, it may be possible that their RMR is reset at a lower level. This will predispose them to more rapid weight gain and will perpetuate the cycle associated with the illness. Work is currently under way to determine the role of thyroid hormone in this process, but as yet there are no systematic data on changes in RMR in patients with bulimia nervosa before and after recovery. (For a more detailed discussion, see Chapter 9.)

5.3 Other

Alteration in nutrition is a significant problem among chronically mentally ill individuals (117). First, weight gain in institutionalized psychiatric patients is widespread and may be associated with increased morbidity. Second, nutritional intake in many psychiatric disorders, both in the community and within institutions, may be impaired for a variety of reasons. Last, patients with psychiatric illness are often prescribed medications that influence energy metabolism, thyroid function, and/or sympathetic nervous system function. This is particularly true of patients with bipolar affective disorder or patients with major depression who have been treated with lithium. The relationship between lithium treatment and changes in thyroid hormone and weight gain is discussed in Chapter 6. Again, there has been very little work in understanding the effects of lithium, or, indeed, most psychotropic medications, on energy balance in patients with bipolar or other psychiatric disorders. Because weight gain is a significant reason for noncompliance to psychotropic medications (102, 118), such studies are certainly indicated.

6. CONCLUSIONS

In the earlier part of this chapter, we described the importance of the interaction between nutrition and energy balance and thyroid function at virtually every level of the hypothalamic-pituitary-thyroid axis and even at a cellular level. Although work has been carried out in control subjects, obese subjects, and patients with a variety of medical illnesses, very little information exists on the possible interaction between thyroid and nutrition in psychiatric populations. Investigations of the interaction of nutrition and thyroid hormones in psychiatric illness may lead to a deeper understanding of the pathophysiology of these disorders. In addition, evaluation of the effects of psychotropic medications on both nutrition and energy metabolism may further our understanding of the mechanisms of actions of these drugs. Furthermore, this understanding may assist in the planning of dietary and nutritional interventions to prevent unwanted changes in body weight and nutrition that accompany treatment with these substances.

REFERENCES

1. Burman KD, Smallridge RC, Osburne R, et al: Nature of suppressed TSH secretion during undernutrition: effect of fasting and refeeding on TSH responses to prolonged TRH infusions. Metabolism 29:46–52, 1980
2. Burman KD, Dimond RC, Harvey GS, et al: Glucose modulation of alterations in serum iodothyronine concentrations induced by fasting. Metabolism 28:291–299, 1979
3. Rojdmark S, Nygren A: Thyrotropin and prolactin responses to thyrotropin-releasing hormone: influence of fasting- and insulin-induced changes in glucose metabolism. Metabolism 32:1013–1018, 1983
4. O'Brian JT, Bybee DE, Burman KD, et al: Thyroid hormone homeostasis in states of relative caloric deprivation. Metabolism 29:721–727, 1980
5. Gardner DF, Kaplan MM, Stanley CA, et al: Effect of triiodothyronine replacement on the metabolic and pituitary responses to starvation. N Engl J Med 300:579–584, 1979
6. Burger AG, Weissel M, Berger M: Starvation induces a partial failure of triiodothyronine to inhibit the thyrotropin response to thyrotropin-releasing hormone. J Clin Endocrinol Metab 51:1064–1067, 1980
7. Croxson MS, Hall TD, Kletzky OA, et al: Decreased serum thyrotropine induced by fasting. J Clin Endocrinol Metab 45:560–568, 1977
8. Carlson HE, Dernick EJ, Chopra IJ, et al: Alterations in basal and TRH-stimulated serum levels of thyrotropin, prolactin, and thyroid hormones in starved obese men. J Clin Endocrinol Metab 45:707–713, 1977
9. Palmblad J, Levi L, Berger A, et al: Effects of total energy withdrawal (fasting) on the levels of growth hormone, thyrotropin, cortisol, adrenaline, noradrenaline, T4, T3, rT3 in healthy males. Acta Medica Scandinavica 201:15–22, 1991

10. Unger J: Fasting induces a decrease in serum thyroglobulin in normal subjects. J Clin Endocrinol Metab 67:1309–1311, 1988
11. Spencer SA, Lum SMC, Wilber JF, et al: Dynamics of serum thyrotropin and thyroid hormone changes in fasting. J Clin Endocrinol Metab 56:883–888, 1983
12. Kelleher PC, Phinney SD, Sims EAH, et al: Effects of carbohydrate-containing and carbohydrate-restricted hypocaloric and eucaloric diets on serum concentrations of retinol-binding protein, thyroxine-binding prealbumin and transferrin. Metabolism 32:95–101, 1983
13. Goodwin GM, Fairburn CG, Keenan JC, et al: The effects of dieting and weight loss upon the stimulation of thyrotropin (TSH) by thyrotropin-releasing hormone (TRH) and suppression of cortisol secretion by dexamethasone in men and women. J Affective Disord 14:137–144, 1988
14. Borst GC, Osburne RC, O'Brian JT, et al: Fasting decreases thyrotropin responsiveness to thyrotropin-releasing hormone: a potential cause of misinterpretation of thyroid function tests in the critically ill. J Clin Endocrinol Metab 57:308–383, 1983
15. Burman KD, Smallridge RC, Burge JR, et al: Ipodate restores the fasting-induced decrement in thyrotropin secretion. J Clin Endocrinol Metab 57:597–602, 1983
16. Koppeschaar SPF, Meinders AE, Schwarz F: The effect of a low-calorie diet alone and in combination with triiodothyronine therapy on weight loss and hypophyseal thyroid function in obesity. Int J Obes 7:123–131, 1983
17. Wilson JHP, Lamberts SWJ: The effect of obesity and drastic caloric restriction on serum prolactin and thyroid stimulating hormone. Int J Obes 5:275–278, 1981
18. Stokholm KH: Decrease in serum free triiodothyronine, thyroxine-binding globulin and thyroxine-binding prealbumin while taking a very-low-calorie diet. Int J Obes 4:133–138, 1980
19. Rabast U, Hahn A, Reiners C, et al: Thyroid hormone changes in obese subjects during fasting and a very-low calorie diet. Int J Obes 5:305–311, 1981
20. Krotkiewski M, Toss L, Bjorntorp P, et al: The effect of a very-low-calorie diet with and without chronic exercise on thyroid and sex hormones, plasma proteins, oxygen uptake, insulin and c peptide concentrations in obese women. Int J Obes 5:287–293, 1981
21. Hill JO, Sparling PB, Shields TW, et al: Effects of exercise and food restriction on body composition and metabolic rate in obese women. Am J Clin Nutr 46:622–630, 1987
22. Utiger RD: Differing thyrotropin responses to increased serum triiodothyronine concentrations produced by overfeeding and by triiodothyronine administration. Metabolism 31:180–183, 1982
23. Danforth E Jr, Horton ES: Dietary-induced alterations in thyroid hormone metabolism during overnutrition. J Clin Invest 64:1336–1347, 1979

24. Danforth EJ, Burger AG: The impact of nutrition on thyroid hormone physiology and action. Ann Rev Nutr 9:201–227, 1989
25. Rojdmark S: Are fasting-induced effects on thyrotropin and prolactin secretion mediated by dopamine? J Clin Endocrinol Metab 56:1266–1270, 1983
26. Saler TM, Yen SSC, Vale W, et al: Inhibition by somatostatin on release of TSH-induced in man by thyrotropin-releasing factor. J Clin Endocrinol Metab 38:742–745, 1974
27. Vale W, Rivier C, Brazeau P, et al: Effects of somatostatin on the secretion of thyrotropin and prolactin. Endocrinology 95:968–973, 1974
28. Azukizawa M, Pekary AE, Hershman JM, et al: Plasma thyrotropin, thyroxine and triiodothyronine relationships in man. J Clin Endocrinol Metab 43:533–542, 1976
29. Brabant G, Ocran K, Ranft U, et al: Physiological regulation of thyrotropin. Biochimie 71:293–301, 1989
30. Paul T, Meyers B, Witorsch RJ, et al: The effect of small increases in dietary iodine on thyroid function in euthyroid subjects. Metabolism 37:121–124, 1988
31. Yoshida K, Kiso Y, Watanabe TK, et al: Erythrocyte zinc in hyperthyroidism: reflection of integrated thyroid hormone levels over the previous few months. Metabolism 39:182–186, 1990
32. Wada L, King JC: Effect of low zinc intakes on basal metabolic rate, thyroid hormones and protein utilization in adult men. J Nutr 116:1045–1053, 1986
33. Dolev E, Deuster PA, Solomon B, et al: Alterations in magnesium and zinc metabolism in thyroid disease. Metabolism 37:61–67, 1988
34. Shibutani Y, Yokota T, Iigima S, et al: Plasma and erythrocyte magnesium concentrations in thyroid disease: relation to thyroid function and the duration of illness. Jpn J Med 28:496–502, 1989
35. Kleiber MM, Boelter DD, Greenberg DM: Fasting catabolism and food utilization of magnesium deficient rats. J Nutr 21:363–368, 1941
36. Joffe RT, Post RM, Ballenger JC, et al: The effects of lithium on neuroendocrine function in affectively ill patients. Acta Psychiatr Scand 73:524–578, 1986
37. Jung RT, Shetty PS, James WPT: Nutritional effects on thyroid and catecholamine metabolism. Clin Sci 58:183–191, 1980
38. Hennemann G: Thyroid hormone deiodination in healthy man, in Thyroid Hormone Metabolism. Edited by Hennemann G. New York, Marcel Dekker, 1986, pp 277–295
39. Engler D, Burger AG: The deiodination of the iodothyronines and of their derivatives in man. Endocr Rev 5:151–184, 1984
40. Leonard JL, Visser TJ: Biochemistry of deiodination, in Thyroid Hormone Metabolism. Edited by Hennemann G. New York, Marcel Dekker, 1986, pp 189–229

41. Visser TJ, Kaplan MM, Leonard JL, et al: Evidence for two pathways of iodo-thyronine 5'-deiodination in rat pituitary that differ in kinetics, propylthi-ouracil sensitivity and response to hyperthyroidism. J Clin Invest 71:992–1002, 1983

42. Kaplan MM: Thyroxine 5'-monodeiodination in rat anterior pituitary ho-mogenates. Endocrinology 106:567–569, 1980

43. Silva JE, Larsen PR: Potential of brown adipose tissue type II thyroxine 5'-deiodinase as a local and systemic source of triiodothyronine in rats. J Clin Invest 76:2296–2305, 1985

44. Vagenakis AG, Portnay GI, Rudolph M, et al: Effect of starvation on the pro-duction and metabolism of thyroxine and triiodothyronine in euthyroid obese patients. J Clin Endocrinol Metab 45:1305–1309, 1977

45. Eisenstein Z, Hagg S, Vagenakis AG, et al: Effect of starvation on the produc-tion and peripheral metabolism of 3,3',5'-triiodothyronine in euthyroid obese subjects. J Clin Endocrinol Metab 47:889–893, 1978

46. Merimee TJ, Finberg ES: Starvation-induced alterations of circulating thy-roid hormone concentrations in man. Metabolism 25:79–83, 1976

47. Suda AK, Pittman CS, Shimizu T, et al: The production and metabolism of 3,5,3'-triiodothyronine and 3,3',5'-triiodothyronine in normal and fasting subjects. J Clin Endocrinol Metab 47:1311–1319, 1978

48. Spaulding SW, Chopra IJ, Sherwin RS, et al: Effect of caloric restriction and dietary composition on serum T3 and reverse T3 in man. J Clin Endocrinol Metab 42:197–200, 1976

49. Mathieson RA, Walberg JL, Gwazdauskas FC, et al: The effect of varying car-bohydrate content of a very-low-caloric diet on resting metabolic rate and thyroid hormones. Metabolism 35:394–398, 1986

50. van der Heyden JTM, Docter R, van Toor H, et al: Effects of caloric depriva-tion on thyroid tissue uptake and generation of low T3 syndrome. Am J Physiol 251:E156–E163, 1986

51. Stokholm KH, Hansen MS: Lowering of serum total T3 during a conven-tional slimming regime. Int J Obes 7:195–199, 1983

52. Barrows K, Snook JT: Effect of a high-protein, very-low calorie diet on rest-ing metabolism, thyroid hormones and energy expenditure of obese middle-aged women. Am J Clin Nutr 45:391–398, 1987

53. Katzeff HL, Yang M-U, Presta E, et al: Calorie restriction iopanoic acid effects on thyroid hormone metabolism. Am J Clin Nutr 52:263–266, 1990

54. Burger AG, O'Connell M, Scheidegger K, et al: Monodeiodination of triio-dothyronine and reverse triiodothyronine during low and high calorie diets. J Clin Endocrinol Metab 65:829–835, 1987

55. Visser TJ, Lamberts SWJ, Wilson JHP, et al: Serum thyroid hormone concen-trations during prolonged reduction of dietary intake. Metabolism 27:405–409, 1978

56. Burman KD, Wartofsky L, Dinterman RE, et al: The effect of T3 and reverse T3 administration on muscle protein catabolism during fasting as measured by 3-methylhistidine excretion. Metabolism 28:805–813, 1979
57. Serog P, Apfelbaum M, Autissier N, et al: Effects of slimming and composition of diet on VO2 and thyroid hormones in healthy subjects. Am J Clin Nutr 35:24–35, 1982
58. Davies HJA, Baird IM, Fowler J, et al: Metabolic responses to low- and very-low-calorie diets. Am J Clin Nutr 49:745–751, 1989
59. Snyder DK, Clemmons DR, Underwood LE: Treatment of obese, diet-restricted subjects with growth hormone for eleven weeks: effects on anabolism, lipolysis and body composition. J Clin Endocrinol Metab 67:54–61, 1988
60. Henson LC, Heber D: Whole body protein breakdown rates and hormonal adaptation in fasted obese subjects. J Clin Endocrinol Metab 57:316–319, 1983
61. Rozen R, Abraham G, Falcou R, et al: The effects of a "physiological" dose of triiodothyronine on obese subjects during a protein-sparing diet. Int J Obes 10:303–312, 1986
62. Wilson JHP, Lamberts SWJ, Swart GR: A metabolic ward study of a high protein, very-low-energy diet. Int J Obes 7:345–352, 1983
63. Wilson JHP, Lamberts WJ: The effect of triiodothyronine on weight loss and nitrogen balance of obese patients on a very-low-calorie liquid-formula diet. Int J Obes 5:279–282, 1981
64. Wadden TA, Mason G, Foster GD, et al: Effects of a very low calorie diet on weight, thyroid hormones and mood. Int J Obes 14:249–258, 1990
65. Chomard P, Vernhes G, Autissier N, et al: Serum concentrations of total and free thyroid hormones in moderately obese women during a six-week slimming cure. Eur J Clin Nutr 42:285–293, 1988
66. Vagenakis AG, Burger A, Portnay GI, et al: Diversion of peripheral thyroxine metabolism from activating to inactivating pathways during complete fasting. J Clin Endocrinol Metab 41:191–194, 1975
67. LoPresti JS, Gray D, Nicoloff JT: Influence of fasting and refeeding on 3,3',5'-triiodothyronine metabolism in man. J Clin Endocrinol Metab 72:103–136, 1991
68. Pasquali R, Parenti M, Mattioli L, et al: Effect of dietary carbohydrates during hypocaloric treatment of obesity on peripheral thyroid hormone metabolism. J Endocrinol Invest 5:47–52, 1982
69. Danforth EJ: Effects of fasting and altered nutrition on thyroid hormone metabolism in man, in Thyroid Hormone Metabolism. Edited by Hennemann G. New York, Marcel Dekker, 1986, pp 335–358
70. Davidson MB, Chopra IJ: Effect of carbohydrate and noncarbohydrate sources of calories on plasma 3,5,3'-triiodothyronine concentrations in man. J Clin Endocrinol Metab 48:277–581, 1979

71. Welle S, O'Connell M, Danforth EJ, et al: Impact of carbohydrate overfeeding on total and free thyroid hormones, thyroid hormone binding proteins, and thermogenesis (abstract). Clin Res 31:279A, 1983
72. Woo R, Daniels-Kush R, Horton ES: Regulation of energy balance. Ann Rev Nutr 5:411–433, 1985
73. Jequier E, Acheson K, Schutz Y: Assessment of energy expenditure and fuel utilization in man. Ann Rev Nutr 7:187–208, 1987
74. Richard D, Rivest S: The role of exercise in thermogenesis and energy balance. Can J Physiol Pharmacol 67:402–409, 1989
75. Kinney JM: Energy metabolism: heat, fuel and life, in Nutrition and Metabolism in Patient Care. Edited by Kinney JM, Jeejeebhoy KN, Hill GL, et al. Philadelphia, PA, WB Saunders, 1988, pp 3–34
76. Danforth EJ: The role of thyroid hormones and insulin in the regulation of energy metabolism. Am J Clin Nutr 38:1006–1017, 1983
77. Guernsey BL, Edelman IS: Regulation of thermogenesis by thyroid hormones, in Molecular Basis of Thyroid Hormone Action. Edited by Oppenheimer JH, Samuels HH. New York, Academic Press, 1983, pp 293–324
78. Abraham RR, Densem JW, Davies P, et al: The effects of triiodothyronine on energy expenditure nitrogen balance and rates of weight and fat loss in obese patients during prolonged caloric restriction. Int J Obes 9:433–442, 1985
79. Nair KS, Halliday D, Ford GC, et al: Effect of triiodothyronine on leucine kinetics metabolic rate glucose concentration and insulin secretion rate during two weeks of fasting in obese women. Int J Obes 13:487–496, 1989
80. Gelfand RA, Hutchinson-Williams KA, Bonde AA, et al: Catabolic effects of thyroid hormone excess: the contribution of adrenergic activity to hypermetabolism and protein breakdown. Metabolism 36:562–569, 1987
81. Piolino V, Acheson KJ, Muller MJ, et al: Thermogenic effect of thyroid hormones: interactions with epinephrine and insulin. Am J Physiol 259:E305–E311, 1990
82. Muller MJ, Burger AG, Ferrannini E, et al: Glucoregulatory function of thyroid hormones: role of pancreatic hormones. Am J Physiol 256:E101–E110, 1989
83. Moore R, Mehrishi JN, Verdoorn C, et al: The role of T3 and its receptor in efficient metabolisers receiving very-low-calorie diets. Int J Obes 5:283–286, 1981
84. Acheson KJ, Burger AJ: A study of the relationship between thermogenesis and thyroid hormones. J Clin Endocrinol Metab 51:84–89, 1980
85. Poehlman ET, Arciero PJ, Melby CL, et al: Resting metabolic rate and postprandial thermogenesis in vegetarians and nonvegetarians. Am J Clin Nutr 48:209–213, 1988
86. Landsberg L, Young JB: The role of the sympathoadrenal system in modulating energy expenditure. Clinics in Endocrinology and Metabolism 13:475–499, 1984

87. Acheson K, Jequier E, Burger A, et al: Thyroid hormones and thermogenesis: the metabolic cost of food and exercise. Metabolism 33:262–265, 1984
88. Phinney SD, LaGrange BM, O'Connell M, et al: Effects of aerobic exercise on energy expenditure and nitrogen balance during very low calorie dieting. Metabolism 37:758–765, 1986
89. Garrell DR, Todd KS, Pugeat MM, et al: Hormonal changes in normal men under marginally negative energy balance. Am J Clin Nutr 39:930–936, 1984
90. McCargar LJ, Clandinin MT, Belcastro AN, et al: Dietary carbohydrate-to-fat ratio: influence on whole-body nitrogen retention, substrate utilization, and hormone response in healthy male subjects. Am J Clin Nutr 49:1169–1178, 1989
91. Ismail-Beigi F, Edelman IS: Mechanism of thyroid calorigenesis: role of active sodium transport. Proc Natl Acad Sci U S A 67:1071–1078, 1970
92. Ismail-Beigi F, Edelman IS: The mechanism of the calorigenic action of thyroid hormone: stimulation of the Na^+ and K^+-activated adenosine triphosphatase activity. J Gen Physiol 57:710–722, 1971
93. Oppenheimer JH: The nuclear receptor-triiodothyronine complex: relationship to thyroid hormone distribution, metabolism, and biological action, in Molecular Basis of Thyroid Hormone Action. Edited by Oppenheimer JH, Samuels HH. New York, Academic Press, 1983, pp 1–34
94. van Hardeveld C: Effects of thyroid hormone on oxygen consumption, heat production and energy economy, in Thyroid Hormone Metabolism. Edited by Hennemann G. New York, Marcel Dekker, 1986, pp 579–608
95. Danforth EJ, Burger A: The role of thyroid hormones in the control of energy expenditure. Clinical Endocrinology and Metabolism 13:581–595, 1984
96. Eaton RP, Steinberg D, Thompson RH: Relationship between free fatty acid turnover and total body oxygen consumption in the euthyroid and hyperthyroid states. J Clin Invest 44:247–260, 1965
97. Okajima F, Ui M: Metabolism of glucose in hyper- and hypothyroid rats in vivo. Biochemistry Journal 182:565–575, 1979
98. Hoppner W, Horst C, Rasmussen UB, et al: Adenine nucleotide translocase: a target of thyroid hormone action? in Molecular Biological Approaches to Thyroid Research. Edited by Loos U, Wartofsky L. Stuttgart, Germany, Theim Publications, 1987, pp 29–33
99. Horst C, Rakos H, Seitz HJ: Rapid stimulation of hepatic oxygen consumption by 3,5-di-iodo-L-thyronine. Biochemistry Journal 261:945–950, 1989
100. Perkins KA, McKenzie SJ, Stoney CM: The relevance of metabolic rate in behavioral medicine research. Behav Modif 11:286–311, 1987
101. Zach J, Ackerman SH: Thyroid function, metabolic regulation, and depression. Psychosom Med 50:454–468, 1988
102. Levitt AJ, Joffe RT, Esche IT, et al: The effect of desipramine on body weight in depression. J Clin Psychiatry 48:27–28, 1987

103. Garland EJ, Remick RA, Zis AP: Weight gain with antidepressants and lithium. J Clin Psychopharmacol 8:323–330, 1988

104. Mezzich JE, Raab ES: Depressive symptomatology across Americas. Arch Gen Psychiatry 37:818–823, 1980

105. Casper RC, Redmond EJ, Katz MM, et al: Somatic symptoms in primary affective disorder. Arch Gen Psychiatry 42:1098–1104, 1985

106. Fernstrom M, McConaha C, Kupfer DJ: Perception of appetite and weight change during treatment for depression. Appetite 13:71–77, 1989

107. Tayek JA, Bistrian BR, Blackburn GL: Improved food intake and weight gain in adults following electroconvulsive therapy for depression. J Am Diet Assoc 88:63–65, 1988

108. Gaist PA, Orbarzinek E, Skwerer RG, et al: Effects of bright light on resting metabolic rate in patients with seasonal affective disorder and control subjects. Biol Psychiatry 28:789–996, 1990

109. Fernstrom MH, Epstein LH, Spiker DG, et al: Resting metabolic rate is reduced in patients treated with antidepressants. Biol Psychiatry 20:692–695, 1985

110. Fernstrom MH, Massoudi M, Kupfer DJ: Fluvoxamine and weight loss. Biol Psychiatry 24:948–949, 1988

111. Esler M, Turbott J, Schwarz R, et al: The peripheral kinetics of norepinephrine in depressive illness. Arch Gen Psychiatry 39:295–300, 1982

112. Golden RN, Markey SP, Risby ED, et al: Antidepressants reduce whole-body norepinephrine turnover while enhancing 6-hydroxymelatonin output. Arch Gen Psychiatry 45:150–154, 1988

113. Gold PW, Goodwin FK, Chrousos GP: The clinical and biochemical manifestations of depression: relation to the neurobiology of stress (part two). N Engl J Med 319:413–420, 1988

114. Fichter MM, Pirke K-M, Holsboer F: Weight loss causes neuroendocrine disturbances: experimental study in healthy starving subjects. Psychiatry Res 17:61–72, 1986

115. Joffe RT: A perspective on the thyroid and depression. Can J Psychiatry 35:754–758, 1990

116. Elliot DL, Goldberg L, Kuehl KS, et al: Sustained depression of the resting metabolic rate after massive weight loss. Am J Clin Nutr 49:93–96, 1989

117. Gopalaswmay AK, Morgan R: Too many chronically mentally disabled patients are too fat. Acta Psychiatr Scand 72:254–258, 1985

118. Berken GH, Weinstein DO, Stern WC: Weight gain: a side effect of tricyclic antidepressants. J Affective Disord 7:133–138, 1984

Chapter 3

Interactions Between Thyroid Hormones and Other Endocrine Systems

Julio Licinio, M.D.
Ma-Li Wong, M.D.
Philip W. Gold, M.D.

CONTENTS

1. INTRODUCTION

Thyroid hormones are the only known biologically active iodine-containing compounds. They are essential for the regulation of normal growth and differentiation, as well as for the maintenance of metabolic stability. Those two broad sets of actions affect the function of virtually every organ system. The interactions between triiodothyronine (T_3), the active thyroid hormone, and target organs occur at the level of the cell nucleus.

In short, the thyroid secretes predominantly thyroxine (T_4), currently seen as a prohormone. Peripherally, T_4 is converted to T_3, the active thyroid hormone. T_3 enters target cells, binds itself to nuclear receptors, and affects DNA transcription. In some tissues this results in an increase in total production of mRNA. In other tissues there is an increase in specific mRNAs, but no overall increase in mRNA synthesis (1,2). In this way, thyroid hormones act directly on the genetic code to modulate the function of a number of physiological systems. In this chapter, we review preclinical and clinical aspects of the interactions of thyroid hormones with other endocrine systems, including the hypothalamic-pituitary-gonadal (HPG) axis, prolactin, cytokines, growth hormone, gastrointestinal hormones, melatonin, and stress-related neuroendocrine systems, such as the hypothalamic-pituitary-adrenal (HPA) axis.

2. REPRODUCTIVE FUNCTION

2.1 Preclinical Studies

The interactions between thyroid hormones and the HPG axis have been well studied. Thyroid hormones affect the HPG axis and are essential for the maintenance of an adult pattern of sexual function. The lack of thyroid hormones in adult female rats seems to produce a reversion of sexual hormones to a prepubertal pattern, whereas T_3 treatment restores normal estrous cycles and ovarian function (3). In amphibians, gonadotropin-releasing hormone (GnRH) administration increases thyroid-stimulating hormone (TSH) secretion (4).

Wang et al. (5) studied the effects of thyroidectomy and T_4 replacement on the release of luteinizing hormone (LH) and GnRH in vitro. Their results suggest that T_4 is inhibitory to the basal and GnRH-stimulated LH release, as well as to the release of GnRH in the absence of ovarian hormones. The same group (6) then studied the interrelationship between estrogen and T_4 on the release of LH and GnRH in vitro. Their results suggest that there is an antagonistic effect between T_4 and estrogen on the response of pituitary LH to GnRH and the release of GnRH.

Maruo et al. (7) studied the role of thyroid hormone directly in ovarian cells. Their findings suggest that thyroid hormones synergize with follicle-stimulating hormone (FSH) to exert direct stimulatory effects on granulosa cell functions, including morphological differentiation, LH–human chorionic gonadotropin receptor formation, and steroidogenic enzyme (3β-hydroxysteroid dehydrogenase and aromatase) induction. Hence, decreases in ovarian functions during the states of hypo- or hyperthyroidism may be at least partially accounted for by a diminished responsiveness of the granulosa cells to FSH.

2.2 Clinical Studies

Clinical studies of HPG axis–thyroid interactions reveal that both hypo- and hyperthyroidism affect the HPG axis. Valenti et al. (8) studied large numbers of patients with either Graves' disease and clinical hyperthyroidism or primary hypothyroidism. Significant changes in HPG function were observed in both states, with increased basal and stimulated values of both gonadotropins. Qualitative and quantitative recovery was seen when the euthyroid state was achieved after treatment of hyper- and hypothyroid patients. The authors concluded that the direct interference with the hypothalamic-pituitary system, rather than the modulation of peripheral estrogen metabolism, is the possible pathogenetic mechanism of abnormal HPG axis in abnormal thyroid status.

McDermott et al. (9) studied the effects of a continuous infusion of thyrotropin-releasing hormone (TRH) on GnRH-stimulated gonadotropin secretion. Their data indicate that a brief TRH infusion, producing mild elevations of thyrotropin and prolactin, affects the HPG axis, predominantly delaying the timing of GnRH-stimulated gonadotropin secretion. In girls with hypothyroidism, Buchanan et al. (10) documented elevated nocturnal levels of FSH, without signs of precocious puberty.

Rojdmark et al. (11) studied the HPG axis in hyperthyroid men. Their subjects had an exaggerated LH and FSH responses to exogenous GnRH, indicating that chronic thyroid hormone excess makes the pituitary gonadotrophs "hypersensitive" to exogenous GnRH. This may in turn explain why human Leydig cells respond more powerfully to exogenous GnRH in thyrotoxic patients than in euthyroid subjects.

In hypothyroidism the reverse seems to occur. Men with hypothyroidism commonly have impotence, decreased LH bioactivity, low serum testosterone, and low testosterone-estradiol–binding globulin concentrations (12). Castro-Magana et al. (13) showed a decreased response to GnRH in hypothyroid boys. Buitrago and Diez (14) documented a negative effect of both hypo- and hyperthyroidism on seminal parameters in men. In addition, thyroid hormones stimulate the in vivo and in vitro production of sex hormone–binding globulin, a plasma protein involved in the transport of sex hormones (15). In conclusion, clinical and preclinical data indicate that normal thyroid status is necessary for the optimal functioning of the HPG axis; both hypothyroidism and hyperthyroidism adversely affect reproductive function.

3. PROLACTIN

TRH is a stimulant of pituitary prolactin secretion. In hyperthyroidism there is a suppression of the plasma prolactin response to TRH. Erfurth and Hedner (16) showed that this phenomenon can be induced in healthy control subjects by exogenous T_4, but not by T_3 administration.

4. CYTOKINES

Cytokines are peptides produced by cells of the immune system. Initially thought to act solely as messengers within cells of the immune system, cytokines have now been found to have a variety of systemic effects and to interact with neuroendocrine systems, including the HPA and HPG axes. Interleukins (ILs), such as IL-1α and IL-1β, have been localized in brain, in areas of importance to the regulation of neuroendocrine function, such as hippocampus and hypothalamus (17,18).

Cytokines also affect energy expenditure and thyroid status. Sato et al.

(19) have demonstrated a number of effects for diverse cytokines on thyroid function. They have shown that IL-1α and IL-1β inhibit iodine-125 (^{125}I) incorporation and ^{125}I-iodothyronine release in a concentration-dependent manner. On electron-microscopic examination there is a marked decrease in lysosome formation in IL-1-treated thyrocytes.

Tumor necrosis factor alpha (TNF-α) and interferon gamma (IFN-γ) also inhibit thyroid function in a concentration-dependent manner. Furthermore, when thyrocytes are cultured with IL-1, TNF-α, and IFN-γ, these cytokines act synergistically to inhibit thyroid function. Kawabe et al. (20) have studied the effects of IL-1 on thyroid tissue and determined that IL-1 regulates the proliferation of thyrocytes. IL-1 modulates thyrotropin-induced thyroglobulin mRNA transcription through a cyclic adenosine monophosphate (cAMP)-dependent mechanism (21). Mooradian et al. (22) have shown that, in humans, increased concentrations of TNF are associated with decreased serum T_3; in their study there was no association between IL-1α levels and thyroid function. Their data, taken together with the previous findings in laboratory animals, suggest that some of the alterations in thyroid hormone levels seen in nonthyroidal illness are associated with elevated serum concentrations of TNF.

5. GROWTH HORMONE

Patients with acromegaly, a state of growth hormone excess, frequently have a goiter. This has been studied by Miyakawa et al. (23). Their data show that somatomedin C–insulin-like growth factor (IGF)-I is one of the factors involved in goiter formation. Individuals with acromegaly also have mild central hypothyroidism, which is not reflected peripherally because of increased peripheral conversion of T_4 to T_3 (24).

In thyroid-deficiency states of various causes, there are decreased levels of growth hormone and decreased responses to various stimuli of growth hormone secretion. In children with primary hypothyroidism, there is decreased nocturnal surge in growth hormone and low somatomedin C–IGF-I levels (25). In endemic cretinism with hypothyroidism, there is a subnormal growth hormone response to clonidine and low somatomedin C–IGF-I levels (26,27). Hypothyroidism is also marked by a decreased growth hormone responsiveness to growth hormone–releasing hormone, which can be corrected after T_4 replacement (28).

6. GASTROINTESTINAL HORMONES

6.1 Insulin

Thyroid hormones affect the function of a number of different gastrointestinal tract hormones. Ikeda et al. (29) have demonstrated that in vitro thyroid hormones do not affect insulin secretion; however, in vivo T_4 substantially increases insulin secretion. As this effect can be blocked by oxprenolol, the authors concluded that thyroid hormone induces hyperinsulinemia via β-adrenergic stimulation. The β-adrenergic stimulation of insulin secretion has been studied in hypo- and hyperthyroid patients (30). Hypothyroid patients had markedly diminished insulin and C-peptide response to the β_2-adrenoceptor agonist terbutaline (125 μg iv), whereas hyperthyroid patients had prompt insulin and C-peptide responses to this test.

In addition to stimulating insulin secretion, T_3 amplifies the effects of insulin in liver cells, stimulating the transcription of the fatty acid synthase gene in hepatocytes in culture (31). Increased transcription of the fatty acid synthase gene precedes the increase in fatty acid synthase mRNA level caused by feeding, which indicates regulation at the level of transcription. The feeding-induced stimulation of fatty acid synthase can be mimicked in culture by incubating hepatocytes with insulin and thyroid hormone (32).

Piolino et al. (33) have shown that, in humans, insulin antagonizes the increase in resting metabolic rate promoted by thyroid hormones. This is probably due to the fact that hyperthyroidism increases hypoinsulinemia-induced increases in lipolysis, free fatty acid recycling, and ketogenesis, without affecting lipid oxidation (34). In hypothyroidism, the peak insulin response to oral glucose is delayed, suggesting impaired pancreatic β-cell response to oral glucose (35). Ikeda et al. (36,37) have shown that the insulin response to glucose in short-term starvation is dependent on the presence of thyroid hormone, with impairment of insulin secretion in the hypothyroid condition.

Muller et al. (38) have studied the role of thyroid hormones on the effects of the enteroinsular axis on insulin secretion. In T_3-induced hyperthyroidism, there are elevated basal and stimulated glucose and insulin levels in rats. The release of gastric inhibitory polypeptide after an oral glucose load is not significantly different between euthyroid and hyperthyroid rats. The insulin response, however, is significantly higher in hyperthyroid animals. It is therefore hypothesized that in hyperthyroidism there is an increased sensitivity to the insulinotropic action of gastric inhibitory polypeptide.

Lenzen and Bailey (39) have comprehensively reviewed the impact of thyroid hormones on pancreatic islet function. Their conclusions are that, overall, thyroid hormones increase the provision of glucose to meet the enhanced energy demands that thyroid hormones impose. Glucose tolerance is decreased by thyroid hormones, and that relates to the enhancement in hepatic glucose production, although the glucose-raising effects of thyroid hormones are partially offset by an increased rate of glucose utilization, especially in the postabsorptive state. The pancreatic β-cell's capacity to secrete insulin is reduced by an excess of thyroid hormones, and the onset of diabetes may be accelerated as pancreatic insulin reserves are depleted.

6.2 Glucagon

Glucagon is another pancreatic islet cell hormone that interacts with thyroid hormones. Kabadi and his group (40,41) demonstrated that hyperglucagonemia causes a decline of T_3 and elevation in reverse triiodothyronine (rT_3). This is a result of glucagon's effects on thyroid hormone metabolism peripherally, not the result of altered release of thyroid hormones. Laurberg and Iversen (42) also documented a lack of effect of glucagon on T_4 and T_3 secretion from perfused dog thyroid lobes.

Clinically, hypothyroid patients have low fasting pancreatic glucagon levels (35). On a molecular level, studies have demonstrated that thyroid hormones oppose some of the effects of glucagon in isolated liver cells, antagonizing glucagon-induced inhibition of S-14 gene transcription (43), antagonizing the glucagon-induced suppression of malic enzyme mRNA levels (44), and antagonizing glucagon suppression of fatty acid synthase mRNA in hepatocytes (32). Because of this antagonism between glucagon and thyroid hormones, the blood glucose response to glucagon (250 μg iv) is greater in hypothyroid than in hyperthyroid patients, but after treatment no difference between the two groups is seen. Intravenous glucagon induces prominent insulin and C-peptide responses of similar magnitude in hyper- and hypothyroid patients before, as well as after, treatment (28).

6.3 Other

Neuropeptide Y (NPY), gastrin, and vasoactive intestinal peptide (VIP) are other hormones present in the gastrointestinal tract that interact with thyroid hormones. NPY is a 36–amino acid member of the pancreatic polypeptide family and is also present in anterior pituitary gland. Furthermore, NPY prohormone mRNA has been identified in the pituitary by Northern blot analysis (45). In hypothyroidism there is a substantial increase in the NPY content of the thyroid gland, whereas in hyperthyroidism there is no change. Sagara et al. (46) studied gastrin levels in thyroid disorders. They found fasting serum gastrin levels measured by radioimmunoassay to be elevated in patients with hyperthyroidism and low in patients with hypothyroidism; treatment of thyroid disorders and achievement of euthyroidism normalized these findings.

In humans, VIP has been found in intrathyroidal nerves and has been shown to stimulate thyroid hormone secretion via a cAMP-dependent mechanism (47–49). Huffman and Hedge (50) demonstrated that thyroid blood flow is, in part, controlled by VIP; their data indicate that changes in thyroid blood flow can occur at doses of VIP that have no apparent effect on circulating thyroid hormone levels. Lam and Reichlin (51) demonstrated that the cell content and basal secretion of VIP in primary rat pituitary cell cultures is increased in hypothyroidism. Recent studies suggest that there is VIP synthesis within the rat anterior pituitary (52). Segerson et al. (53) demonstrated that thyroid hormone regulates VIP mRNA levels in the rat anterior pituitary gland and that the content of rat pituitary VIP increases in hypothyroidism.

7. MELATONIN

Chronic melatonin infusion in animals results in a decrease in thyroid function. In humans with thyroid disease, circadian rhythms of melatonin have been studied. Both hypo- and hyperthyroidism are associated with normal melatonin levels and rhythmicity (54).

8. HYPOTHALAMIC-PITUITARY-ADRENAL (HPA) AXIS

Thyroid hormones interact with hormones of the HPA axis (2). Gluco-corticoids inhibit TRH and TSH secretion (55), diminish T_3 production, decrease thyroid-binding globulin concentrations, and increase thyroid-binding prealbumin concentrations (56). In states with glucocorticoid excess there is a blunted TSH response to TRH and normal T_4, but subnormal levels of circulating T_3, secondary to decreased peripheral conversion of T_4 to T_3 and increased conversion of T_4 to rT_3. Grubeck-Loebenstein et al. (57) showed that in adrenal insufficiency there are increased T_3 levels and decreased T_3 levels.

In hypothyroidism there are increased cortisol levels. Kamilaris et al. (58) showed that thyroid hormone deficiency increases corticotroph sensitivity to corticotropin-releasing hormone (CRH), diminishes the plasma adrenocorticotropic releasing hormone (ACTH) response to metyrapone-induced hypocortisolemia, and has no apparent effect on the acute adrenal response to ACTH. Their data suggest that the release of hypothalamic CRH and/or other ACTH secretagogues is decreased in hypothyroidism. Kamilaris et al. (59) confirmed this finding at a molecular level by demonstrating that long-standing hypothyroidism is associated with reduced stress-stimulated CRH mRNA levels. Iranmanesh et al. (60) used hormone-deconvolution techniques to determine that the hypercortisolemia in primary hypothyroidism is due mostly to decreased metabolic clearance of cortisol and a decrease in the negative feedback effect of cortisol on the hypothalamic-pituitary axis. In hyperthyroidism there is a decrease in the concentration of cytosolic glucocorticoid receptors in the hippocampus and increased peripheral levels of ACTH and corticosterone, suggesting hyperactivity of the HPA axis secondary to decreased negative feedback of glucocorticoids on the central components of the HPA axis (61).

9. CONCLUSIONS

In summary, normal thyroid status is essential for the optimal function of most hormonal systems. In vitro and animal studies have well documented the effects of thyroid hormones in practically all other endocrine systems. Clinically, patients with hypo- or hyperthyroidism have a variety of clinical and biochemical abnormalities in essential systems such as the HPG and HPA axes, growth regulation, cytokines, and the gastroenteroinsular axis.

A careful assessment of thyroid function is of importance in psychiatry because hypothyroidism and hyperthyroidism can mimic psychiatric disorders as diverse as depression, organic brain syndrome, panic disorder, and generalized anxiety disorder (see Chapter 5). Furthermore, as thyroid augmentation of antidepressant medication is used clinically in medication-refractory depressed patients (see Chapter 6), it is important for the psychiatrist prescribing thyroid hormones to be well informed of the effects of thyroid hormones on other endocrine systems.

REFERENCES

1. Oppenheimer JH: Thyroid hormone action at the nuclear level. Ann Intern Med 102:374–384, 1985
2. Utiger RD: The thyroid: physiology, hyperthyroidism, hypothyroidism, and the painful thyroid, in Endocrinology and Metabolism, 2nd Edition. Edited by Felig P, Baxter JD, Broadus AE, et al. New York, McGraw-Hill, 1986, pp 389–472
3. Ortega E, Rodriguez E, Ruiz E, et al: Activity of the hypothalamo-pituitary ovarian axis in thyroid rats with or without triiodothyronine replacement. Life Sci 46:391–395, 1990
4. Denver RJ: Several hypothalamic peptides stimulate in vitro thyrotropin secretion by pituitaries of anuran amphibians. Gen Comp Endocrinol 72:383–393, 1988
5. Wang SW, Pu HF, Chiang ST, et al: Effects of thyroidectomy and thyroxine replacement on the release of luteinizing hormone and gonadotropin-releasing hormone in vitro. Horm Res 25:215–222, 1987
6. Wang PS, Chao HT, Wang SW: Interrelationship between estrogen and thyroxine on the release of luteinizing hormone and gonadotropin-releasing hormone in vitro. J Steroid Biochem 28:691–696, 1987
7. Maruo T, Hayashi M, Matsuo H, et al: The role of thyroid hormone as a biological amplifier of the actions of follicle-stimulating hormone in the functional differentiation of cultured porcine granulosa cells. Endocrinology 121:1233–1241, 1987
8. Valenti G, Ceda GP, Denti L, et al: Gonadotropin secretion in hyperthyroidism and hypothyroidism. Ric Clin Lab 14:53–63, 1984
9. McDermott MT, Sjoberg RJ, Hofeldt FD, et al: Effects of a continuous thyrotropin-releasing hormone infusion on gonadotropin-releasing hormone-stimulated gonadotropin secretion. J Lab Clin Med 116:187–190, 1990
10. Buchanan CR, Stanhope R, Adlard P, et al: Gonadotropin, growth hormone and prolactin secretion in children with primary hypothyroidism. Clin Endocrinol (Oxf) 29:427–436, 1988

11. Rojdmark S, Berg A, Kallner G: Hypothalamic-pituitary-testicular axis in patients with hyperthyroidism. Horm Res 29:185–190, 1988

12. Wortsman J, Rosner W, Dufau ML: Abnormal testicular function in men with primary hypothyroidism. Am J Med 82:207–212, 1987

13. Castro-Magana M, Angulo M, Canas A, et al: Hypothalamic-pituitary gonadal axis in boys with primary hypothyroidism and macroorchidism. J Pediatr 112:397–402, 1988

14. Buitrago JM, Diez LC: Serum hormones and seminal parameters in males with thyroid disturbance. Andrologia 19:37–41, 1987

15. Plymate SR, Hoop RC, Jones RE, et al: Regulation of sex hormone-binding globulin production by growth factors. Metabolism 39:967–970, 1990

16. Erfurth EM, Hedner P: Suppressed plasma prolactin response to thyrotropin releasing hormone in hyperthyroidism reproduced by thyroxine but not by triiodothyronine administration to normal subjects. Acta Endocrinol (Copenh) 117:241–248, 1988

17. Breder CD, Dinarello CA, Saper CB: Interleukin-1 immunoreactive innervation of the human hypothalamus. Science 240:321–324, 1988

18. Licinio J, Wong M-L, Smith MA, et al: Localization of interleukin 1 mRNA in rat brain. Society of Neuroscience Abstracts 16(ii):971, 1990

19. Sato K, Satoh T, Shizume K, et al: Inhibition of 125I organification and thyroid hormone release by interleukin-1, tumor necrosis factor-alpha, and interferon-gamma in human thyrocytes in suspension culture. J Clin Endocrinol Metab 70:1735–1743, 1990

20. Kawabe Y, Eguchi K, Shimomura C, et al: Interleukin-1 production and action in thyroid tissue. J Clin Endocrinol Metab 68:1174–1183, 1989

21. Kung AW, Lau KS: Interleukin-1 beta modulates thyrotropin-induced thyroglobulin mRNA transcription through 3', 5'-cyclic adenosine monophosphate. Endocrinology 127:1369–1374, 1990

22. Mooradian AD, Reed RL, Osterweil D, et al: Decreased serum triiodothyronine is associated with increased concentrations of tumor necrosis factor. J Clin Endocrinol Metab 71:1239–1242, 1990

23. Miyakawa M, Saji M, Tsushima T, et al: Thyroid volume and serum thyroglobulin levels in patients with acromegaly: correlation with plasma insulin-like growth factor I levels. J Clin Endocrinol Metab 67:973–978, 1988

24. Eskildsen PC, Kruse A, Kirkegaard C: The pituitary-thyroid axis in acromegaly. Horm Metab Res 20:755–757, 1988

25. Chernausek SD, Turner R: Attenuation of spontaneous, nocturnal growth hormone secretion in children with hypothyroidism and its correlation with plasma insulin-like growth factor I concentrations. J Pediatr 114:968–972, 1989

26. Cavaliere H, Knobel M, Medeiros-Neto G: Effect of thyroid hormone therapy on plasma insulin-like growth factor I levels in normal subjects, hypothyroid patients and endemic cretins. Horm Res 25:132–139, 1987

27. Martins MC, Knobel M, Medeiros-Neto G: Decreased growth hormone (GH) response to oral clonidine in endemic cretinism: effect of L-T$_3$ therapy. J Endocrinol Invest 11:477–481, 1988

28. Valcavi R, Dieguez C, Preece M, et al: Effect of thyroxine replacement therapy on plasma insulin-like growth factor 1 levels and growth hormone responses to growth hormone releasing factor in hypothyroid patients. Clin Endocrinol (Oxf) 27:85–90, 1987

29. Ikeda T, Fujiyama K, Hoshino T, et al: Acute effect of thyroid hormone on insulin secretion in rats. Biochem Pharmacol 40:1769–1771, 1990

30. Ahren B, Lundquist I, Hedner P, et al: Glucose tolerance and insulin and C-peptide responses after various insulin secretory stimuli in hyper- and hypothyroid subjects before and after treatment. Diabetes Res 2:95–103, 1985

31. Stapleton SR, Mitchell DA, Salati LM, et al: Triiodothyronine stimulates transcription of the fatty acid synthase gene in chick embryo hepatocytes in culture: insulin and insulin-like growth factor amplify that effect. J Biol Chem 265:18442–18446, 1990

32. Goodridge AG: Regulation of the gene for fatty acid synthase. Federation Proceedings 45:2399–2405, 1986

33. Piolino V, Acheson KJ, Muller JM, et al: Thermogenic effect of thyroid hormones: interactions with epinephrine and insulin. Am J Physiol 259:E305–E311, 1990

34. Muller MJ, Acheson KJ, Jequier E, et al: Thyroid hormone action on lipid metabolism in humans: a role for endogenous insulin. Metabolism 39:480–485, 1990

35. Kung AW, Lam KS, Pun KK, et al: Circulating somoatostatin after oral glucose in hypothyroidism. J Endocrinol Invest 13:403–406, 1990

36. Ikeda T, Mokuda O, Tominaga M, et al: Glucose intolerance in thyrotoxic rats: role of insulin, glucagon, and epinephrine. Am J Physiol 255:E843–E849, 1988

37. Ikeda T, Fujiyama K, Hoshino T, et al: Thyroidal dependence of glucose-induced insulin secretion in starved rats. Biochem Med Metab Biol 42:220–223, 1989

38. Muller MK, Hellwig J, Schafer A, et al: Effect of GIP on insulin release to intravenous glucose infusion in hyperthyroid rats. Horm Metabol Res 18:163–166, 1986

39. Lenzen S, Bailey CJ: Thyroid hormones, gonadal and adrenocortical steroids and the function of the islets of Langerhans. Endocr Rev 5:411–434, 1984

40. Kabadi UM, Premachandra BN: Lowering of T$_3$ and rise in reverse T$_3$ induced by hyperglucagonemia: altered thyroid hormone metabolism, not altered release of thyroid hormones. Horm Metab Res 19:486–489, 1987

41. Kabadi UM, Premachandra BN: Decline of T$_3$ and elevation in reverse T$_3$ induced by hyperglucagonemia: changes in thyroid hormone metabolism, not altered release of thyroid hormones. Horm Metab Res 20:513–516, 1988

42. Laurberg P, Iversen E: Lack of effect of glucagon on T_4 and T_3 secretion from perfused dog thyroid lobes. Horm Metab Res 19:451–454, 1987

43. Kinlaw WB, Schwartz HL, Hamblin PS, et al: Triiodothyronine rapidly reverses inhibition of S14 gene transcription by glucagon. Endocrinology 123:2255–2260, 1988

44. Back DW, Wilson SB, Morris SM Jr, et al: Hormonal regulation of lipogenic enzymes in chick embryo hepatocytes in culture: thyroid hormone and glucagon regulate malic enzyme mRNA level at post-transcriptional steps. J Biol Chem 261:12555–12561, 1986

45. Jones RH, Chap Z, Pena J, et al: Fasting and postabsorptive hepatic glucose and insulin metabolism in hyperthyroidism. Am J Physiol 256:E159–E166, 1989

46. Sagara K, Shimada T, Fujiyama S, et al: Serum gastrin levels in patients with thyroid dysfunction. Gastroenterol Jpn 18:79–83, 1983

47. Toccafondi RS, Brandi ML, Melander A: Vasoactive intestinal peptide stimulation of human thyroid cell function. J Clin Endocrinol Metab 58:157–160, 1984

48. Laurberg P: VIP and hormone secretion from thyroidal follicular and C-cells. Horm Metab Res 18:230–233, 1986

49. Ahren B, Hedner P: Effects of VIP and helodermin on thyroid hormone secretion in the mouse. Neuropeptides 13:59–64, 1989

50. Huffman L, Hedge GA: Effects of vasoactive intestinal peptide on thyroid blood flow and circulating thyroid hormone levels in the rat. Endocrinology 118:550–557, 1986

51. Lam KS, Reichlin S: Pituitary vasoactive intestinal peptide regulates prolactin secretion in the hypothyroid rat. Neuroendocrinology 50:524–528, 1989

52. Jones PM, Ghatei MA, Steel J, O'Halloran D, et al: Evidence for neuropeptide Y synthesis in the rat anterior pituitary and the influence of thyroid hormone status: comparison with vasoactive intestinal peptide, substance P, and neurotensin. Endocrinology 125:334–341, 1989

53. Segerson TP, Lam KS, Cacicedo L, et al: Thyroid hormone regulates vasoactive intestinal peptide (VIP) mRNA levels in the rat anterior pituitary gland. Endocrinology 125:2221–2223, 1989

54. Soszynski P, Zgliczynski S, Pucilowska J: The circadian rhythm of melatonin in hypothyroidism and hyperthyroidism. Acta Endocrinol (Copenh) 119:240–244, 1988

55. Otsuki M, Dakoda M, Baba S: Influence of glucocorticoids on TRF-induced TSH response in man. J Clin Endocrinol Metab 36:95–102, 1973

56. Gamstedt A, Jarnerot G, Kagedal B: Dose related effects of betamethasone on iodothyronines and thyroid hormone-binding proteins in serum. Acta Endocrinol (Copenh) 96:484–490, 1981

57. Grubeck-Loebenstein B, Vierhapper H, Waldhausl W, et al: Thyroid function in adrenocortical insufficiency during withdrawal and re-administration of glucocorticoid substitution. Acta Endocrinol (Copenh) 103:254–258, 1983

58. Kamilaris TC, DeBold CR, Pavlou SN, et al: Effect of altered thyroid hormone levels on hypothalamic-pituitary-adrenal function. J Clin Endocrinol Metab 65:994–999, 1987

59. Kamilaris TC, Redwine J, Smith M, et al: Effect of short and long duration hypothyroidism and hyperthyroidism on hypothalamic corticotropin-releasing hormone mRNA responses to stress. Society of Neuroscience Abstracts 16(i):91, 1990

60. Iranmanesh A, Lizarralde G, Johnson ML, et al: Dynamics of 24-hour endogenous cortisol secretion and clearance in primary hypothyroidism assessed before and after partial thyroid hormone replacement. J Clin Endocrinol Metab 70:155–161, 1990

61. Johnson EO, Calogero AE, Rabin DR, et al: Modulation of hippocampal glucocorticoid receptors in adult rats by altered thyroid status. Society of Neuroscience Abstracts 16(ii):1071, 1990

Chapter 4

The Hypothalamic-Pituitary-Thyroid Axis: Clinical and Theoretical Principles

Betty L. Chan, M.D.
William Singer, M.D.

CONTENTS

1. INTRODUCTION

The endocrine diseases most frequently encountered by a psychiatrist are disorders of the thyroid gland. Both acute psychiatric illness (1) and medications such as lithium and tricyclic antidepressants (2) can affect thyroid function. Conversely, thyroid dysfunction may manifest occasionally as isolated psychiatric disorders (see Chapter 5). Although florid cases of thyroid disorders are readily recognized, the diagnosis of subtler instances of dysfunction requires a basic understanding of the physiology of the hypothalamic-pituitary-thyroid axis and the proper interpretation of modern laboratory tests for thyroid function. In this chapter, we review the clinical and theoretical aspects of these topics (which serves as a summary of Part I and an introduction to Part II of this book).

2. PHYSIOLOGY OF THE THYROID GLAND

2.1 Biosynthesis and Metabolism

The thyroid gland, as a distinct histological entity capable of synthesizing thyroxine (T₄) and triiodothyronine (T₃), is found only in vertebrates. The human thyroid gland develops from a primordium in the midventral floor of the pharynx. At about 73–80 days of gestation, the human thyroid gland becomes capable of concentrating iodine and synthesizing T₄. The basic functional unit of the thyroid gland is the follicle, which consists of a single layer of epithelial cells enclosing colloid and surrounded by a bed of blood and lymphatic vessels. Thyroid hormone is synthesized in the epithelial cells as thyroglobulin, a prohormone, and exported to the colloid for storage. The thyroid gland is unique among endocrine organs in its large storage capacity and relatively slow release of hormone; the gland normally contains about 8 mg of iodine, a reserve sufficient for about 3 months.

The main features of the biosynthesis and metabolism of thyroid hormones are outlined below. Approximately 150 μg of inorganic iodine ingested daily in food and water is absorbed into the blood. The iodine is then actively concentrated in the thyroid epithelial cells to a level 30–100 times its concentration in plasma. This step can be competitively inhibited by thiocyanate and perchlorate, which accounts for the antithyroid action of these drugs. Because iodine is a nonthreshold substance being readily excreted by the kidney, in a sense the renal-excretory mechanism is in competition with the thyroid-concentrating mechanism.

Within minutes after entering the thyroid, inorganic iodide is oxidized to iodine or hypoiodite in a peroxidase-dependent fashion near the apex of the cells. This step is indistinguishable from the next step in which iodine is incorporated into tyrosine residues within the thyroglobulin molecule. Thyroglobulin is a large glycoprotein with a molecular weight of 700,000; 20% of this contains carbohydrate residues. Like all other secretory proteins, thyroglobulin is synthesized on the ribosomes of follicular cells with a signal peptide that allows its insertion into the rough endoplasmic reticulum. Glycosylation begins in the rough endoplasmic reticulum and is completed in the Golgi complex where the terminal sialic acid residues are added and thyroglobulin is processed in exocytotic vesicles for transport to the apical plasma membrane (3,4). Glycosylation is necessary for secretion of thyroglobulin into the colloid (5). The iodination of thyroglobulin requires four components—thyroglobulin, iodine, peroxidase, and hydrogen peroxide—and careful studies indicate that the process takes place at the apical plasma membrane. The resultant monoiodotyrosine (MIT) and diiodotyrosine (DIT) are brought into close proximity and coupled through an ether linkage to form T_4 and T_3, the principal hormones secreted by the thyroid gland.

Both the iodination of thyroglobulin and the coupling of MIT and

DIT can be inhibited by thiourea derivatives like propylthiouracil and methimazole, which is the basis of the antithyroid action of these drugs. Besides thyroglobulin, the thyroid contains a small amount of thyralbumin (similar to albumin), another iodoprotein, which is increased in many hyperfunctioning thyroids and in some neoplasms, but whose function is unclear.

Release of hormone from the thyroid gland is stimulated by thyroid-stimulating hormone (TSH), released by the anterior pituitary in response to low circulating levels of free (i.e., not protein-bound) thyroid hormones. Under the influence of TSH, thyroglobulin is endocytosed from the colloid to the apical portion of the follicular cell. The colloid-containing droplets fuse with lysosomes and are hydrolyzed, releasing T_4 and T_3 into the circulation. This proteolytic step is inhibited by iodine and probably accounts for the antithyroid action of pharmacological doses of iodine (6). Lithium also inhibits proteolysis of thyroglobulin, but at a site different from that of iodine, and the antithyroid action of lithium and iodine may be additive.

The two active circulating thyroid hormones in serum are T_4 and T_3. Even though recent studies have clearly identified other circulating iodothyronines including $3,3',5'$-L-triiodothyronine (or reverse triiodothyronine [rT_3]), the acetic and propionic acid derivatives of T_4 and T_3, and trace quantities of various forms of deiodinated thyronines and deaminated and ether-cleaved products (7), current data do not suggest a major biological function for these products.

Of the T_4 in circulation, 99.95% is bound to protein (Table 4–1). An interalpha globulin, thyroxine-binding globulin (TBG), acts as a carrier for 75% of the T_4, and the remainder is bound less tightly to thyroxine-binding prealbumin (TBPA) and to albumin. Unbound, or "free," thyroxine (FT_4) accounts for approximately 0.04% and is in equilibrium with the bound form. T_3 is 99.5% bound and 0.5% free.

Table 4–1.   Plasma protein binding of thyroxine (T_4) and triiodothyronine (T_3)

	T_4 (%)	T_3 (%)
Thyroxine-binding globulin (TBG)	75	38
Thyroxine-binding prealbumin (TBPA)	15	27
Albumin	10	35

It is more loosely bound to TBG than is T_4; this is reflected in the half-life of T_4 in the circulation (about 7 days versus 1 day for T_3).

In human serum, the concentration of total T_4 in most laboratories ranges from 60 to 140 mM/L, for T_3 from 1.3 to 2.8 mM/L. Because only free thyroid hormone is metabolically active, the most sensitive indicator of altered hormonal activity is a change in the FT_4 level. Only 15%–20% of circulating T_3 is secreted by the thyroid; the rest is derived peripherally from monodeiodination. In both hypo- and hyperthyroidism, a larger percentage of circulating T_3 is derived directly from the thyroid. It is estimated that about 20% of the T_4 secreted by the thyroid undergoes monodeiodination in the peripheral tissues to produce about 30 μg/day of T_3. Because T_3 is about four times more active than T_4 metabolically, it follows that most thyroid hormonal activity is attributable to T_3 rather than to T_4.

Monodeiodination can remove either the iodine at the 5′ position to yield biologically active T_3 or the iodine at the 5 position to yield the inactive rT_3. In a number of conditions (e.g., uremia, acute and chronic illness, stress, malnutrition, and steroid therapy), rT_3 level rises and T_3 level falls. Although the biological significance of these changes is not clear, they are clinically relevant, because, in the conditions listed above, a low serum T_3 cannot be interpreted as evidence of hypothyroidism if the serum T_4 and TSH are normal (discussed in more detail below).

2.2 Biological Action

a. Growth and development

The physiological effects of thyroid hormone are numerous and by no means confined to those associated with the overt manifestations of hyperthyroidism or hypothyroidism. One of the earliest recognized developmental roles was its control of amphibian metamorphosis. Thyroidectomized tadpoles do not develop into frogs, but the addition of T_4 to the water induces all the changes for development to a terrestrial adult (7). These morphological changes are accompanied by various biochemical developments (e.g., a change from larval to adult hemoglobin, changes in retinal pigments, an increase in lysosomal hydrolases, and synthesis of urea cycle enzymes). As most of these changes require new protein synthesis, the site of thyroid hormone action appears to be at a transcriptional or translational level.

The developmental effects of thyroid hormone so dramatically apparent in amphibians also play an important role in the autogenesis of higher vertebrates. In humans, there is recent evidence that transplacental transfer of thyroid hormone from the mother is important for normal brain development in the fetus, whose own gland does not start production until about 12 weeks of gestation (8). At that stage, TSH also becomes detectable in the fetal pituitary gland. In mammals, thyroid hormones appear to influence the secretion of growth hormone as well as of various tissue growth factors. The effect on fetal brain has been studied in rats who show cortical neuronal deficiency with diminished synapse formation and a defect in myelination. In humans, delay in treatment of hypothyroidism beyond a few weeks after birth causes irreversible brain damage.

b. Thermoregulation

It had been proposed that thyroid hormones augment oxygen consumption and heat generation by uncoupling oxidative phosphorylation. This hypothesis has been discarded, however, because it could not be experimentally verified. In recent years, it has been shown that thyroid hormone increases hepatic S-14 gene transcription, which appears to have an important role in regulation of lipogenesis and may play a key role in the action of thyroid hormone on energy metabolism (9). It is postulated that thyroid hormone, by augmenting the induction of S-14 and other lipogenic enzymes, stimulates the formation of fatty acid from carbohydrate. At the same time, thyroid hormone also stimulates increased entrance of fatty acid into the mitochondria to undergo oxidation, resulting in water, carbon dioxide, and energy. The energy generated is used to synthesize fatty acid again.

Thyroid hormones have a stimulatory effect on Na^+/K^+-dependent ATPase, controlling active extrusion and, indirectly, passive entry of Na^+ across cell membranes (see Chapter 3). Thyroid hormones appear to enhance futile metabolic cycles, which result in an increase in oxidation of fatty acids and dissipation of heat without concomitant generation of "useful" work (10). Thus in hyperthyroidism, there may be excessive futile cycling with dissipation of body fuels as heat, resulting in the symptoms of heat intolerance and weight loss, whereas the opposite effect is seen in hypothyroidism. Of interest is the fact that the role of thyroid hormone in thermogenesis is a recent evolutionary acquisition with the appearance of homeotherms about 200 million years ago. Nonhomeotherms, such as trout and reptiles, have thyroid hormones and nuclear T3 receptors, suggesting that in earlier vertebrates thyroid hormone served other purposes (e.g, differentiation and development) and that as homeotherms evolved the hormone was co-opted for thermoregulation (11). (This topic is more extensively dealt with in Chapter 2.)

c. Central nervous system function

Even more interesting is the absence of increased oxygen consumption and associated rise in enzymes involved in fatty acid oxidation in the brain in response to thyroid hormone. It can be speculated that the role of thyroid hormone in the brain may be different from that in peripheral tissues. In rat brain, the density of nuclear T_3 receptor shows a caudocranial pattern with the highest density in the phylogenetically newer regions concerned with higher mental function (12). In rats rendered hypothyroid with propylthiouracil, there is increased cerebral dopamine content and tyrosine hydroxylase activity (13), whereas in hyperthyroid rats there is a decrease in the brain tyrosine hydroxylase activity. The putative role of biogenic amines in psychiatric illness is well documented. Whether similar changes in brain biogenic amines mediate the psychiatric manifestation of hypo- and/or hyperthyroidism in humans remains to be determined.

d. Cardiac function

It has been speculated that the inotropic and chronotropic cardiac manifestations of hypo- and hyperthyroidism may be mediated through the effect of thyroid hormone on the β-adrenergic system. In general, hyperthyroidism increases β-receptor–mediated force and rate responses, whereas hyperthyroidism has opposite effects (14). These changes can be partially explained by parallel changes in the density of β-adrenergic receptors (14). Thyroid hormone appears also to play a role in the regulation of vascular tone through its modulation of the β-adrenergic system (15). This may explain why clinical hypothyroidism may be associated with labile and difficult-to-control blood pressure during anesthesia. Thyroid hormone may also mediate its effect on the heart and skeletal muscle through its major role in the regulation of myosin gene expression (16).

2.3   Intracellular Transport

Circulating T_4 and T_3 are taken up by all tissues in varying amounts. It has been postulated that thyroid hormones, being rather polar molecules, enter cells via a special transporter. A temperature-dependent, energy-requiring, saturable, and stereospecific L-T_3 uptake mechanism has been demonstrated in myoblast (17), fibroblast (18), and rat pituitary cell lines (19). It has also been suggested that the operation of a stereospecific, energy-dependent transport system is responsible for the accumulation of T_3 in the nucleus (19). Both the L and D enantiomers bind with comparable affinities to isolated nuclei and to solubilized receptor preparations, yet D-T_3 is a very weak thyromimetic. This difference in biological activities between the two enantiomers can be accounted for by the preferential accumulation of L-T_3 in the nucleus as a result of the operation of a stereospecific nuclear uptake mechanism.

2.4   Thyroid Hormone Receptor

The effects of thyroid hormone are mediated through the binding of T_3 to nuclear receptor proteins that modulate the transcription of specific genes in target cells (20). Although several investigators in the past have suggested that thyroid hormones can initiate cellular responses through an interaction with extranuclear components (21, 22), there is no entirely convincing evidence to date that the binding of T_3 to extranuclear sites results in significant changes in physiological function (23). Intrinsic to the nuclear-initiating hypothesis of thyroid hormone action is the recognition that T_3 is the active hormone and that T_4 largely serves as a prohormone (24,25).

Thyroid hormone receptors are nonhistone DNA-binding proteins present in the nucleus (20,26). Unlike estrogen and glucocorticoid receptors, thyroid hormone receptors can enter the cell nucleus in the absence of T_3 and are found predominantly in the nucleus and not in the cytosol. They are characterized by a sedimentation coefficient of 3.7 S and a molecular weight of about 49,000, although a variety of studies (27–31) suggest that two forms, with molecular weights of 47,000 and 57,000, are present. Thyroid hormone receptors bind L-T_3 with an association constant of 1.3 M in vitro and a binding capacity of about 1 pmol/mg DNA (23). Thus thyroid hormone receptors have the characteristics expected of receptors (i.e., high affinity and low capacity). Thyroid hormone receptors have been identified in all vertebrate species that contain significant concentration of T_3 in their serum. In humans, thyroid hormone receptors have been identified in practically all tissues including heart, brain, liver, kidney, and gonads. Concerted efforts to isolate the T_3 receptor using conventional chromatographic techniques have not been successful.

In the mid-1980s, the scene was dramatically altered with the advent of molecular biological techniques. By that time, both the estrogen and glucocorticoid receptors had been purified and cloned and shown to have sequence homology to the viral oncogene *erb* A (32–34). Weinberger et al. (35) and Sap et al. (36) probed cDNA libraries for v-*erb* A–related cDNAs, reasoning that other hormones that act on the nucleus might be structurally related. Serendipitously, Weinberger et al. (35) recovered a human cDNA (classified now as a "beta" type), and Sap et al. (36) recovered an "alpha" type from a chicken cDNA library. When these cDNAs were transcribed and translated in vitro, they coded for proteins that bound T_3 and other thyroid hormone analogues with an affinity similar to that of the native thyroid hormone receptor molecule. Subsequent studies in rats and humans have isolated four c-*erb* A gene products, three of which, c-*erb* Aα1 (on chromosome 17 in humans), c-*erb* Aβ1 (on chromosome 3), and c-*erb* Aβ2 (also on chromosome 3, generated by alternative splicing) encode biologically active T_3 receptors. The fourth, c-*erb* Aα2 may play an inhibitory role in T_3 action (37,38).

There are several possible advantages to having multiple receptors for thyroid hormone. One possibility is that they may be expressed in a tissue-specific fashion. This has been confirmed by the identification of the c-*erb* Aα2 gene product as the predominant thyroid receptor in the brain and the c-*erb* Aβ2 gene product to be specific to the pituitary gland (39). Second, it is possible that they respond differently to thyroid hormones and their metabolites. Hodin et al. (40) showed that rats rendered hypothyroid with propylthiouracil responded to T_3 with differential and tissue-specific changes in the expression of the four c-*erb* A mRNAs. Of note is the uniform unresponsiveness of the brain *erb* A mRNA level and the uniqueness of the pituitary gland in its decrease in *erb* Aβ2 expression in response to thyroid hormone. Third, because their DNA-binding domains differ slightly, they might activate an overlapping, yet partially distinct, genetic network. Finally, multiple thyroid receptor genes might be responsive to distinct metabolic or hormonal regulators (32). The brain thyroid hormone receptor (40) may act as a modulator of the brain's response to thyroidal status by inhibiting T_3 action.

Despite the fact that thyroid and steroid hormones are neither structurally nor biosynthetically related, they share a common structure for their receptors. This supports the proposal that there is a large superfamily of genes whose products are hormone-responsive transcriptional factors. Receptors for other hormones including progesterone, aldosterone, vitamin D_3, and retinoic acid have been identified as belonging to this superfamily (see Table 4–2). All genes in this fam-

Table 4–2. Evidence for a superfamily of hormonal receptors

Receptor glucocorticoid	Homology to domain C of glucocorticoid receptor (%)	Homology to domain E of glucocorticoid receptor (%)
Mineralocorticoid	94	57
Progesterone	90	55
Estrogen	52	30
Thyroid	47	17
(T_3Rα)	47	17
(T_3Rβ)	47	17
v-*erb* A	47	17
Retinoic acid	45	15

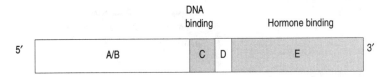

Figure 4–1. Basic structure of the gene for the superfamily of hormonal receptors.

ily can be divided into four regions: A/B, C, D, and E (Figure 4–1). C and E encode functional domains mediating DNA and ligand binding, respectively. Domain C is highly conserved among members of the family. The common biological action shared by all these hormones is their intimate involvement in regulation of growth, differentiation, and morphogenesis. Therefore, the identification of this superfamily of receptor genes represents a critical advance because it suggests a unifying hypothesis for receptor structure and function (41,42).

Although for many decades it has been understood that sex steroids can influence behavior, the role of other hormones in neurological function remains controversial. Since the classic description by Thomas Addison in 1855 of adrenal insufficiency, glucocorticoids have been associated with inability to concentrate, restlessness, insomnia, anxiety, disturbed sleep, and frank psychotic episodes. Hyperthyroidism can also be associated with similar symptoms. The effects of thyroid hormone on central nervous system development and behavior and the high level of thyroid hormone receptors in the brain lead to the prediction that aberrant hormonal production, variation in receptor expression, or receptor mutations could mediate aberrant metabolic effects in the central nervous system (43). Thus an important area of future research is the contribution of thyroid receptors to the etiology of psychiatric illness.

3. REGULATION OF THYROID HORMONE FUNCTION

The synthesis and release of thyroid hormones is under the control of TSH, among other factors (Figure 4–2). TSH itself is controlled by negative feedback of thyroid hormones and stimulation by thyrotropin-releasing hormone (TRH) from the hypothalamus.

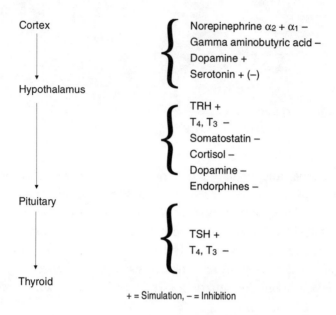

Figure 4–2. Regulation of thyroid hormone secretion. TRH = thyrotropin-releasing hormone; T_4 = thyroxine; T_3 = triiodothyronine; TSH = thyroid-stimulating hormone.

3.1 Thyroid-Stimulating Hormone (TSH)

TSH is a heterodimer with an alpha chain, which it shares with luteinizing hormone and follicle-stimulating hormone, and a beta chain, which confers specificity to the molecule. It is a glycoprotein with a carbohydrate moiety constituting about 20% of the molecule. The carbohydrate tail is essential for the bioactivity of the molecule.

Thyrotrophs normally constitute about 5% of pituitary cells but multiply severalfold in primary hypothyroidism because of a lack of negative feedback. Although both T_4 and T_3 act on the thyrotrophs, T_4 is processed preferentially (i.e., the thyrotrophs appear to prefer deiodinating T_4 in situ to preformed T_3). This negative feedback by the thyroid hormones overrides the stimulation by TRH; even small amounts of T_4 or T_3 will attenuate the TSH response to TRH.

TSH acts on thyroid cells by attaching itself to specific cell membrane receptors, which then elicits a rise in adenyl cyclase activity, and this in turn acts as the second messenger to cause thyroid hormone synthesis and release. Various pathological receptor antibodies may be present that will modulate the role of TSH on thyroid cells. Some of these antibodies mimic the effect of TSH by stimulating the cells, but lack the negative feedback mechanism to get turned off (as is the case in the etiology of Graves' disease). Others block the receptor site and cause hypothyroidism. The assay of these antibodies is useful, particularly in the diagnosis of Graves' disease, but especially in predicting intrauterine or neonatal hyper- or hypothyroidism.

The TSH response to TRH is influenced by numerous factors that mediate the frequently attenuated response seen in various physical and psychological diseases. TSH has a diurnal pattern with a small peak between 7 and 11 P.M. and a nadir at around 11 A.M. The significance of this is unclear, but in certain species (e.g., rats) this is more marked.

3.2 Thyrotropin-Releasing Hormone (TRH)

TRH is a tripeptide that is widely distributed in the central nervous system. Hypothalamic TRH stimulates the synthesis and release of both TSH and prolactin. Under certain circumstances, it also stimulates the release (and possibly the synthesis) of other pituitary hormones such as growth hormone in most acromegalic individuals. This may be an atavistic action because TRH normally regulates growth hormone secretion in birds.

TRH secretion is modulated by various neurotransmitters, as well as by thyroid hormones that have recently been shown to reduce TRH gene expression. No convincing evidence of TSH feedback on TRH has been published. TRH uses calcium rather than adenyl cyclase as its second messenger. As a result, certain drugs that modulate calcium channels may also alter the TSH response to TRH. The effect of TRH on prolactin is completely divorced from its effect on TSH. However, the hyperprolactinemia at times found in primary hypothyroidism is probably caused by TRH elevation in response to lack of negative feedback. Finally, TRH in other parts of the brain and spinal cord is probably an important neurotransmitter or neuromodulator. Large amounts of TRH have been shown to limit damage in experimental spinal injuries and have also resulted in improvement in patients with amyotrophic lateral sclerosis.

3.3 Autonomous Thyroid Secretion

The thyroid gland secretes low amounts of hormone even when TSH is apparently absent. Thyroid cell replication has also been considered to be regulated in part, at least, by local growth factors.

4. THYROID FUNCTION TESTS

The accurate measurement of thyroid hormone levels in the blood is complicated by the fact that there are several binding proteins that may be altered by a variety of drugs and disease states in a rather nonspecific way (Table 4–3). Only the free, unbound hormones are physiologically active, and they constitute 0.04% of total T_4 and 0.5% of total T_3. In the discussion that follows, we consider the most common thyroid function tests.

4.1 Thyroxine (T_4)

In view of the frequency of binding protein changes, measuring just the serum T_4 has a large margin of diagnostic error. To derive the physiologically active, free fraction of T_4, it is necessary to either measure simultaneously the T_3 resin uptake (T_3RU), which is inversely proportional to the unoccupied building sites on the TBG molecule, or to measure the FT_4 directly by dialysis (which is laborious) or by other appropriate methods, each having its own drawbacks. These methods offer, in our opinion, no real advantage over the calculated free thyroxine index (FT_4I), but are increasingly in vogue.

4.2 Triiodothyronine (T_3)

T_3 is also affected by binding protein alterations, albeit to a somewhat lesser degree than is T_4. If dialysis of the sample or use of one of the other methods to estimate the free-hormone fraction is not desired,

Table 4–3. Conditions influencing thyroxine-binding globulin levels

Increase	Decrease
Neonates	Androgens
Estrogens (including pregnancy)	Glucocorticoids
Hepatitis	Cirrhosis
Familial	Nephrotic syndrome
Porphyria	Familial asparaginase deficiency
Perphenazine	

the free triiodothyronine index (FT$_3$I) can be derived from the formula

$$T_3 \times T_3RU = FT_3I$$

which correlates well with direct measurement. (The same formula allows the calculation of the FT$_4$I.)

4.3   Reverse Triiodothyronine (rT$_3$)

In certain stress conditions, physical or psychological, the proportions of T$_3$ and rT$_3$ change as a result of either altered deiodination of T$_4$ or clearance of T$_3$, rT$_3$, or both. The concentrations of these two T$_4$ metabolites usually have a reciprocal relationship to one another (i.e., when the T$_3$ level is low the rT$_3$ level tends to be elevated). It is rarely clinically useful to measure rT$_3$.

4.4   Thyroid-Stimulating Hormone (TSH)

The serum TSH is the most accurate measure of primary hypothyroidism and will normally be elevated even when the T$_4$ and T$_3$ levels are still normal. There is an inverse relationship between these thyroid hormones and TSH levels in both the pathological and euthyroid range. TSH measures may be influenced by a diurnal rhythm, but are not affected by ambient temperature in adults.

With the advent of very sensitive assays of TSH (sTSHs), levels as low as 0.01 U/L can be measured. sTSHs have been touted as the ideal screening tests for both hypo- and hyperthyroidism. However, up to 15% of nonhyperthyroid patients have low levels, especially those in a hospital setting. Some commercial assays lack specificity, which makes proper interpretation at the lower end difficult. The value of the TSH assays lies in the diagnosis of early primary hypothyroidism, in confirming hyperthyroidism, in titrating the optimal replacement therapy of T$_4$, and in testing pituitary responsiveness to TRH.

4.5   TRH-TSH Test

As can be seen in Figure 4–2, various factors may influence the TSH response to TRH. Thus in a variety of physical and psychological stress conditions, the response is blunted, probably principally due to modulation by adrenergic neurotransmitters and hypercortisolemia, but also due to other factors. With the advent of the sTSHs, the TRH test is largely obviated, as a low TSH level usually denotes that a hypo-response to TRH will be found, but this is not always the case.

4.6   Radioiodine Uptake (RIU)

The radioiodine uptake (RIU) test is useful in differentiating hyper-thyroxinemia due to Graves' disease from subacute thyroiditis or io-dine or thyroid hormone ingestion. Tables 4–4 and 4–5 detail changes in RIU in different conditions.

5.   DIAGNOSIS OF THYROID DYSFUNCTIONAL STATES

5.1   Hyperthyroidism

Table 4–4 lists the common causes of hyperthyroidism and the tests that will help differentiate them. In elderly patients, the diagnosis is frequently difficult, as an apathetic presentation is the rule (see Chap-ter 5). In addition, there may be other associated illnesses (e.g., heart failure) that may depress the T_3 level and thus give a picture of T_4-toxicosis. Iodine-containing medications such as amiodarone may precipitate either hyper- or hypothyroidism, and over-the-counter kelp or other iodine-containing compounds may do the same.

   The frequently seen transient hyperthyroxinemia in acute psychi-atric conditions can at times be difficult to distinguish from Graves' disease. It is a common phenomenon affecting up to 25% of patients. Both T_4 and T_3 may be elevated, although often there is only T_4 eleva-tion. In a recent study (44) using an sTSH assay, 17% of subjects also had an elevated TSH; only 1% had a suppressed TSH. This normal or elevated TSH in this condition is the clue to a correct diagnosis. The underlying cause is likely a suprahypothalamic stimulus to increased TRH and TSH secretion. The prevalence of this condition in non-psychiatric patients has not been established, but it may be more com-mon than is presently appreciated.

5.2   Hypothyroidism

Table 4–5 lists the common causes of hypothyroidism and their bio-chemical diagnostic evaluation. Postpartum thyroiditis may present

Table 4–4. Diagnostic tests in hyperthyroidism

	FT$_4$I	FT$_3$I	TSH	RIU	TG
Graves' disease	Increase	Increase	Decrease	Increase	Nondiagnostic
Silent subacute thyroiditis	Increase	Increase or normal	Decrease	Decrease	Nondiagnostic
Postpartum thyroiditis	Increase	Increase or normal	Decrease	Decrease	Nondiagnostic
de Quervain's thyroiditis	Increase	Increase or normal	Decrease	Decrease	Nondiagnostic
Iodine induced	Increase	Increase	Decrease	0	Nondiagnostic
Hydatidiform mole	Increase	Increase	Decrease	Increase	Nondiagnostic
Thyroxine overdose	Increase	Increase	Decrease	0	Decrease
Triiodothyronine overdose	Decrease	Increase	Decrease	0	Decrease
Acute psychiatric states	Increase	Normal	Decrease or Normal	Decrease or Normal	Nondiagnostic

Note. FT$_4$I = free thyroxine index; FT$_3$I = free triiodothyronine index; TSH = thyroid-stimulating hormone; RIU = radioiodine uptake; TG = serum thyroglobulin.

Table 4–5. Diagnostic tests in hypothyroidism

	TSH	FT$_4$	RIU	MAb
Hashimoto's thyroiditis	Increase	Decrease or low normal	Increase, decrease, or normal	Increase
Postthyroidectomy	Increase	Decrease or low normal	Decrease or normal	Variable
Post-^{131}I treatment	Increase	Decrease or low normal	Decrease or normal	Variable
Subacute thyroiditis (late phase)	Increase	Decrease or low normal	Low normal	Variable
Postpartum thyroiditis	Increase	Decrease or low normal	Low normal	Variable
Iodine ingestion	Increase	Decrease or low normal	0	Variable
Lithium	Increase	Decrease or low normal	Decrease or normal	Variable
Hypopituitarism	Increase	Decrease or low normal	Decrease or normal	0

Note. TSH = thyroid-stimulating hormone; FT$_4$ = free thyroxine; RIU = radioiodine uptake; MAb = Antimicrosomal antibodies (antiperoxidase).

with hypothyroidism without going through a phase of hyperthyroidism and may not remit. Even for patients in whom it remits (usually those with hyperthyroidism), the thyroiditis tends to recur after subsequent deliveries, but it does not appear to correlate with postpartum depression. Mild TSH elevation with normal thyroid hormone levels has been termed *mild, subclinical,* or *compensated* hypothyroidism. TSH levels usually vary from 4 to 20 U/L. The question is when to treat these patients. Those with a sizable goiter, documented progressive TSH elevation, or an FT_4I toward the lower end of normal should be given the benefit of T_4 treatment. Those whose TSH and microsomal antibodies are elevated have a 5% per annum chance of becoming overtly hypothyroid.

The upper limit of normal for TSH may be a little higher for older people, and there is little point in treating this group when the TSH elevation is limited. Isolated secondary hypothyroidism due to pituitary dysfunction is very unusual, and there are often other clinical and biochemical markers implicating other pituitary hormones as well.

5.3 Sick Euthyroid Syndrome

Acute or chronic illness can lead to what has been termed the *sick euthyroid syndrome,* which may mimic either hypo- or hyperthyroidism. The hallmark of this syndrome is the finding of low serum T_3 and FT_3I levels. Patients with the syndrome can be divided into two groups. Patients in the first group have a variety of moderately severe illnesses with a low T_3 level and usually low-normal TSH levels. They clearly require no treatment and their tests return to normal pari passu with their improvement from the underlying illness. They may have a raised rT_3 level, largely due to decreased clearance as a result of decreased 5' deiodinase activity. Patients in the second group have more serious illness. In such patients, both T_3 and T_4 levels are decreased, in part due to impaired hormone binding caused by unknown mechanisms. This decreased binding leads to an increased metabolic clearance. The rT_3 is elevated, and the TSH is usually normal or slightly elevated. The TRH test is unhelpful because the response is impaired in severe illness. An appropriately elevated cortisol level will virtually rule out hypopituitarism because selective TSH deficiency or nonfamilial TRH deficiency is very rare. Attempts at treating sick euthyroid syndrome patients with T_3 or T_4 are usually not successful. The prognosis is usually very poor in patients showing both low T_3 and T_4 levels.

6. CONCLUSIONS

In this chapter, we have attempted to present an overview of the regulation of thyroid function in normal and abnormal conditions. We have also tried to outline a rational approach to testing thyroid function. There is increasing evidence that thyroid hormones and their regulating peptides play an important, if subtle, role on brain function outside the diagnostic constraints of clinical hyper- or hypothyroidism. The recent advances showing the characterization and study of different thyroid receptors in neurons will, we hope, shed further light on the thyroid-psychiatry interface.

REFERENCES

1. Reus V: Behavioural disturbances associated with endocrine disorders. Annu Rev Med 37:205–214, 1986
2. Joffe RT, Roy-Byrne PP, Uhde TW, et al: The thyroid and affective illness: a reappraisal. Biol Psychiatry 19:1685–1691, 1984
3. Alvino CG, Tasso V, Polistina C, et al: The segregation into microsomal vesicles and core glycosylation in vitro of a 300-K Da rat thyroglobulin subunit. Eur J Biochem 125:15–19, 1982
4. Monaco F, Salvatore G, Robbins J: The site of sialic acid incorporation into thyroglobulin in the thyroid gland. J Biol Chem 250:1595–1599, 1975
5. Eggo MC, Burrow GN: Glycosylation of thyroglobulin: its role in secretion, iodination and stability. Endocrinology 113:1655–1663, 1983
6. Vagenakis AG, Downs P, Braverman LE, et al: Control of thyroid hormone secretion in normal subjects receiving iodides. J Clin Invest 52:528–532, 1973
7. Galton VA: Thyroid hormone action in amphibian metamorphosis, in Molecular Basis of Thyroid Hormone Action. Edited by Oppenheimer JH, Samuels HH. New York, Academic Press, 1983, pp 445–483
8. Morreale de Escobar G, Calvo R, Obregon MJ, et al: Contribution of maternal thyroxine to fetal thyroxine pools in normal rats near term. Endocrinology 126:2765–2767, 1990

9. Freake HC, Oppenheimer JH: Stimulation of MRNA-S14 and lipogenesis in brown fat by hypothyroidism, cold exposure and cafeteria feeding: evidence supporting a general role for S14 in lipogenesis and lipogenesis in the maintenance of thermoregulation. Proc Natl Acad Sci U S A 34:3070–3074, 1987

10. Oppenheimer JH: Tissue and cellular effects of thyroid hormones and their mechanism of action, in Thyroid Function and Disease. Edited by Burrows GN, Oppenheimer JH, Volpe R. Philadelphia, PA, WB Saunders, 1989, pp 95–97

11. Ichikawa K, Hashizume K, Mivamoto T, et al: Differences in nuclear thyroid hormone receptors among species. Gen Comp Endocrinol 74:68–76, 1989

12. Gullo D, Sinha A, Bashir A, et al: Differences in nuclear triiodothyronine binding in rat brain cells suggest phylogenetic specialization of neuronal functions. Endocrinology 120:2398–2403, 1987

13. Sata AT, Imura E, Murata A, et al: Thyroid hormone: catecholamine interrelationship during cold acclimation in rats: compensatory role of catecholamine for altered thyroid states. Acta Endocrinol (Copenh) 113:536–542, 1986

14. Bilezikian JP, Loeb JN: The influence of hyperthyroidism and hypothyroidism on alpha-and beta-adrenergic receptor systems and adrenergic responsiveness. Endocr Rev 4:378–388, 1983

15. Rioux F, Berkowitz BA: Role of the thyroid gland in the development and maintenance of spontaneous hypertension in rats. Circ Res 40:306–312, 1977

16. Gustafson TA, Markham BE, Morkin E: Effects of thyroid hormone on alpha-actin and myosin heavy chain gene expression in cardiac and skeletal muscles of rate: measurement of mRNA content using synthetic oligonucleotide probes. Circ Res 59:194–201, 1986

17. Pontecorvi A, Lakshmanan M, Robbina J: Intracellular transport of 3.5.3′-tri-iodo-L-thyronine in rat skeletal myoblast. Endocrinology 121:2145–2152, 1987

18. Cheng SY, Maxfield FR, Robins J, et al: Receptor mediated uptake of 3,3′,5-tri-iodothyronine by cultured fibroblasts. Proc Natl Acad Sci U S A 77:3425–3426, 1980

19. Freake HC, Mooradian AD, Schwartz HL, et al: Stereospecific transport of triiodothyronine to cytoplasm and nucleus in GHI cells. Mol Cell Endocrinol 44:25–35, 1986

20. DeGroot LJ, Nakai A, Sakurai A, et al: The molecular basis of thyroid hormone action (review). J Endocrinol Invest 12:843–861, 1989

21. Sterling K: Thyroid hormone action at the cell level. N Engl J Med 300:117–123, 1979

22. Davis PJ, Blas SD: In vitro stimulation of human red blood cell Ca(2+)-ATPase by thyroid hormone. Biochem Biophys Res Commun 99:1073–1080, 1981

23. Oppenheimer JH, Schwartz HL, Mariash DN, et al: Advances in our understanding of thyroid hormone action at the cellular level (review). Endocr Rev 8:298–308, 1987

24. Oppenheimer JH: The nuclear receptor-triiodothyronine complex: relationship to thyroid hormone distribution, metabolism and biological action, in Molecular Basis of Thyroid Hormone Action. Edited by Oppenheimer JH, Samuels HH. New York, Academic Press, 1983, pp 1–35

25. Samuels HH: Identification and characterization of thyroid hormone receptors and action using cell culture techniques, in Molecular Basis of Thyroid Hormone Action. Edited by Oppenheimer JH, Samuels HH. New York, Academic Press, 1983, pp 36–66

26. DeGroot LJ, Refetoff S, Strausser JL, et al: Nuclear triiodothyronine binding protein: partial characterization and binding to chromatin. Proc Natl Acad Sci U S A 71:4042–4046, 1974

27. Latham KR, Ring JC, Baxter JD: Solubilized nuclear "receptors" for thyroid hormones: physical properties and binding properties, evidence for multiple forms. J Biol Chem 251:7388–7397, 1976

28. Pascual A, Casanova J, Samuels HH: Photoaffinity labelling of thyroid hormone nuclear receptors in intact cells. J Biol Chem 257:9640–9647, 1982

29. David-Inouye Y, Somack R, Nordeen SK, et al: Photoaffinity labelling of the rat liver nuclear thyroid hormone receptor with 125I triiodothyronine. Endocrinology 111:1758–1760, 1982

30. Ichikawa K, DeGroot LJ: Purification and characterization of rat liver nuclear thyroid hormone receptors. Proc Natl Acad Sci U S A 84:3420–3424, 1987

31. Van Der Walt B, Nikodem JM, Cahnmann HJ: Use of underivatized thyroid hormones for photoaffinity labelling of binding proteins. Proc Natl Acad Sci U S A 79:3508–3512, 1982

32. Hollenberg SM, Weinberger C, Ong E, et al: Primary structure and expression of a functional human glucocorticoid receptor cDNA. Nature 315:635–641, 1985

33. Weinberger C, Hollenberg S, Rosenfeld M, et al: Domain structure of human glucocorticoid receptor and its relationship to the V-*erb* A oncogene product. Nature 318:670–672, 1985

34. Debuire B, Henry C, Bernissa M, et al: Sequencing the *erb* A gene of avian erythroblastosis virus reveals a new type of oncogene. Science 224:1456–1459, 1984

35. Weinberger C, Thompson CC, Ong ES, et al: The C-*erb*-A gene encodes a thyroid hormone receptor. Nature 324:18–31,641–646, 1986

36. Sap J, Munez A, Damm K, et al: The C-*erb*-A protein is a high-affinity receptor for thyroid hormone. Nature (London) 324:635–640, 1986

37. Mitsuhashi T, Tennyson GE, Nikodem VM: Alternative splicing generates messages encoding rat c-*erb*-A proteins that do not bind thyroid hormone. Proc Natl Acad Sci U S A 85:5804–5808, 1988

38. Thompson CC, Weinberger C, Lebo R, et al: Identification of a novel thyroid hormone receptor expressed in the mammalian central nervous system. Science 237:1610–1614, 1987

39. Bradley DJ, Young WS III, Weinberger C: Differential expression of alpha and beta thyroid hormone receptor genes in rat brain and pituitary. Proc Natl Acad Sci U S A 86:7250–7254, 1989

40. Hodin RA, Lazar MA, Chin WW: Differential and tissue-specific regulation of the multiple rat C-*erb* A messenger RNA species by thyroid hormone. J Clin Invest 95:101–105, 1990

41. Evans RM: The steroid and thyroid hormone receptor superfamily. Science 240:889–895, 1988

42. Robertson M: Towards a biochemistry of morphogenesis (review). Nature 330:420–421, 1988

43. Sapolsky RM: Glucocorticoid toxicity in the hippocampus: reversal by supplementation with brain fuels. J Neurol Sci 6:2240–2244, 1986

44. Chopra IJ, Solomon DH, Huang TS: Serum thyrotropin in hospitalized psychiatric patients: evidence for hyperthyrotropinemia as measured by an ultrasensitive thyrotropin assay. Metabolism 39:538–543, 1990

PART II

Clinical Principles

Chapter 5

Psychiatric Aspects
of Thyroid Disease

Victor I. Reus, M.D.

CONTENTS

1. INTRODUCTION

Underdiagnosis of medical illness in psychiatric patients remains a serious problem in health care. Several recent controlled studies have indicated that endocrine disorders, in general, and thyroid diseases, in particular, are the most frequent medical conditions causing or exacerbating behavioral symptomatology (1). In individuals lacking a family or personal psychiatric history, the appearance of behavioral change in association with gross perturbations in thyroid hormone level and the disappearance of same with normalization in function allows a causal relationship to be hypothesized. More often, however, psychiatric symptoms antedate or postdate clinical thyroid pathology or occur in association with very subtle changes in thyroid economy. When "nonclinical" thyroid abnormalities occur in patients with primary psychiatric diagnoses, the question arises as to whether these changes are simply nonspecific signs of alteration in central neurotransmitter systems or represent a primary defect in thyroid regulation (2–4). The inability to measure thyroid hormone activity in the central nervous system (CNS) in vivo and the absence of an adequate physiological indicator of thyroid hormone effect in the periphery have hampered understanding of the mechanisms through which perturbations in thyroid function affect behavior. Interpretation of the available literature is further confounded by difficulties in separating behavioral changes associated with the natural course of the disease from those induced iatrogenically by medical or surgical intervention.

In the sections that follow, I review the psychiatric pathology observed in thyroid disease. In general, such alterations are classified according to traditional conceptions of the gross metabolic state of the individual (i.e., either hyper- or hypothyroid) and not specifically to the underlying etiology. Because in recent years most thyroid disease has been found to have an autoimmune etiology, associated with some degree of genetic vulnerability (5,6), specific attention is paid to those reports in which the underlying endocrine pathology is more clearly described. Recognition that patients with autoimmune disease may have individually unique populations of aberrant antibodies, directed at separate target sites, and that dysregulation in components of immune response may itself have behavioral consequence, makes it possible that behavioral pathology occurs in autoimmune thyroid disease even in the "euthyroid" state (7,8).

2. HYPERTHYROIDISM

Behavioral symptomatology has been recognized as a cardinal manifestation of hyperthyroid states since Caleb Parry's original report in 1786 (cited in 9). Parry identified fear as a precipitating cause and noted that patients with hyperthyroidism had "a propensity to morbid determinations." These observations were echoed by Graves a decade later in a lecture linking alterations in thyroid function and volume to the diagnosis of globus hystericus in women (10). The development of the discipline of psychosomatic medicine in the early 1900s brought with it the belief that in many cases the endocrinologic perturbation was brought on by extreme stress. In perhaps the most extensive series, Bram in 1927 found a clear history of "psychic traumas as an exciting cause" in 85% of 3,343 cases of exophthalmic goiter (cited in 11). Modern anecdotal reports also exist (12, 13), but systematic and controlled longitudinal studies are lacking. It has not been possible thus far to construct an animal model in which hyperthyroidism is produced by stress, and possible pathophysiological mechanisms through which emotional stimuli might precipitate prolonged endocrine alteration remain highly speculative. In addition, hyperthyroid states are not usually found to be associated with elevations in pituitary release of thyroid-stimulating hormone (TSH), as had originally been believed (14–16).

Hyperthyroid patients frequently complain of weakness, fatigue, emotional lability, irritability, restlessness, and sleep disturbance, in addition to overt somatic symptoms (17–20). Excessive vigilance and hyperreactivity may also be observed. Cognitive complaints of decreased attention span and intellectual impairment are not uncommon and have been objectively documented (21–23). Overall, the presenting symptomatology of the organic affective disorder associated with hyperthyroidism is most suggestive of an agitated depression. In some cases, particularly in older patients, an "apathetic" rather than agitated presentation may be paramount. Such symptoms are usually secondary to severe thyrotoxic-induced myopathy and weight loss and can be found in patients who otherwise lack the typical clinical features of thyrotoxicosis (with the exception of tachycardia). Because apathetic hyperthyroidism may result in significant morbidity, including coma and death, it is important to investigate thyroid function in elderly patients who present with dementia, delirium, or significant psychomotor retardation. Thus far, biological markers such as response to the dexamethasone suppression test and sleep electroencephalogram (EEG) seem to offer little help in differential diagnosis (24).

Thyroid storm, though increasingly rare, signifies an acute medical emergency in which the usual signs and symptoms of thyrotoxicosis are exacerbated, usually by concurrent infection or trauma. Psychotic reactions and frank delirium are frequently found, in association with hyperpyrexia, extreme agitation, and tachycardia. There are no pathognomonic attributes of the psychotic state that may be associated with thyroid storm or less severe hyperthyroid states, but paranoid features have been frequently recorded (10).

Pharmacological treatment of the thought and mood impairments associated with hyperthyroid states remains controversial. It is generally agreed that tricyclic antidepressants are contraindicated and increase the risk of CNS toxicity (25). In many patients, the behavioral symptomatology is closely linked to circulating thyroid hormone levels and abates when the hyperthyroid state is treated with either radioactive or surgical ablative therapy or propylthiouracil (25,26). Neuroleptics are sometimes required in reduced dosage, although haloperidol, in particular, should be avoided on the basis of a series of case reports documenting enhanced neurotoxicity and possible precipitation of thyroid storm (27–29). Lithium is also problematic in such cases and may result in progression of exophthalmos. Adjunctive usage of β-blockers, such as propranolol, is sometimes found helpful in decreasing symptoms of anxiety and agitation.

Interestingly, improvement in these thought and mood impairments can occur without associated change in thyroid hormone level. One recent longitudinal study (30) investigating propranolol response in Graves' disease found improvement in the symptoms of depression, as well as anxiety, but no significant beneficial effect on alterations in memory or attention after 2 weeks of treatment. Iatrogenic thyrotoxicosis associated with pharmacological thyroid hormone treatment usually resolves with decrease or discontinuation of the supplemental hormonal treatment (31). In some cases, however, thyrotoxicosis is associated with a vitamin B_{12} deficiency, necessitating concomitant diagnosis and treatment for psychiatric symptomatology (32). A positive response to electroconvulsive therapy (ECT) has also been reported anecdotally, with thyroid hormone indices normalizing and anxious depressive symptomatology resolving after three ECT treatments (33).

Difficulties in diagnosis and treatment may arise when hyperthyroidism occurs in the context of psychoactive drug dependence. In one reported case (34), hyperthyroidism was overlooked because of attribution of the behavioral disturbance to an associated sedative withdrawal and a diagnosis of possible bipolar disorder. In addition to complicating diagnoses, it has been suggested that cocaine usage itself can precipitate thyroid toxicity, a phenomenon that has also been reported for amphetamine (35,36).

Unusual manifestations of thyrotoxicosis may occur (37). One such example involved a 48-year-old woman who presented with anorexia nervosa secondary to a refusal of treatment for thyrotoxicosis in an attempt to keep her weight low (38). In general, it should be recognized that any singular somatic correlate of the hyperthyroid state may erroneously be interpreted as a sign or symptom of a primary psychiatric disorder or in some way complicate the assessment or treatment of a preexisting psychiatric condition. This is particularly true for movement disorders. Hyperthyroid chorea, a rare presentation of thyrotoxicosis, has been mistaken as a psychiatric illness (39) and has confounded recognition of an underlying tardive dyskinesia (40).

The relationship of thyroid disease to "organic anxiety syndrome" is of some interest. Although generalized anxiety is perhaps most common, formal agoraphobia, social phobia, and classic panic attacks have been reported in patients with thyrotoxicosis (23, 41–44). In subjects presenting with a primary diagnosis of panic disorder, however, thyroid dysfunction is rarely found, although there is some evidence of a higher prevalence of thyroid illness in personal and family history (45). An association is theoretically more likely in patients with documented mitral valve prolapse, given its markedly increased independent occurrence in both panic and autoimmune thyroid disorders (46).

Hyperthyroidism sometimes presents coincidently with bipolar disorder. Although it is possible that these two relatively common illnesses occur together by chance, in certain cases recurrent episodes of mania clearly coincide with those of hyperthyroidism (47). Mania has also been observed as a concomitant of rapid-replacement therapy in hypothyroid patients (48). In the retrospective reviews and case reports that have appeared, women and patients with a personal or family history of mental disorder seem to be at increased risk, the mania usually occurring 4–7 days after aggressive initiation of thyroid hormone treatment. In most cases the manic symptomatology is transient, lasting 1–2 weeks and resolving without sequelae.

The means by which thyroid hormone excess might result in the behavioral pathology noted remains speculative. Although many peripheral signs of thyrotoxicosis are consistent with noradrenergic hyperfunction and are ameliorated by β-adrenergic antagonists, thyrotoxicosis is generally associated with increased β-adrenergic receptor binding, increased α_2-adrenergic receptor binding, and decreased norepinephrine turnover (49–51). Investigators using experimental models of hyperthyroidism achieved through exogenous hormone administration have also reported decreased desipramine binding (51). Alternative links to the neurochemistry of mood are possible, however, given findings that thyroid hormones inhibit γ-aminobutyric acid (GABA) uptake, facilitating GABAergic neurotransmission and theoretically affecting other neurotransmitter systems that may be interrelated, such as that involving dopamine (52). One problem in the interpretation of such findings and in postulating an association to individual psychiatric symptoms is that thyroid hormone effects on receptor complexes are clearly dependent on the target tissue studied. Thus altered thyroid status may produce an increase, a decrease, or no change in receptor number, depending on the animal model and organ studied (53). It is also clear that thyroid hormone affects postreceptor second messenger activity.

An alternative conception of the way in which thyroid disease and noradrenergic function are linked derives from evidence that norepinephrine serves as a neurotransmitter that regulates immune responsiveness. Either through acting directly on lymphocyte or macrophage receptors or by modulating the release of lymphokine or other regulatory hormones or through indirect mechanisms, changes in norepinephrine transmission clearly alter immune responsiveness and, in turn, are affected by it (54). It is possible that such feedback loops underlie episodic recurrences in autoimmune thyroid disease and the behavioral symptomatology observed.

3. THYROID NODULES AND THYROIDECTOMY

Thyroid nodules are quite common, occurring in 4%–7% of the general population (55). Transformation into malignancy is rare, and the prognosis of occult carcinoma is relatively benign (56). In some individuals with "hot" nodules (i.e., increased radioactive uptake relative to surrounding tissue), behavioral symptomatology has been observed even in the face of euthyroidism (57). Several early reports (58,59) found an association between thyroid "hot spots" and social change and postulated that thyrotoxicosis could result from conditions of prolonged stress. When hyperthyroidism occurs secondary to an adenoma, the clinical symptomatology is indistinguishable from that reported for individuals having a clearer autoimmune etiology. In one case (60) reported in the endocrinology literature, a 36-year-old woman with nodular goiter, "nervousness," and tachycardia became clinically euthyroid and asymptomatic once domestic problems resolved. Classical manic symptoms may appear when the hyperthyroid state is terminated precipitously with radioactive-iodine treatment.

Partial or total removal of the thyroid gland is sometimes used therapeutically in treatment of thyrotoxicosis, nontoxic goiter, and malignancy. Transient hyperthyroidism, sustained hypothyroidism, and hypocalcemia are possible adverse sequelae of surgical intervention and possible concomitant damage to the parathyroid gland. Thyroidectomy has, however, been used beneficially in the treatment of severe Hashimoto's thyroiditis, resulting in the disappearance of antithyroid autoantibodies (61). Numerous reports (62–65) in the literature detail adverse behavioral responses to thyroidectomy, although most of these do not provide sufficient endocrine data to evaluate whether replacement therapy was sufficient or whether parathyroid insufficiency was involved. The clinical picture is generally mixed, with confusion, thought disorder, and variations in mood ranging from depression to elation. ECT, in addition to hormonal replacement, is of little therapeutic benefit. Alternatively, some individuals who present with behavioral disturbance prior to thyroidectomy exhibit an improved course postsurgery.

Investigations of possibly different responses or course in patients undergoing total, as opposed to partial, thyroidectomy have been inconclusive, and psychiatric morbidity can occur in the absence of hypocalcemia or hypoparathyroidism. In one particularly well-documented case (66), rapid-cycling affective illness developed after subtotal thyroidectomy and responded only partially to lithium carbonate treatment. Treatment with thyroxine (T_4), however, decreased both the frequency and amplitude of the mood cycling, eventually resulting in a normalization of mental status. Abnormal, but regular, cycles in behavior and metabolism can be produced in rats undergoing partial radiothyroidectomy (67). Lithium reverses these effects, lengthening the free-running circadian periods (68), whereas triiodothyronine (T_3) or T_4 restitution has been shown to counteract thyroidectomy-induced decrease in dopamine and increase in norepinephrine level and utilization in the hypothalamus (69).

4. PRECLINICAL HYPERTHYROIDISM

The term *preclinical hyperthyroidism* has been used operationally to desig-
nate patients without nodular goiter who are clinically euthyroid, show
normal laboratory values of T_4 and T_3, and have no radiological evidence
for an autonomous adenoma, despite a relatively blunted or absent TSH
response to thyrotropin-releasing hormone (TRH) infusion. Such a con-
stellation of signs has been described following the treatment of Graves'
disease, in early stages of recurrent hyperthyroidism, and in depressed
individuals with no other observable thyroid pathology (70). These metabolic characteristics may have some physiological significance, but investigators of one study (71) were unable to find differences in systolic time
intervals, sex hormone–binding globulin, and ankle reflex time between
such patients and a group of healthy control subjects. Interestingly, patients showing this endocrine profile have behavioral and somatic complaints quite similar to those with definite hyperthyroidism; symptoms of
anxiety, malaise, and irritability occur in association with decreased attention and concentration, palpitations, tremor, and tachycardia (72).

5. EUTHYROID HYPERTHYROXINEMIA

Isolated hyperthyroxinemia is a frequent biochemical finding in medical
patients with varying diagnosis (73,74). In the absence of thyroid disease,
the hypermetabolic state observed may clinically mimic hyperthyroidism,
but is usually of no specific clinical consequence. In general, the condition
is associated with impairments in peripheral conversion of T_4 to T_3 and
changes in metabolism of T_4 (the elevation in T_4 being a compensatory
response to low circulating T_3 levels). However, it has been demonstrated
that some patients presenting with transient hyperthyroidism have chronic lymphocytic thyroiditis, a condition that, in the absence of goiter and
neck pain, has been termed *painless thyroiditis* or *hyperthyroiditis* (74,75).
Euthyroid familial hyperthyroxinemia has also been reported to be caused
by genetic alterations in thyroid hormone–binding proteins (76,77).

In several of the cases in the literature the presenting symptomatology
is predominantly behavioral, with anxiety and fatigue most common in
the brief descriptions available (76). Although both thyrotoxic and euthyroid hyperthyroxinemia are not usually associated with increased TSH secretion, inappropriate release of thyrotropin occurs (78). In one such case,

inappropriate TSH secretion with abnormal in vitro sensitivity to dopamine was found in a male schizophrenic patient, suggesting a possible linkage between the two syndromes in this patient.

Transient hyperthyroxinemia exists in patients with acute psychiatric disorders, being characterized by an elevation in free T_4 index that remits on follow-up evaluation in several weeks time. Serum T_3 is generally normal, but minor deviations are possible. Although several studies (79,80) have found elevations in serum T_4 levels in 15%–33% of acute psychiatric patients studied, more recent reports (81) have suggested a somewhat lower prevalence. The evanescent nature of the state makes true prevalence assessments problematic. One dramatic presentation, followed longitudinally, involved a 32-year-old woman who experienced 19 affective episodes and six hospital admissions within 34 months, the manic episodes always being associated with a hyperthyroxinemia that resolved as the psychosis cleared with pharmacological intervention (82).

Understanding of the role of elevations in free T_4 in the psychiatric population remains limited. It is possible that such individuals have an underlying abnormality in plasma membrane thyroid hormone transport or T_3 nuclear binding, resulting in a mild thyroid hormone resistance syndrome. Some authors have argued for transient TRH hypersecretion, but convincing biochemical data are lacking. Whether the various abnormalities represent a primary defect or an adaptive response is unclear. Whybrow and Prange (83) have suggested that compensatory elevations in thyroid hormone level are therapeutic in depression, beneficially increasing β-adrenergic activity in the face of low norepinephrine levels.

6. AUTOIMMUNE THYROIDITIS

In 1912 Hashimoto described chronic lymphocytic infiltration of the thyroid gland, a condition later found to be autoimmune in origin (84). The incidence of autoimmune thyroiditis has increased in recent decades, possibly secondary to viruses, dietary change, or other environmental stimuli, to the point where it is now the most frequent thyroid disorder in the general population. The disease is six- to eightfold more prevalent in women than in men, and is most likely to occur between the ages of 30 and 50.

From a functional perspective, autoimmune thyroiditis presents with either hyperthyroidism or hypothyroidism, and assumes a course that either waxes or wanes or is chronically progressive toward diminished thyroid functioning as chronic inflammation results in fibrosis and destruction of the thyroid follicles (5). The progression to hypothyroidism has been graded by Evered et al. (85) on a continuum, the earliest perturbation being defined by an augmented TSH response to TRH infusion in the face of normal T_4 and TSH values.

From an endocrinologic perspective, individuals with autoimmune thyroiditis have been considered "symptomless," and most current recommendations call for suppressive treatment with thyroid hormones only if marked clinical complaint or goiter occurs. In select cases, however, psychiatric symptoms present in the absence of clinical or subclinical hypothyroidism. Depression, impairments in concentration, and irritability are most common, with mania and psychotic thought disorder also possible (86–88). Such patients seem resistant to traditional psychopharmacological treatment of their behavioral pathology, but in general respond rapidly to thyroid replacement therapy (89). Several, but not all, groups report a somewhat greater prevalence of antithyroid antibodies in psychiatric patients presenting with primary mood disorders (90,91). No specific relationship has been found with panic disorder (92).

Although controversy continues, it is quite clear that the presence of circulating autoantibodies in thyroid disease has considerable import in both diagnosis and prognosis, the functional and structural character of the gland itself being dependent on the integrated balance among them. Levels of thyroid hormones measured in the peripheral circulation provide only a statistical and crude relationship to metabolic activity, and any given target tissue may be functionally either hypo- or hyperthyroid in the context of "normal" levels of circulating thyroid hormones. Even if serum T_4 levels are normal, antimicrosomal antibody determination may be appropriate in the general screening of a population at risk because of evidence that it serves, together with functional evidence of subclinical hypothyroidism, as a good predictor of the development of formal hypothyroidism and allows a conceptual integration of signs and symptoms such as depression, fatigue, response to antidepressants, impaired cognition, and decreased libido (8). Presence of antithyroid antibodies does not in itself guarantee impairment in thyroid function; however, studies have shown 50%–70% of patients with symptomless autoimmune thyroiditis will have evidence of decreased thyroid reserve (93).

Postpartum autoimmune lymphocytic thyroiditis is a common disorder with a prevalence of 2%–11%, depending on the population studied (94–96). In most cases, the course of the syndrome involves a transient thyrotoxicosis that coincides with rising antithyroid antibody titers and a return to normal function several months after delivery. Many patients will become transiently hypothyroid, and a few will go on to develop chronic hypothyroidism. The existence of such changes has led some investigators to speculate a possible relationship to the behavioral syndromes of postpartum "blues" and postpartum depression or psychosis. Hamilton (97) and colleagues observed a decreased basal metabolic rate in patients hospitalized for postpartum psychiatric disorders, and found that thyroid replacement had a marked antidepressant effect in the majority of cases. In the endocrinologic literature, Amino and Miyai (94) reported three cases of psychosis in a sample of 28 women with postpartum thyroiditis, whereas Jansson et al. (95) found symptoms of anxiety and depression in some women at the time thyroid dysfunction was reported. Similar findings of "mild depression" or "nervousness" also exist (96,98). The presence of antibodies by itself does not clearly increase the risk of such symptomatology, but further controlled investigation is indicated (99, 100).

7. SUBCLINICAL HYPOTHYROIDISM

Subclinical hypothyroidism, defined operationally as an elevated resting level of TSH in the context of normal T_3 and T_4 levels, is present in about 5% of the general population, with a reported prevalence in women over age 60 of 15% (101–103). Gold et al. (104) and others (105,106) have published data linking subclinical hypothyroidism and depressive symptomatology, but whether this represents a chance or rare association remains open to opinion. Still others (107), studying a mixed patient and volunteer population, have enumerated a negative correlation between sensation seeking and higher levels of TSH. In the best controlled study to date, Cooper et al. (108) described common symptoms of malaise, involving principally decreased energy and lassitude, which responded to L-thyroxine therapy. Occult thyroid dysfunction has also been reported in refractory depression, the mood state responding to thyroid replacement (109–112). One cross-sectional study, however, which explored the relationship between subclinical hypothyroidism and depressive symptomatology in 16 nursing home residents, found no association between degree of elevation in TSH and psychological depressive symptomatology (113).

In some individuals, there is evidence that marginal hypothyroidism, if sustained for a long enough period, might produce irreversible cognitive dysfunction (114) and possibly alteration in ventricular volume (115). It is interesting to note in this regard that prior to the ability to measure TSH directly, paroxysmal slowing on EEG was reported in subclinical hypothyroidism (116).

Formal prevalence studies of subclinical hypothyroidism in the affective disorder population are rare. In the most comprehensive study, Gold et al. (117) assessed thyroid function in 250 consecutively admitted patients who complained of depression and/or loss of energy and noted that approximately 8% "had some degree of hypothyroidism"; 3.6% had elevation of basal TSH, and 4% were identified solely on the basis of an augmented TSH response to TRH. In succeeding papers, Extein et al. (118) noted comparable findings on prevalence, as have other research groups.

Winokur et al. (119), for example, observed an exaggerated TSH response in 9% of their depressed patients; Calabrese and Gulledge (120) noted an 8.3% rate of augmented TSH responses in 24 consecutive inpatients referred for treatment of depression. Hatotani et al. (121), using a somewhat more liberal standard of augmented response, chronicled a rate of approximately 14% in the general depressed population, a figure that rose to 20% if one limited the population to females. Targum et al. (122) published a comparable rate of approximately 15% in a study of unipolar endogenously depressed patients, and Calloway et al. (123) showed that 6 out of 68 patients with primary depression had an augmented response. Again, it should be noted that all of the patients found to have an augmented response were female. Finally, Kathol et al. (124) uncovered an exaggerated TSH response to TRH in 9 of 28 recovered depressed patients. Interpretation of these studies is complicated by an inconsistent documentation of prior lithium treatment (125–127).

It has been suggested that subclinical hypothyroidism either contributes to the expression of or is involved in affecting the course of rapid-cycling bipolar mood disorder. O'Shannick and Ellinwood (128) described two women with rapid-cycling bipolar disorder who had elevated levels of TSH and noted in a retrospective review of other women with parallel clinical and laboratory presentations. Similar observations have been made by

Cowdry et al. (129) and others (130,131). One potentially confounding aspect of these papers is that elevation in basal TSH may have been induced by prior lithium treatment. There is some initial evidence that pharmacological doses of thyroid hormone help to stabilize the mood dysfunction either alone or in combination with traditional mood-stabilizing medication (132,133). Somewhat confounding any clear understanding of the mechanisms involved, however, treatment response in the latter investigation was not dependent on previous thyroid status.

8. HYPOTHYROIDISM

Sir William Gull (134), in addressing the Clinical Society of London in 1873, became the first physician to comment specifically on the mental status of the hypothyroid patient, mentioning an apparent slowness in thought and affective instability and reflecting that "the nervous power is upon the whole lessened, and hence have arisen the changes in temper, and the attacks which have been described to me" (p. 183). In 1878, William Ord (135) put forth the concept of "myxedema," implying by this that the observed torpor and lassitude and "a tendency to slovenly attitude," were secondary to a "jelly-like swelling of the connective tissue," and a "overgrowth of the mucus-yielding cement by which the fibrils of the white element are held together" (p. 71). In its classic 1888 report on myxedema, the Clinical Society of London itself pointed out that 16 of 45 myxedematous patients carried a diagnosis of insanity, most exhibiting delusions and hallucinations. In the case reports and reviews that followed, "myxedema madness" encompassed a broad range of psychiatric presentation, from personality disturbance to frank psychosis. In certain circumstances, severe behavioral change developed in the absence of classical signs and symptoms of hypothyroidism, and although recovery from neuropsychiatric dysfunction was usually observed with proper diagnosis and treatment, it was by no means complete in all cases (136,137).

As many as 5%–15% of myxedematous patients may have signs of psychosis (138,139). Thyroid hormone treatment usually results in improvement within a week of treatment, but initial exacerbation is also possible. There is no significant difference in treatment effect between T_4 and T_3 when depression and anxiety are alleviated (140). A similar course and response has been reported for mania, which, paradoxically, may be the presenting behavioral state rather than depression (141–143).

Gross hypothyroidism is common in the general population, with a prevalence of 4.4% demonstrated among patients older than 60 years in the Framingham population. In a manner parallel to subclinical hypothyroidism, gross hypothyroidism serves as a risk factor in the development of rapid-cycling bipolar affective disorder. In a group of 24 patients with rapid-cycling bipolar affective disorder, 51% were classified as having grade I hypothyroidism, and an additional 41% had elevations in basal TSH (129). One hypothesis put forth at the conclusion of this investigation was that a relative central thyroid hormone deficit predisposes to rapid cycling, even in the presence of a normal serum L-T_4 level. Evidence for comparatively increased levels in reverse triiodothyronine (rT_3) in a population of individuals with unipolar depression has also been interpreted as possibly reflective of a "selective central hypothyroidism." Primary hypothalamic hypothyroidism is a rare disorder, but significant behavioral complaint is apparent in several cases reported in the literature (144–146).

The behavioral changes wrought by hypothyroidism theoretically involve a decreased responsivity of central β-adrenergic receptors, as postulated previously, but may derive from alterations in cerebral blood flow, oxygenation, or glucose usage, and, in some cases, subsequent neuronal damage (147–149). It is also possible that electrophysiological effects are of import. Hypothyroid states increase seizure activity, and cyclical relationships between thyroid function parameters and recurrent complex partial seizures have been demonstrated (150). Such findings would not be incompatible with current "kindling" conceptions of cycling in bipolar mood disorder.

9. THYROID EFFECTS ON BEHAVIORAL DEVELOPMENT

It is clear that gross disturbances in maternal thyroid function adversely affect development in the fetal central and peripheral nervous system, with sustained impairments in behavior the subsequent result. To date, the human studies that have been completed in regions where iodine deficiency is endemic indicate a fairly positive prognosis if replacement therapy is instituted promptly (151). Even in the absence of clinical cretinism in the child or gross abnormality in maternal thyroid state, however, subtle deficits in motor and cognitive performance may be observed (152).

To date, the developmental studies that have been completed focus almost entirely on intelligence, despite animal studies that would indicate that exploratory behavior, avoidance learning, and stress responsivity are particularly sensitive to thyroid status during critical periods of neuronal development (153). Perinatal hypothyroidism in these models has severe adverse consequences for sympathetic nervous system activity in maturation, affecting both tonic control and response during acute challenge (154). Adrenocortical stress response and development of regulatory hippocampal glucocorticoid receptors are also markedly influenced by thyroid hormone concentration during early postnatal life (155). Because fetal thyroid function may be affected by nonspecific factors such as smoking during pregnancy or maternal ethanol intake, as well as by diet and genetic factors, more sophisticated behavioral assessments of possible populations at risk are indicated (156,157).

10. CONCLUSIONS

Although considerations of mechanism must remain speculative, it is clear that thyroid diseases frequently present with psychiatric symptomatology (Table 5–1). Recognition of such features is important, not only for correct diagnosis, but also for early intervention in those presentations in which changes in mood and mentation antedate gross changes in thyroid function. Although no specific behavioral profile has been delineated, the predictability of behavioral change in thyroid disease supports the view that

Table 5–1.   Behavioral symptoms and syndromes associated with thyroid disease

Thyroid disease	Symptoms and syndromes
Hyperthyroidism	
Mild	Anxiety, emotional lability, irritability, vigilance, hyperactivity
Severe	Cognitive impairment, delusions/hallucinations, agitation, mania, paranoia
"Subclinical" hyperthyroidism	Anxiety, irritability, impaired concentration
"Apathetic" hyperthyroidism	Psychomotor retardation, delirium, dementia
Hypothyroidism	
Mild	Lethargy, mental sluggishness, depression
Severe	Delusions, hallucinations, paranoia, disorientation, agitated depression, rapid-cycling mood disorder
"Subclinical" hypothyroidism	Malaise, impaired memory, depression

such states may represent the best naturally occurring model for investigation of the biology of mood and mentation (158,159).

REFERENCES

1. Hall RCW, Gardner ER, Stickney SK, et al: Physical illness manifesting as psychiatric disease, II: analysis of a state hospital inpatient population. Arch Gen Psychiatry 37:989–995, 1980
2. Mason JW, Kennedy JL, Kosten TR, et al: Serum thyroxine levels in schizophrenia and affective disorder diagnostic subgroups. J Nerv Ment Dis 177:351–358, 1989
3. Southwick S, Mason JW, Giller EL, et al: Serum thyroxine change and clinical recovery in psychiatric inpatients. Biol Psychiatry 25:67–74, 1989
4. Tollefson G, Valentine R, Hoffmann N, et al: Thyroxine binding and TSH in recurrent depressive episodes. J Clin Psychiatry 46:267–272, 1985
5. Adams DD: Autoimmune mechanisms, in Autoimmune Endocrine Disease. Edited by Davies TF. New York, Wiley, 1983, pp 1–38
6. Tunbridge WMG: The epidemiology of hypothyroidism. Clinics in Endocrinology and Metabolism 8:21–27, 1979
7. Baker GHB: Invited review: psychological factors and immunity. J Psychosom Res 31:1–10, 1987
8. Reus VI, Freimer N: Antithyroid antibodies: behavioral significance, in Neuropsychopharmacology. Edited by Bunney WE Jr, Hippius H, Laakmann G, et al. Berlin, Germany, Springer-Verlag, 1990, pp 362–370
9. Davis AT: Psychotic states associated with disorders of thyroid function. Int J Psychiatry Med 19:47–56, 1989
10. Weiner H: Psychobiology and Human Disease. New York, Elsevier, 1977
11. Mason JW: A review of psychoendocrine research on the pituitary-thyroid system. Psychosom Med 30:666–681, 1968
12. Burch EA Jr, Messervy TW: Psychiatric symptoms in medical illness: hyperthyroidism revisited. Psychosomatics 19:71–75, 1978
13. Martin JB, Reichlin S: Endocrine response to stress and psychiatric disease, in Clinical Neuroendocrinology, 2nd Edition. Edited by Martin J, Reichlin S, Brown G. Philadelphia, PA, FA Davis, 1987, pp 669–694
14. Loosen PT: Hormones of the hypothalamic-pituitary-thyroid axis: a psychoneuroendocrine perspective. Pharmacopsychiatry 19:401–415, 1986
15. Wilson WH, Jefferson JW: Thyroid disease, behavior, and psychopharmacology. Psychosomatics 26:481–492, 1985
16. Zach J, Ackerman SH: Thyroid function, metabolic regulation, and depression. Psychosom Med 50:454–468, 1988
17. Fava GA, Sonino N, Morphy MA: Major depression associated with endocrine disease. Psychiatr Dev 4:321–348, 1987

18. Folks DG: Organic affective disorder and underlying thyrotoxicosis. Psychosomatics 25:243–245, 1984
19. Gabrilove JL: Neurologic and psychiatric manifestations in the classic endocrine syndromes, in Endocrines and the Central Nervous System. Edited by the Association for Research in Nervous and Mental Disease. Baltimore, MD, Williams & Wilkins, 1966, pp 419–441
20. Walter-Ryan WG, Fahs JJ: The problem with parsimony: mania and hyperthyroidism. J Clin Psychiatry 48:289–290, 1987
21. MacCrimmon DJ, Wallace JE, Goldberg WM, et al: Emotional disturbance and cognitive deficits in hyperthyroidism. Psychosom Med 41:331–340, 1979
22. Perrild H, Hansen JM, Arnung K, et al: Intellectual impairment after hyperthyroidism. Acta Endocrinol 112:185–191, 1986
23. Weller MPI: Agoraphobia and hyperthyroidism. Br J Psychiatry 144:553–554, 1984
24. Kronfol Z, Greden JF, Condon M, et al: Application of biological markers in depression secondary to thyrotoxicosis. Am J Psychiatry 129:1319–1322, 1982
25. Kathol RG, Turner R, Delahunt J: Depression and anxiety associated with hyperthyroidism: response to antithyroid therapy. Psychosomatics 27:501–505, 1986
26. Young LD: Organic affective disorder associated with thyrotoxicosis. Psychosomatics 25:490–492, 1984
27. Jefferson JW: Haldol decanoate and thyroid disease. J Clin Psychiatry 49:457–458, 1988
28. Kamlana SH, Holms L: Paranoid reaction and underlying thyrotoxicosis. Br J Psychiatry 149:376–377, 1986
29. Weiner MF: Haloperidol, hyperthyroidism, and sudden death. Am J Psychiatry 136:717–718, 1979
30. Trzepacz PT, McCue M, Klein I, et al: Psychiatric and neuropsychological response to propranolol in Graves' disease. Biol Psychiatry 23:678–688, 1988
31. Josephson AM, MacKenzie TB: Thyroid-induced mania in hypothyroid patients. Br J Psychiatry 137:222–228, 1980
32. Lassen E, Ewald H: Acute organic psychosis caused by thyrotoxicosis and vitamin B12 deficiency: case report. J Clin Psychiatry 46:106–107, 1985
33. Diaz-Cabal R, Pearlman C, Kawecki A: Hyperthyroidism in a patient with agitated depression: resolution after electroconvulsive therapy. J Clin Psychiatry 47:322–323, 1986
34. Fishman B, Barasch A: Diagnostic dilemma: drug withdrawal, borderline personality, and hyperthyroidism. Psychosomatics 27:370–372, 1986
35. Burton KR, Martin CA, Murray FT, et al: Hyperthyroidism in a cocaine-dependent patient. J Clin Psychiatry 50:305-306, 1989

36. Nakashima M, Kajita S, Otsuki S: Reduction of rat striatal thyrotropin-releasing hormone receptor produced by repeated methamphetamine administration. Biol Psychiatry 25:191–199, 1989

37. Giannandrea PF: The depressed hyperthyroid patient. Gen Hosp Psychiatry 9:71–73, 1987

38. Rolla AR, El-Hajj GA, Goldstein HH: Untreated thyrotoxicosis as a manifestation of anorexia nervosa. Am J Med 81:163–165, 1986

39. Van Uitert RL, Russakoff LM: Hyperthyroid chorea mimicking psychiatric disease. Am J Psychiatry 139:1208–1209, 1979

40. Munetz MR, Ginchereau EH, Toenniessen LM: Tardive dyskinesia complicated by hyperthyroidism. Psychosomatics 28:553–555, 1987

41. Orenstein H, Peskind A, Raskind MA: Thyroid disorders in female psychiatric patients with panic disorder or agoraphobia. Am J Psychiatry 145:1428–1430, 1988

42. Raj A, Sheehan DV: Medical evaluation of panic attacks. J Clin Psychiatry 48:309–313, 1987

43. Stein MB: Panic disorder and medical illness. Psychosomatics 27:833–840, 1986

44. Turner TH: Agoraphobia and hyperthyroidism. Br J Psychiatry 145:215–216, 1984

45. Lesser IM, Rubin RT, Lydiard RB: Past and current thyroid function in subjects with panic disorder. J Clin Psychiatry 48:473–476, 1987

46. Matuzas W, Al-Sadir J, Uhlenhuth EH, et al: Mitral valve prolapse and thyroid abnormalities in patients with panic attacks. Am J Psychiatry 144:493–496, 1987

47. Corn TH, Checkley SA: A case of recurrent mania with recurrent hyperthyroidism. Br J Psychiatry 143:74–76, 1983

48. Josephson AM, MacKenzie TB: Appearance of manic psychosis following rapid normalization of thyroid states. Am J Psychiatry 136:846–847, 1979

49. Atterwill CK, Bunn SJ, Atkinson DJ, et al: Effects of thyroid status on presynaptic alpha2-adrenoceptor function and β-adrenoceptor binding in the rat brain. J Neural Transm 59:43–55, 1984

50. Strombom U, Svensson TH, Jackson DM, et al: Hyperthyroidism: specifically increased response to central NA-(alpha-) receptor stimulation and generally increased monoamine turnover in brain. J Neural Transm 41:73–92, 1977

51. Swann AC: Thyroid hormone and norepinephrine: effects on alpha-2, beta, and reuptake sites in cerebral cortex and heart. J Neural Transm 71:195–205, 1988

52. Crocker AD, Overstreet DH, Crocker JM: Hypothyroidism leads to increased dopamine receptor sensitivity. Pharmacol Biochem Behav 24:1593–1597, 1986

53. Bilezikian JP, Loeb JN: The influence of hyperthyroidism and hypothyroidism on alpha- and β-adrenergic receptor systems and adrenergic responsiveness. Endocr Rev 4:378–388, 1983

54. Felten DL, Felten SY, Bellinger DL, et al: Noradrenergic sympathetic neural interactions with the immune system: structure and function. Immunol Rev 100:225–260, 1987

55. Gharib H, James EM, Charboneau W, et al: Suppressive therapy with levothyroxine for solitary thyroid nodules. N Engl J Med 317:70–75, 1987

56. Rojeski MT, Gharib H: Nodular thyroid disease. N Engl J Med 313:428–436, 1985

57. Wallerstein RS, Holzman PS, Voth HM, et al: Thyroid "hot spots": a psychophysiological study. Psychosom Med 27:508–523, 1965

58. Morillo E, Gardner LI: Bereavement as an antecedent factor in thyrotoxicosis of childhood: four case studies with survey of possible metabolic pathways. Psychosom Med 41:545–555, 1979

59. Voth HM, Holzman PS, Katz JB, et al: Thyroid "hot spots": their relationship to life stress. Psychosom Med 32:561–568, 1970

60. Wu S-Y, Green WL: Triiodothyronine (T3)-binding immunoglobulins in a euthyroid woman: effects on measurement of T3 (RIA) and on T3 turnover. J Clin Endocrinol Metab 42:640–652, 1976

61. Timsit J, Karsenty G, Monteiro R, et al: Hashimoto's thyroiditis with a monoclonal antithyroglobulin autoantibody: disappearance of the monoclonal antibody after thyroidectomy. J Clin Endocrinol Metab 66:880–884, 1988

62. Berrios GE, Leysen A, Samuel C, et al: Psychiatric morbidity following total and partial thyroidectomy. Acta Psychiatr Scand 72:369–373, 1985

63. Brockman DD, Whitman RM: Post-thyroidectomy psychosis. J Nerv Ment Dis 116:340–345, 1952

64. Carpelan H: Mental Disorder in Thyroidectomized Patients. Copenhagen, Ejnar Munksgaard, 1957

65. Howard MQ, Ziegler LH: Psychoses and allied states occurring subsequent to thyroidectomy. Am J Psychiatry 98:745–749, 1942

66. Bauer MS, Whybrow PC: The effect of changing thyroid function on cyclic affective illness in a human subject. Am J Psychiatry 143:633–636, 1986

67. Richter CP, Jones GS, Biswanger L: Periodic phenomena and the thyroid. Archives of Neurology and Psychiatry 81:117–139, 1959

68. Schull J, McEachron DL, Adler NT, et al: Effects of thyroidectomy, parathyroidectomy and lithium on circadian wheelrunning in rats. Physiol Behav 42:33–39, 1988

69. Andersson K, Eneroth P: Thyroidectomy and cental catecholamine neurons of the male rat. Neuroendocrinology 45:14–27, 1987

70. Boutin JM, Matte R, D'Amour D, et al: Characteristics of patients with normal T3 and T4 and a low TSH response to TRH. Clin Endocrinol 25:579–588, 1986

71. Staub JJ, Grani R, Birkhauser M, et al: Evaluation of "preclinical hyperthyroidism" using oral TSH, metoclopramide, systolic time intervals, sex-hormone-binding globulin and T4-suppression test. Journal of Molecular Medicine 4:49–58, 1980

190   *The Thyroid Axis and Psychiatric Illness*

72. Rockel M, Teuber J, Schmidt R, et al: Korrelation einer "Latenten Hyper-thyreose" mit psychischen und somatischen Veranderungen. Klin Wochen-schr 65:264–273, 1987
73. Gavin LA, Rosenthal M, Cavalieri RR: The diagnostic dilemma of isolated hyperthyroxinemia in acute illness. JAMA 242:251–253, 1979
74. McConnon JK: Thirty-five cases of transient hyperthyroidism. Can Med Assoc J 130:1159–1161, 1984
75. Nikolai TF, Brosseau J, Kettrick MA, et al: Lymphocytic thyroiditis with spontaneously resolving hyperthyroidism (silent thyroiditis). Arch Intern Med 140:478–482, 1980
76. Maxon HR, Burman KD, Premachandra BN, et al: Familial elevations of total and free thyroxine in healthy, euthyroid subjects without detectable binding protein abnormalities. Acta Endocrinol 100:224–230, 1982
77. Premachandra BN, Gossain VV, Perlstein IB: Increased free thyroxine in a euthyroid patient with thyroxine-binding globulin deficiency. J Clin Endo-crinol Metab 42:309–318, 1976
78. Drucker D, Josse R: Inappropriate TSH secretion with abnormal thyrotroph sensitivity to dopamine. Clin Invest Med 8:117–120, 1985
79. Cohen KL, Swigar ME: Thyroid function screening in psychiatric patients. JAMA 242:254–255, 1979
80. Spratt DI, Pont A, Miller MB, et al: Hyperthyroxinemia in patients with acute psychiatric disorders. Am J Med 78:41–48, 1982
81. Kramlinger KG, Gharib H, Swanson DQ: Normal serum thyroxine values in patients with acute psychiatric illness. Am J Med 76:779–801, 1984
82. Alarcon RD, Shirriff JR, Kern EE III: Euthyroid hyperthyroxinemia and rapid-cycling affective disorder: case report. J Clin Psychiatry 46:61–63, 1985
83. Whybrow PC, Prange AJ Jr: A hypothesis of thyroid-catecholamine-receptor interaction: its relevance to affective illness. Arch Gen Psychiatry 38:106–113, 1981
84. McGregor AM: Immunoendocrine interactions and autoimmunity. N Engl J Med 322: 1739–1741, 1990
85. Evered DC, Ormston BJ, Smith PA, et al: Grades of hypothyroidism. Br Med J 1:657–662, 1973
86. Hall RCW, Popkin MK, DeVaul R, et al: Psychiatric manifestations of Hashi-moto's thyroiditis. Psychosomatics 23:337–342, 1982
87. Henderson LM, Behan PO: The neuropsychiatric manifestations of Hashi-moto's disease: an unrecognized syndrome (abstract). Neurology 37:111, 1987
88. Sandler AP, Thompson J, Putney D: Symptomatic thyroiditis and schizo-phrenia in a six-year-old girl. J Clin Psychiatry 45:36–37, 1984
89. Schmidt PJ, Rosenfeld D, Muller KL, et al: A case of autoimmune thyroiditis presenting as menstrual related mood disorder. J Clin Psychiatry 51:434–436, 1990

90. Gold MS, Herridge P, Hapworth WE: Depression and "symptomless" autoimmune thyroiditis. Psychiatric Annals 17:750–757, 1987
91. Gold MS, Pottash ALC, Extein I: "Symptomless" autoimmune thyroiditis in depression. Psychiatry Res 6:261–269, 1982
92. Stein MB, Uhde TW: Autoimmune thyroiditis and panic disorder. Am J Psychiatry 146:259–260, 1989
93. De Boel S, Bonnyns M, Jonckheer M, et al: Thyroid hormone reserve in asymptomatic autoimmune thyroiditis. Acta Endocrinol 114:336–339, 1987
94. Amino N, Miyai K: Postpartum autoimmune endocrine syndromes, in Autoimmune Endocrine Disease. Edited by Davies TF. New York, Wiley, 1983, pp 247–272
95. Jansson R, Bernander S, Karlsson A, et al: Autoimmune thyroid dysfunction in the postpartum period. J Clin Endocrinol Metab 58:681–687, 1984
96. Lervang H-H, Pryds O, Kristensen PO: Thyroid dysfunction after delivery: incidence and clinical course. Acta Medica Scandinavica 222:369–374, 1987
97. Hamilton JA: Postpartum Psychiatric Problems. Saint Louis, MO, CV Mosby, 1962, pp 112–125
98. Nikolai TF, Turney SL, Roberts RC: Postpartum lymphocytic thyroiditis. Arch Intern Med 147:221–224, 1987
99. Harris B, Fung H, Johns S, et al: Transient post-partum thyroid dysfunction and postnatal depression. J Affective Disord 17:243–249, 1989
100. Stewart DE, Addison AM, Robinson GE, et al: Thyroid function in psychosis following childbirth. Am J Psychiatry 145:1579–1581, 1988
101. Cooper DS: Subclinical hypothyroidism. JAMA 258:246–247, 1987
102. Editorial: Subclinical hypothyroidism. Lancet 1:251–252, 1986
103. Reus VI: Behavioral aspects of thyroid disease in women. Psychiatr Clin North Am 12:153–165, 1989
104. Gold MS, Pottash AC, Mueller EA III, et al: Grades of thyroid failure in 100 depressed and anergic psychiatric inpatients. Am J Psychiatry 138:253–255, 1981
105. Krahn DD: Affective disorder associated with subclinical hypothyroidism. Psychosomatics 28:440–441, 1987
106. McNamara ME, Southwick SM, Fogel BS: Sleep apnea and hypothyroidism presenting as depression in two patients. J Clin Psychiatry 48:164–165, 1987
107. Arque JM, Segura R, Torrubia R: Correlation of thyroxine and thyroid-stimulating hormone with personality measurements: a study in psychosomatic patients and healthy subjects. Neuropsychobiology 18:127–133, 1987
108. Cooper DS, Halpern R, Wood LC, et al: L-thyroxine therapy in subclinical hypothyroidism. Ann Intern Med 101:18–24, 1984
109. Baruch P, Jouvent R, Widlocher D: Increased TSH response to TRH in refractory depressed women (letter). Am J Psychiatry 142:145–146, 1985
110. Gewirtz GR, Malaspina D, Hatterer JA: Occult thyroid dysfunction in patients with refractory depression. Am J Psychiatry 145:1012–1014, 1988

111. Russ MJ, Ackerman SH: Antidepressant treatment response in depressed hypothyroid patients. Hosp Community Psychiatry 40:954–956, 1989
112. Zach J: Occult thyroid dysfunction in refractory depression. Am J Psychiatry 146:280–281, 1989
113. Drinka PJ, Voeks SK: Psychological depressive symptoms in grade II hypothyroidism in a nursing home. Psychiatry Res 21:199–204
114. Haggerty JJ, Evans DL, Prange AJ Jr: Organic brain syndrome associated with marginal hypothyroidism. Am J Psychiatry 143:785–786, 1986
115. Johnstone EC, Owens DGC, Crow TJ, et al: Hypothyroidism as a correlate of lateral ventricular enlargement in manic-depressive and neurotic illness. Br J Psychiatry 148:317–321, 1986
116. Fader BW, Struve FA: The possible value of the electroencephalogram in detecting subclinical hypothyroidism associated with agitated depression: a case study. Clin Electroencephalogr 3:94–101, 1972
117. Gold MS, Pottash ALC, Extein I: Hypothyroidism and depression. JAMA 245:1919–1221, 1981
118. Extein I, Pottash ALC, Gold MS: The TRH test in affective disorders: experience in a private clinical setting. Psychosomatics 25:379–389, 1984
119. Winokur A, Amsterdam JD, Oler J, et al: Multiple hormonal responses to protirelin (TRH) in depressed patients. Arch Gen Psychiatry 40:525–531, 1983
120. Calabrese J, Gulledge AD: Depression and hypothyroidism (letter). JAMA 11:2470–2471, 1983
121. Hatotani N, Nomura J, Tamaguchi T, et al: Clinical and experimental studies on the pathogenesis of depression. Psychoneuroendocrinology 2:115–130, 1977
122. Targum SD, Byrnes SM, Sullivan AC: The TRH stimulation test in subtypes of unipolar depression. J Affective Disord 4:29–34, 1982
123. Calloway SP, Dolan RJ, Fonagy P, et al: Endocrine changes in clinical profiles in depression, II: the thyrotropin-releasing hormone test. Psychol Med 14:759–765, 1984
124. Kathol RG, Winokur G, Sherman BM, et al: Provocative endocrine testing in recovered depressives. Psychoneuroendocrinology 9:57–67, 1984
125. Joffe RT, Kutcher S, MacDonald C: Thyroid function and bipolar affective disorder. Psychiatry Res 25:117–121, 1988
126. Perrild H, Hegedus L, Baastrup PC, et al: Thyroid function and ultrasonically determined thyroid size in patients receiving long-term lithium treatment. Am J Psychiatry 147:1518–1521, 1990
127. Shader RI, Greenblatt DJ: Back to basics--diagnosis before treatment: homelessness, hypothyroidism, aging, and lithium (editorial). J Clin Psychopharmacol 7:375, 1987
128. O'Shanick GJ, Ellinwood EH Jr: Persistent elevation of thyroid-stimulating hormone in women with bipolar affective disorder. Am J Psychiatry 139:513–514, 1982

129. Cowdry RW, Wehr TA, Zis AP, et al: Thyroid abnormalities associated with rapid-cycling bipolar illness. Arch Gen Psychiatry 40:414–420, 1983

130. Extein I, Pottash ALC, Gold MS: Does subclinical hypothyroidism predispose to tricyclic-induced rapid mood cycles? J Clin Psychiatry 43:290–291, 1982

131. Tapp A: Affective cycling in thyroid disease. J Clin Psychiatry 49:199–200, 1988

132. Bauer MS, Whybrow PC: Rapid-cycling bipolar affective disorder, II. Arch Gen Psychiatry 47:435–440, 1990

133. Bauer MS, Whybrow PC, Winokur A: Rapid-cycling bipolar affective disorder, I. Arch Gen Psychiatry 47:427–432, 1990

134. Gull WW: On a cretinoid state supervening in adult life in women, in Transactions of the Clinical Society of London, Vol 7. London, Longmans, Green & Company, 1874, pp 180–185

135. Ord WM: On myxedema: a term proposed to be applied to an essential condition in the "cretinoid" affection occasionally observed in middle-aged women. Royal Medical and Chirurgal Society Transaction 61:57–78, 1878

136. Reed K, Bland RC: Masked "myxedema madness." Acta Psychiatr Scand 56:421–426, 1977

137. Tachman ML, Guthrie GP Jr: Hypothyroidism: diversity of presentation. Endocr Rev 5:456–465, 1984

138. Nordgren L, von Scheele C: Myxedematous madness without myxedema. Acta Medica Scandinavica 199:233–236, 1976

139. Darko DF: The diagnostic dilemma of myxedema and madness, axis I and axis II: a longitudinal case report. Int J Psychiatry Med 18:263–270, 1988

140. Denicoff KD, Joffe RT, Lakshmanan MC, et al: Neuropsychiatric manifestations of altered thyroid state. Am J Psychiatry 147:94–99, 1990

141. Balldin J, Berggren U, Rybo E, et al: Treatment-resistant mania with primary hypothyroidism: a case of recovery after levothyroxine. J Clin Psychiatry 48:490–491, 1987

142. Shaw E, Halper J, Yi PE, et al: Diagnosis of "myxedema madness" (letter). Am J Psychiatry 142:655, 1985

143. Zolese G, Henryk-Gutt R: Mania induced by biochemical imbalance resulting from low energy diet in a patient with undiagnosed myxoedema. Br Med J 295:1026–1027, 1987

144. Gharib H, Abboud CF: Primary idiopathic hypothalamic hypothyroidism. Am J Med 83:171–174, 1987

145. Linnoila M, Cowdry R, Lamberg B-A, et al: CSF triiodothyronine (rT$_3$) levels in patients with affective disorders. Biol Psychiatry 18:1489–1492, 1983

146. Rippere V: Hypothalamic hypothyroidism with end-organ resistance: further personal observations. Med Hypotheses 2:241–248, 1986

147. Comer CP, Norton S: Behavioral consequences of perinatal hypothyroidism in postnatal and adult rats. Pharmacol Biochem Behav 22:605–611, 1985

148. Gottesfeld Z, Butler IJ, Findley WE: Prenatal and postnatal hypothyroidism abolishes lesion-induced noradrenergic sprouting in the adult rat. J Neurosci Res 14:61–69, 1985

149. Gravel C, Hawkes R: Thyroid hormone modulates the expression of a neurofilament antigen in the cerebellar cortex: premature induction and overexpression by basket cells in hyperthyroidism and a critical period for the correction of hypothyroidism. Brain Res 422:327–335, 1987

150. Tauboll E, Stokke KT, Gjerstad L, et al: Association between regularly occurring complex partial seizures and thyroid function parameters. Epilepsia 27:419–422, 1986

151. Dussault JH, Ruel J: Thyroid hormones and brain development. Annu Rev Physiol 49:321–334, 1987

152. Pharoah POD, Connolly KJ, Ekins RP, et al: Maternal thyroid hormone levels in pregnancy and the subsequent cognitive and motor performance of the children. Clin Endocrinol 21:265–270, 1984

153. Tamasy V, Meisami E, Du J-Z, et al: Exploratory behavior, learning ability, and thyroid hormonal responses to stress in female rats rehabilitating from postnatal hypothyroidism. Dev Psychobiol 19:537–553, 1986

154. Slotkin TA, Slepetis RJ: Obligatory role of thyroid hormones in development of peripheral sympathetic and central nervous system catecholaminergic neurons: effects of propylthiouracil-induced hypothyroidism on transmitter levels, turnover and release. J Pharmacol Exp Ther 230:53–61, 1984

155. Meaney MJ, Aitken DH, Sapolsky RM: Thyroid hormone influence the development of hippocampal glucocorticoid receptors in the rat: a mechanism for the effects of postnatal handling on the development of the adrenocortical stress response. Neuroendocrinology 45:278–283, 1987

156. Meberg A, Marstein S: Smoking during pregnancy: effects on the fetal thyroid function. Acta Paediatr Scand 75:762–766, 1986

157. Weiner N, Disbrow JK, French TA, et al: The influence of catecholamine systems and thyroid function on the actions of ethanol in long-sleep (LS) and short-sleep (SS) mice. Ann N Y Acad Sci 492:375–383, 1987

158. Fundaro A, Molinengo L: Emotional behaviour in relation to hypothyroidism and hyperthyroidism in the rat. Medical Sciences Research 15:253–254, 1987

159. Nemeroff CB: Clinical significance of psychoneuroendocrinology in psychiatry: focus on the thyroid and adrenal. J Clin Psychiatry 50:13–20, 1989

Chapter 6

The Thyroid and Depression

Russell T. Joffe, M.D.
Anthony J. Levitt, M.D.

CONTENTS

---

1. INTRODUCTION

It has long been known that there is an association between abnormalities of thyroid function and psychiatric symptoms, particularly disorders of mood. In the early part of the last century, Parry (1) described the occurrence of psychiatric symptoms associated with hyperthyroidism. Later, an association between melancholia and hypothyroidism was described both by the Clinical Society of London (2) and in the classical longitudinal observations of Asher (3). The consistent descriptions of an association between clinical thyroid disorders and psychiatric, particularly affective, morbidity led to the assumption that thyroid hormones may be important in the regulation of mood and in the pathophysiology of primary affective illness.

Over the past quarter of a century, there has been an extensive research effort to identify potential abnormalities of thyroid function in patients with various affective disorders. The resultant literature can be divided up into three broad categories: *1)* the evaluation of a variety of thyroid function tests in patients with affective illness, *2)* the effect of different antidepressant treatments on thyroid function tests, and *3)* the use of various thyroid hormones in the treatment of patients with primary affective illness. Our aim in this chapter is to provide a comprehensive and critical review of these three main areas of study of the thyroid axis in affective illness. For the purposes of discussion, we deal with each of these areas separately, although it is clear that they are closely interrelated.

2. PERIPHERAL THYROID HORMONE LEVELS

Many studies have measured circulating thyroid hormone levels in patients with a variety of affective disorders. Some of these are summarized in Table 6–1. Although there is great variability in the results of these studies, there is general consensus that the vast majority of patients with primary affective illness have thyroid function tests within the euthyroid range (4–6). In the sections that follow, we consider each of the thyroid hormones separately.

2.1 Thyroxine (T_4)

Studies that have examined circulating levels of thyroxine (T_4) or free thyroxine (FT_4) have produced inconsistent findings (7–21) (Table 6–1). Several studies (8,9,11,14,15,18) have shown measures of T_4 to be in the upper range of normal or significantly higher in depressed patients compared with those in healthy or psychiatric control groups. However, other studies (10,13,16) have reported lower levels of T_4 or triiodothyronine (T_3) in depressed patients compared with control subjects. It is difficult to reconcile these apparently opposite findings. However, methodological limitations in these studies preclude definitive conclusions being drawn from their observations.

Table 6–1. Circulating thyroid hormone levels in depression

Study	N patients	PBI	T_4	FT_4	T_3RU	T_3	FT_3	TSH
Board et al. 1959 (7)	33	0						
Dewhurst et al. 1968 (8)	15		+					
Whybrow et al. 1972 (9)	30	0		+	0			
Rybakowski and Sowinski 1973 (10)	9		−	−	0			
Takahashi et al. 1974 (11)	36		+					
Yamaguchi et al. 1975 (12)	16		−					
Kolakowska and Swigar 1977 (13)	115		+					
Hatotani et al. 1977 (14)	36		+					
Rinieris et al. 1978 (15)	40		−	−	0			
Linnoila et al. 1979 (16)	12		0			−		
Nordgren and van Scheele 1981 (17)	25		0		0			
Targum et al. 1982 (18)	54		+					
Joffe et al. 1985 (19)	11		0	0				
Orsulak et al. 1985 (20)	32		0					
Wahby et al. 1989 (21)	27		0	0				

Note. PBI = protein-bound iodine; T_4 = thyroxine; FT_4 = measure of free thryoxine; T_3RU = triiodothyronine resin uptake; T_3 = triiodothyronine; FT_3 = measure of free triiodothyronine; TSH = thyroid-stimulating hormone.
+ = increase; − = decrease; 0 = no change.

These limitations include small sample sizes, variable definitions of depression, and technical differences in the measurement of T_4, particularly in the earlier studies.

In contrast to the studies that have examined T_4 levels in depressed patients versus control subjects, there is remarkable consistency in studies in which measures of T_4 were examined before and after recovery in depressed patients. These studies (7,9,12,22–36), involving a sample size of at least 10 patients, are summarized in Table 6–2. Of these 18 studies, 17 demonstrated a significant reduction in one or more measures of T_4 after clinical recovery from depression. Earlier studies that were negative (e.g, 17) involved very small sample sizes. Because the reductions in T_4, although substantial, are limited, levels before and after antidepressant treatment usually fall within the normal range reported for clinical thyroid disorders. In the only negative

Table 6–2.   Longitudinal studies of thyroid hormone levels in affective illness

Study	PBI	T_4	FT_4	T_3	rT_3	TSH
		Change with recovery				
Board et al. 1959 (7)	−					
Gibbons et al. 1960 (22)	−					
Whybrow et al. 1972 (9)		−				
Ferrari 1973 (23)	−					
Kirkegaard et al. 1975 (24)		−	−			
Kirkegaard et al. 1975 (25)		−	−			
Yamaguchi et al. 1975 (12)		−				
Kirkegaard et al. 1977 (26)		−	−			
Kirkegaard and Faber 1981 (27)		−	−			
Roy-Byrne et al. 1984[a] (28)		−	−	−		
Kirkegaard and Faber 1986 (29)		−	−		−	
Unden et al. 1986 (30)		−			−	+
Joffe and Singer 1987 (31)		0				
Baumgartner et al. 1988[a] (32)		−	−			
Muller and Boning 1988 (33)		−	−	−		
Brady and Anton 1989 (34)			−			−
Mason et al. 1989 (35)		−	−			
Joffe and Singer 1990[a] (36)		−	−			

Note.   PBI = protein-bound iodine; T_4 = thyroxine; FT_4 = measure of free thyroxine; T_3 = triiodothyronine; rT_3 = reverse triiodothyronine, TSH = thyroid-stimulating hormone.
− = decrease; + = increase; 0 = no change.
[a]Related to antidepressant response.

longitudinal study to date (31), no significant reduction in T_4 levels was observed in 16 patients with primary major depression who were treated with the monoamine oxidase inhibitor phenelzine. However, the sample size was small, thus creating the possibility of insufficient statistical power to demonstrate an effect on thyroid hormones with treatment. Furthermore, the small sample size did not allow for a meaningful statistical comparison of T_4 levels before and after treatment in patients who responded to treatment versus those who did not respond.

Three studies to date (28,32,36) have examined changes in measures of T_4 in relationship to antidepressant response. In all three studies, patients who responded to several antidepressant treatments were found to have substantially greater reductions in T_4 and measures of FT_4 compared with those who did not respond. Roy-Byrne et al. (28) were the first to observe a relationship between decrements in T_4 and therapeutic response in 50 patients with primary affective illness who were treated with carbamazepine. Further, Baumgartner et al. (32) found that decreases in measures of T_4 were substantially correlated with antidepressant response in 31 patients treated with either chlorimipramine or maprotiline. In a recent study (36) of patients with primary major depression, we observed a substantial reduction in mean levels of T_4 and FT_4 index in 16 patients who responded but not in 12 who did not respond to desipramine treatment.

In summary, with regard to measures of T_4, although cross-sectional comparisons with control groups are inconclusive (Table 6–1), longitudinal studies are remarkably consistent in showing decrements in T_4 levels after recovery from depression. We have suggested that, although these decreases are within the normal range, they may be of pathophysiological significance in primary affective illness (37).

Whereas most studies in depressed patients demonstrate changes in T_4 within the normal range, several studies (38–46) have reported abnormal elevations of T_4 in psychiatric patients with a variety of diagnoses (Table 6–3). Combined, these studies suggest that from none to 33% of psychiatric patients recently admitted to an inpatient unit are reported to have elevations of T_4 with or without increases in FT_4. These patients do not have any clinical evidence of hyperthyroidism, and the abnormality of T_4 is usually transient and normalizes after 2–3 weeks (39,42,46).

Transient hyperthyroxinemia occurs in a variety of psychiatric patients in general, and it was observed in 12% of 99 subjects admitted to an inpatient unit with the diagnosis of primary affective disorder (45). Although it has been suggested that the phenomenon of transient elevations of T_4 is only observed in recently admitted inpatients, we have found that 7% of 125 outpatients with primary major depressive disorder exhibited this abnormality of thyroid function (R. T. Joffe, A. J. Levitt, unpublished data, March 1990). The pathophysiological significance of transient hyperthyroxinemia is uncertain. It has been suggested that it may be due to the stress associated with acute psychiatric illness and hospitalization (4) or to altered peripheral conversion of T_4 to T_3 (45). One study (46) showed that, in many cases, the transient elevations of serum T_4 were associated with increases in serum thyroid-stimulating hormone (TSH) (or thyrotropin) using a sensitive TSH assay, suggesting that transient hyperthyroxinemia may be the result of a central nervous system abnormality in regulation of the thyroid axis. Although the etiology of this phenomenon remains to be clarified, it is of clinical relevance because it has to be distinguished from cases of hyperthyroidism associated with psychiatric symptoms. Transient hyperthyroxinemia can, however, be identified

Table 6–3. Transient hyperthyroxinemia in psychiatric illness

Study	N patients	Diagnosis	Status	Prevalence (%)
McLarty et al. 1978 (38)	1,206	Mixed	Inpatient	2.5
Cohen and Swigar 1979 (39)	480	Mixed	Inpatient	9
Levy et al. 1981 (40)	150	Mixed	Inpatient	7
Morley and Shafer 1982 (41)	386	Mixed	Inpatient	19
Spratt et al. 1982 (42)	645	Mixed	Inpatient	33
Caplan et al. 1982/83 (43)	100	Mixed	Inpatient	5
Kramlinger et al. 1984 (44)	278	Mixed	Inpatient	0.003
Chopra et al. 1990 (46)	84	Mixed	Inpatient	24
Styra et al. 1991 (45)	99	Primary affective	Inpatient	12
Joffe and Levitt. 1990 (unpublished data)	125	Major depression	Outpatient	7

by the absence of clinical signs and symptoms of thyroid disease and the return to normal T_4 levels within a few weeks.

2.2 Triiodothyronine (T_3)

The findings with T_3 are more consistent than those with T_4. Several studies (17,19,20,21) suggest that mean T_3 or free triiodothyronine (FT_3) levels in depressed patients are decreased compared with those in control subjects (Table 6–1). However, in the longitudinal studies (Table 6–2), consistent changes in T_3 levels have not been observed. As with the studies examining T_4, methodological difficulties such as sensitivity of hormone assays, inadequate sample sizes, and variable definition of depression may account for some of the inconsistency of findings. The clinical definition of depression and occurrence of associated symptomatology may be particularly important factors in the variability in T_3 measures observed, as we (47) have recently shown that patients with psychotic depression have significantly lower T_3 levels than do subjects with nonpsychotic unipolar depression. This finding is consistent with an increasing body of literature suggesting a relationship between particular abnormalities of thyroid function and specific psychiatric symptoms in patients with depression (48).

The data on T_3, therefore, suggest that there are no consistent alterations of T_3 levels observed in patients with primary depression. These data taken together with data on T_4 levels suggest that there may be a significant change in the ratio of T_4 to T_3 after clinical recovery in depressed patients, which may be of significance in understanding the biological basis of depression (37).

2.3 Reverse Triiodothyronine (rT_3)

Reverse triiodothyronine (rT_3) is formed from the monodeiodination of T_4. There is a reciprocal relationship between the amount of T_3 and rT_3 formed from the metabolism of T_4 (49). Under usual physiological conditions, rT_3 does not have an effect on the regulation of the hypothalamic-pituitary-thyroid axis (50). However, after experimental infusion of T_4, the cerebral cortex of the rat produces about 20 times more rT_3 than T_3 (51). Moreover, it has been shown that concentrations of rT_3 are about 20 times higher in human cerebrospinal fluid than in serum (52). Therefore, measurement of rT_3 in patients with affective illness has been of considerable interest. These studies (27,53–55) are summarized in Table 6–4. The data suggest that serum rT_3 levels are increased in the depressed state and normalize with clinical recovery (53,56). Although Linnoila et al. (53) observed increased serum rT_3 levels in mania and unipolar depression as compared with those in bipolar depression, their study involved small sample sizes and has not been replicated (56). In the only study to date that has examined cerebrospinal fluid rT_3 levels (54), these levels were found to be increased in unipolar depression as compared with those in bipolar depression or mania.

Taken together, studies of T_4, T_3, and rT_3 levels may suggest some alteration in thyroid hormone metabolism, particularly of T_4, in depression. However, the pathophysiological significance for affective illness remains uncertain. Clearly, the potential role of rT_3 in brain function and, therefore, in depression remains to be clarified before any potential significance of these findings (53–56) can be further evaluated.

Table 6–4.   Reverse triiodothyronine (rT_3) levels in affective illness

Study	Population	Sample	Result
Kirkegaard and Faber 1981 (27)	80 endogenous depression patients	Blood	Increased rT_3 normalized with recovery
Linnoila et al. 1982 (53)	13 depression patients 7 mania patients 8 healthy control subjects	Blood	rT_3 increased in mania and unipolar depression as compared with bipolar depression and controls
Linnoila et al. 1983 (54)	34 depression patients 11 mania patients	CSF	rT_3 increased in unipolar depression as compared with bipolar depression or mania
Kjellman et al. 1983 (55)	32 major depression patients (26 studied after recovery) 22 healthy control subjects 16 recovered depression patients	Blood	No significant difference in rT_3 between groups; however, significant decrease in rT_3 between depressed and recovered patients

Note.   CSF = cerebrospinal fluid.

2.4   Thyroid-Stimulating Hormone (TSH)

In most studies involving depressed patients, either as compared with healthy control subjects or over the course of antidepressant treatment, abnormalities of TSH have not usually been observed (see Tables 6–1 and 6–2). However, TSH is a very sensitive indicator of varying degrees of thyroid failure. In recent years, the definitions of various degrees of hypothyroidism have been standardized (57). Grade I, or clinical, hypothyroidism is characterized by clinical symptoms of thyroid underactivity and is associated with abnormally decreased levels of T_4 and T_3, elevated TSH levels, and an augmented TSH response to thyrotropin-releasing hormone (TRH). In grade II hypothyroidism, peripheral thyroid hormone levels are within normal limits, but basal and TRH-stimulated TSH levels are abnormally elevated. Patients with grade II hypothyroidism do not have classical symptoms of clinical hypothyroidism. Patients with grade III hypothyroidism have no clinical stigmata of hypothyroidism and have normal circulating T_4, T_3, and basal TSH levels but an abnormally elevated TSH response to TRH stimulation (57).

"Subclinical" hypothyroidism, defined as grade II or III hypothyroidism, may arise from a variety of causes. These include iodine deficiency and ablative treatment of clinical hyperthyroidism (58). However, the most common cause of subclinical hypothyroidism is autoimmune thyroiditis (59). Autoimmune thyroiditis is itself a heterogeneous group of disorders characterized by destruction of the thyroid gland and the development of various types of antithyroid antibodies. It is estimated that approximately 5% of the general population has subclinical hypothyroidism, although the frequency may increase to 10%–15% in women over age 60 (60,61).

The medical consequences of subclinical hypothyroidism are uncertain. The studies that have examined this issue refer largely to grade II hypothyroidism. Some studies (62,63) suggest that patients with this condition have alterations in physiological parameters such as myocardial contractility that are reversed by L-thyroxine (L-T_4) replacement therapy. Furthermore, other studies (e.g., 60) have reported that grade II hypothyroidism may be a risk factor for coronary artery disease due to alterations in serum lipoproteins. The clinical importance of these observations (60,62,63) remains to be clarified. However, follow-up studies indicate that subclinical hypothyroidism in the presence of antithyroid antibodies will progress to clinical hypothyroidism at the rate of 5%–8% per year (60).

The psychiatric sequelae of subclinical hypothyroidism are also controversial. Gold et al. (64,65) reported that approximately 9% of patients who present to a psychiatric clinic with complaints of depression and anergia have biochemical evidence of subclinical hypothyroidism. It still remains to be clarified, however, what proportion of unselected patients with primary major depressive disorder have evidence of subclinical hypothyroidism. Moreover, the clinical and treatment correlates of major depression associated with subclinical hypothyroidism have received limited attention in the literature.

There are some preliminary data showing that depression associated with subclinical hypothyroidism is less likely to respond to conventional antidepressants (reviewed in 58). In our study (48), we evaluated 139 patients with unipolar, nonpsychotic major depression, 19 of whom were found to have grade II hypothyroidism. Subjects with subclinical hypothyroidism were much less likely than the remainder of the cohort to respond to the first tricyclic antidepressant used for their current episode. It was also observed that patients with subclinical hypothyroidism were substantially more likely to have a concurrent panic disorder diagnosis. Although this group of patients may be more resistant to conventional antidepressants, it is unknown whether patients with subclinical hypothyroidism may have an antidepressant response to thyroid hormones alone or in addition to standard antidepressants. There are preliminary data showing that patients with major depression and subclinical hypothyroidism have an antidepressant response to either thyroid hormone replacement (66) or to T_3 augmentation of their antidepressant (67). These studies (66,67) are preliminary in nature and involve only small numbers of patients without adequate controls. Therefore, they require confirmation in further studies involving larger sample sizes and more attention to experimental design.

The relationship between subclinical hypothyroidism and major depression requires further study. However, such a relationship may be more relevant to bipolar affective disorder, particularly the rapid-cycling form. Several studies (68–72) have examined the prevalence of varying degrees of hypothyroidism in patients with rapid-cycling bipolar affective disorder (Table 6–5).

Cho et al. (68) were the first to report a high prevalence of clinical hypothyroidism in female patients with rapid-cycling affective illness. In a later study, Cowdry et al. (69) reported that 92% of rapid-cycling patients versus 52% of non-rapid-cycling patients had evidence of varying degrees of hypothyroidism. Although Wehr et al. (70) also found a high proportion of bipolar patients with clinical thyroid disease, they did not find an excess prevalence in those subjects with the rapid-cycling form of illness. In our own study (71), we found that the prevalence of varying degrees of hypothyroidism was more related to duration of lithium treatment rather than to the course of affective illness. In a recent report, Bauer et al. (72), who examined only rapid-cycling patients, found that there was a higher prevalence of all grades of hypothyroidism in their study group compared with previously published frequencies of thyroid dysfunction in non-rapid-cycling bipolar patients. In the light of the previous study from Wehr et al. (70), the conclusions of this more recent study (72) are limited by the absence of a non-rapid-cycling control group.

Although the studies to date suggest that varying degrees of hypo-

Table 6–5. Thyroid function and rapid-cycling bipolar affective disorder

| | | | | | Prevalence (%) of hypothyroidism | | | | | |
| | n patients | | Percent female | | Grade I | | Grade II | | Grade III | |
Study	R	NR	R	NR	R	NR	R	NR	R	NR
Cho et al. 1979 (68)	16	99	100	100	31.7	2.1	—	—	—	—
Cowdry et al. 1983 (69)	24	19	83	53	50	0	42	32	—	—
Wehr et al. 1988 (70)	51	19	92	100	47	39	—	—	—	—
Joffe et al. 1988 (71)	17	25	41	80	0	20	0	12	—	—
Bauer et al. 1990 (72)	30	—	83	—	23	—	27	—	10	—

Note. R = rapid cycling; NR = non-rapid cycling.

thyroidism are common in patients with bipolar affective disorder, the specificity of these abnormalities for the rapid-cycling form of illness and their relationship to particulars of lithium treatment remain to be clarified. Nonetheless, these observations (Table 6–5) have provided some of the rationale for the use of hypermetabolic doses of T_4 for the treatment of patients with bipolar disorder, particularly the rapid-cycling form.

Recent studies have examined the prevalence of antithyroid antibodies in depressed patients. These studies derive from the fact that autoimmune disorders are the most common cause of subclinical forms of hypothyroidism (58). Studies (73–77) that have examined the frequency of antithyroid antibodies in depressed patients are summarized in Table 6–6. These studies have shown that between 8% and 20% of patients with depression have positive antithyroid antibody titers. Although studies to date suggest that a high proportion of patients with affective illness may have subtle degrees of thyroid hypofunction, the data should be interpreted with caution for two reasons. First, most of these studies (73,74,76) have lacked any control group. In the one study (77) in which a non-affective psychiatric disorder control group was used, there was no difference in the frequency of antithyroid antibodies between the two groups (9% in patients with affective disorder versus 10% in those with non-affective psychiatric disorder). Second, in several of the studies, the

Table 6–6. Antithyroid antibodies in major depression

Study	N patients	Population	Prevalence n	Prevalence %
Gold et al. 1982 (73)	100	Patients with depression and/or anergia	9	9
Nemeroff et al. 1985 (74)	45	Affective disorder patients	9	20
Reus et al. 1986 (75)	170	Patients with multiple psychiatric diagnoses (n with depression unspecified)	—	25
Joffe 1987 (76)	58	Major depression patients	5	8.6
Haggerty et al. 1990 (77)	99	Affective disorder patients	9	9
	68	Non-affective psychiatric disorder patients	7	10

prevalence rates of 9% (73,77) and 8.6% (76) are not substantially different from the prevalence of positive antithyroid antibody titers of 6.8% observed in the general population (78).

In summary, varying degrees of clinical and subclinical hypothyroidism as well as positive antithyroid antibody titers, suggestive of asymptomatic autoimmune thyroiditis (58), have been observed in patients with depression and, particularly, in those with bipolar affective disorder. The specificity of these findings for patients with affective illness and their importance for choice of treatment require further study.

2.5 Circadian Rhythms

It has been well established that there is a circadian variation of serum TSH levels (79,80). Most studies report that levels of TSH increase during the night, although peak TSH levels have been reported to occur anywhere between midnight and 6 A.M. (79,80). A circadian rhythm of peripheral thyroid hormones is less well established. However, two studies (81,82) have reported an inverse relationship in the circadian patterns of T_4 compared with TSH in healthy control subjects. As the circadian variation of TSH in control subjects has been relatively well described, several studies (30,83–87) have attempted to elucidate whether abnormalities of the circadian variation in thyroid hormones occur in depression (Table 6–7).

In an initial uncontrolled study, Weeke and Weeke (83) reported that decreased nocturnal secretion of TSH was related to severity of depression. In a subsequent study (84) they found that although the diurnal pattern of TSH did not reliably distinguish depressed patients from healthy control subjects, there was a substantial decrease in mean and maximum 24-hour TSH secretion between depression and recovery within the same patients. These data strongly suggest that diminished circadian variation of TSH is associated with primary depression. Although the pathophysiological significance of this observation is uncertain, it may be consistent with other abnormalities of thyroid function observed in depression, such as relative increases in circulating T_4 levels and a blunted TSH response to TRH (see section 3.2). Furthermore, this abnormality may also be consistent with dis-

Table 6–7. Circadian variation in thyroid function tests in depression

Study	Population	Control subjects	Measurement	Result
Weeke and Weeke 1978 (83)	19 endogenous depression patients (11 unmedicated, 8 given tricyclics)	None	T_4, T_3, FT_4, FT_3, TSH at 2 P.M. and midnight	Absence of diurnal variation in TSH and free hormones related to severity of depression
Weeke and Weeke 1980 (84)	4 endogenous depression patients	None	T_3, TSH every 1 hour for 24 hours	No different from that for healthy people
Golstein et al. 1980 (85)	13 depression patients (5 bipolar patients, 8 unipolar; all medication free)	6 healthy volunteers	TSH only every 30 minutes for 24 hours	Decreased mean 24-hour TSH and absent nocturnal TSH rise in unipolar patients
Kijne et al. 1982 (86)	9 endogenous depression patients (mean age 72 years)	Before and after recovery	T_4, T_3, TSH every 4 hours; extra sample between midnight and 4 A.M.	No difference between depression and recovery
Kjellman et al. 1984 (87)	32 major depression patients	26 paired data on recovery 32 healthy volunteers 17 recovered depression	TSH every 2 hours for 24 hours	Lower mean 24-hour and maximum TSH in depression control subjects; normalized with recovery
Unden et al. 1986 (30)	31 major depression patients	32 healthy control subjects 23 partially or completely remitted subjects	T_4, T_3, TSH every 4 hours, but every 2 hours midnight to 8 A.M.	Mean 24-hour TSH decreased in depressed compared with recovered and healthy subjects

Note. T_4 = thyroxine; T_3 = triiodothyronine; FT_4 = free thyroxine; FT_3 = free triiodothyronine, TSH = thyroid-stimulating hormone.

turbance of circadian variation reported for several other endocrine and biological parameters in primary affective disorder.

3. THE THYROID AXIS

3.1 Thyrotropin-Releasing Hormone (TRH)

The tripeptide, TRH, is widely distributed throughout the central nervous system (88). In addition to its stimulatory effect on the pituitary thyrotrophs leading to TSH secretion, TRH appears to have widespread neurotransmitter and neuromodulatory effects (89,90). Consequently, several studies have examined TRH levels in relationship to affective illness. With regard to animal studies, several of these have examined the effects of antidepressant treatments on TRH levels in rat brain. These studies have been largely inconclusive. Lighton et al. (89) reported that electroconvulsive shock led to decreased TRH levels in rat spinal cord and nucleus accumbens. In contrast, Przegalinski and Jaworska (91) found that amitriptyline, but not imipramine, caused increased TRH levels in rat striatum and nucleus accumbens. The differential effects of these various treatments, particularly the two tricyclics, on TRH led to the conclusion that the antidepressant effects of these drugs in humans are likely not related to their effects on TRH (89,91).

Two studies have examined levels of TRH in the cerebrospinal fluid of depressed subjects. Kirkegaard et al. (92) compared cerebrospinal fluid TRH levels in 15 patients with endogenous depression and 20 subjects with neurological disease. They found that the mean TRH levels were higher both before and after recovery in the affectively ill patient group compared with the neurological control subjects. Moreover, the mean TRH level did not differ significantly before and after treatment. Banki et al. (93) reported much higher cerebrospinal fluid TRH concentration in depressed patients compared with other patient groups. Furthermore, subjects with violent suicidal behavior had a tendency toward a particularly high level of TRH within the depressed group of patients. Although findings from these two studies (92,93) are relatively consistent, the potential importance of elevated TRH levels as a state versus trait marker, as well as its relationship to other abnormalities of thyroid function tests observed in depressed patients, remain to be clarified. In a postmortem study, Biggins et al. (94) reported no significant difference in the TRH levels in the amygdala of subjects with schizophrenia and Alzheimer's disease compared with those of subjects with depression. This study, taking into account all the limitations of a postmortem study, suggests that the specificity of alterations of TRH levels in the central nervous system for depression requires further study.

In summary, there is an extensive, often conflicting, literature on thyroid hormone levels in depressed patients. Despite the apparently inconclusive data, there are certain consistent findings that emerge. First, most patients with primary affective illness have circulating thyroid hormone levels that are in the euthyroid range. Only a minority of patients have evidence of clinical or subclinical hypothyroidism. Second, only in a minority of patients does subclinical hypothyroidism contribute to the pathophysiology and treatment of primary affective disorder. Furthermore, subclinical hypothyroidism may be more relevant to patients with bipolar rather than unipolar disorder. Last, the substantial decrements in T_4 and FT_4 that occur with antidepressant treatment are the most consistently observed alteration in thyroid function tests in patients with primary affective illness. This finding has been observed in almost all of the studies to date (see Table 6–2).

Decrements in measures of T_4 may be particularly relevant to patients with unipolar disorder, and the opposite effect may occur in subjects with bipolar disorder in which increases in peripheral thyroid function tests may be associated with treatment response (95). This potential difference in changes in thyroid function tests with treatment between unipolar and bipolar depression would not be inconsistent with a whole range of biological variables that distinguish bipolar from unipolar affective disorder (96). Furthermore, it may explain potential discrepancies in understanding the use of various thyroid hormones to augment response to antidepressant and mood-stabilizing treatments (see section 5).

Although the decrements in thyroid function tests are substantial, they occur within the euthyroid range. Nonetheless, these changes may be of importance to the regulation of cerebral function and, therefore, alterations of mood. Recent studies suggest that thyroid hormones have a direct and important effect on mature brain function. Furthermore, small changes in thyroid hormone levels, within the euthyroid range for peripheral organs such as liver and kidney, may have significant effects on cerebral thyroid function, which may manifest as alterations in mood, behavior, and cognition.

The evidence for a direct effect of thyroid hormone on brain is as follows. First, the nuclear T_3 receptor, the site of initiation of thyroid hormone action, occurs widely throughout mature brain (97). Second, Dratman and her co-workers (98,99) have shown that thyroid hormones are concentrated in discrete regions of the brain in synaptosomes, suggesting that they may have important modulatory effects on neurotransmission. Last, homeostatic mechanisms, mediated by both brain and liver, have been described that are extremely sensitive to small changes in cerebral thyroid hormone levels (100–106). Because the brain appears to be responsive to small changes in thyroid hormone levels, it can be assumed that the changes in thyroid function with antidepressant treatments would have significant effects on cerebral function.

However, the pathophysiological significance of these data has been interpreted in different ways, leading to two opposing hypotheses about the role of thyroid hormones in the etiology of affective illness (5,6). According to the first hypothesis, the increases in measures of T_4 observed in depression are a compensatory response on the part of the thyroid axis that occurs in order to maintain affective homeostasis. This theory, proposed by Bauer and Whybrow (5), maintains that thyroid hormones are mobilized during the depressed phase so as to allow for normalization of depressed mood. This hypothesis is based on the assumption that increases in thyroid function favor recovery from depression and are consistent with the observations from patients with clinical thyroid disorders (1–3). The early clinical findings were that hypothyroidism was associated with depression and that thyroid replacement resulted in alleviation of the psychiatric symptoms (2,3). This has led to the widely accepted hypothesis that decreases in thyroid hormones increase vulnerability to depression whereas increases in thyroid hormone promote recovery from depression (107).

Bauer and Whybrow (5) have proposed several observations from the accumulated research data to support their hypothesis. First, they point to the many previous studies that show relative increases in measures of T_4 in depressed patients (Tables 6–1 and 6–2). Second, earlier studies from their group reported that increases in tissue indicators of thyroid hormone activity predict response to antidepressants (9). This finding suggests that mobilization of T_4 is required for antidepressant response (9). Last, the consensus of studies showing that measures of T_4 decrease with antidepressant treatment (Table 6–2) also supports their formulation that increased mobilization of thyroid activity during depression is both a promoter and a predictor of favorable response to antidepressant treatment (5).

We have suggested an alternative hypothesis (37) based on similar data used to argue for the hypothesis of Bauer and Whybrow (5). We have proposed that depression is a state of relative hyperthyroidism and that the depressed state is associated with relative increases in circulating levels of T_4. We have also proposed that substantial, but limited, decrements in circulating T_4 are required for antidepressant response (37). In other words, the relative increases in T_4 in depression are interpreted as being compensatory according to the first hypothesis (5) and pathological according to our theory (37). The results of the three studies (28,32,36) that show that greater decrements in T_4 and measures of FT_4 occur in patients who respond compared with those who do not respond to antidepressants are consistent with our hypothesis. Our theory (37) only explains the alterations in thyroid function tests that occur in the euthyroid range. It does not attempt to directly explain the well-described association between clinical hypothyroidism and depression (2,3). Nonetheless, patients with clinical thyroid disorders suffer from profound metabolic and hormonal derangements, and the resultant effects on cerebral function may not necessarily be directly comparable to the subtle clinical effects that occur with smaller changes in cerebral thyroid function with depression and with antidepressant response.

Further studies are required to evaluate both these conflicting hypotheses (5,37). These studies should involve several strategies, including longitudinal clinical studies in which the relationship between changes in thyroid function tests and alterations in mood are evaluated in a careful, prospective manner. In addition, the effect of pharmacological agents that increase or decrease thyroid function without necessarily having specific psychotropic effects should be examined to evaluate their effects on mood and cognition. Regardless of which hypothesis clarifies the role of thyroid hormones in the pathophysiology of mood disorders, several studies in humans confirm that small alterations in thyroid function are of significance. A 1984 study (108) showed that, in healthy volunteers, the normal variations in thyroid hormone levels are closely related to alterations in specific cognitive and electrophysiological parameters. Another study (109) showed that alteration of carbohydrate intake in the diet may lead to small alterations in thyroid function that lead to changes in mood. Furthermore, investigators (110,111) have found that patients with grade II or III subclinical hypothyroidism have been observed to have significant impairment of memory and other cognitive functions.

3.2 Thyrotropin-Releasing Hormone (TRH) Test

The TRH test is the measurement of serum TSH levels following the administration of TRH. This is a widely used, standard endocrine procedure. In recent years, it has become extensively used in psychiatric patients, particularly in those patients with affective disorders (104,112–114).

a. Technique

The technique used in psychiatric patients follows the general principles established for endocrine patients (115,116). Therefore, the TRH is usually administered intravenously over about 1 minute to a patient who is in the recumbent position at approximately 9 A.M. after an overnight fast (113–116). The dose of TRH administered is usually 500 μg, although this has varied between 200 and 500 μg in the various studies. A dose of 500 μg was suggested in order to provide a dose that produces a slightly supramaximal stimulus to TSH because there appears to be a linear TSH response to TRH between doses of 100 and 400 μg, above which a plateau in response is reached (117,118). This supramaximal dose is proposed to have two advantages. First, it provides the opportunity of observing a behavioral effect of the administration of TRH. Second, it avoids the possibility of observing a false-positive blunting of the TSH response by using a submaximal dose.

The interpretation of the TRH test has also been quite variable in the psychiatric literature. The most useful approach appears to be to define the frequency of blunting of the TSH response to TRH in a particular sample. The comparison of mean TSH responses between various groups does not appear to be particularly helpful as it does not clearly distinguish different diagnostic groups and does not firmly establish that an abnormality of this test exists in patients with primary affective disorder. In fact, two studies (119,120) have shown that although group means in TSH levels did not clearly differentiate depressed patients from control subjects, the frequency of blunting of the TRH test clearly distinguished these groups. In the original studies (113,114), it was suggested that a maximum change in TSH response of less than 5 units should be defined as a blunted response. This definition of blunting was said to reliably distinguish depressed patients from healthy control subjects (114,115). However, in the large number of studies that have examined the TRH test in depression, the definition of blunting has varied widely. The definition of blunting used by investigators has ranged from a maximum TSH response of less than 2 μU/ml to one of less than 7μU/ml.

b. **Factors affecting the thyrotropin-releasing hormone (TRH) test**

Several factors may affect the interpretation of the TRH test. With regard to demographic variables, increasing age (120,121) and male sex (122) may diminish the TSH response. Several medical conditions may also reduce the TSH response regardless of psychiatric diagnosis, including fasting (123), renal failure (124), hepatic failure (125), and Klinefelter's syndrome (125). In addition, various hormones and neurochemicals may also cause blunting of this test, including administration of dopamine (126,127), glucocorticoids (128), and the peptides, neurotensin (129) and somatostatin (130). Of course, administration of thyroid hormones may also normalize the TRH-stimulated TSH response in both healthy control subjects and patients with psychiatric and endocrine disorders (128). Drugs such as lithium, the anticonvulsants, and even the antipsychotics may also affect the interpretation of this test (124).

In addition to these various factors that may affect the TRH test, there are technical difficulties in its interpretation. In particular, until recently, the TSH radioimmunoassay was not particularly sensitive at these low levels of measurement, which could account for some of the variance observed in the results of research studies to date. Recently, a more sensitive immunoradiometric TSH assay has been developed that allows for greater sensitivity in measurement of very low serum levels of TSH.

c. **Diagnosis of depression**

A large number of studies involving several thousand patients have examined the frequency of a blunted TRH test response in depressed patients (for reviews, see 113,114). By the various definitions of blunting used in these studies, approximately 25%–30% of depressed patients have been reported to have a blunted TSH response to TRH.

Studies have clearly shown that the blunted TRH-stimulated TSH levels are not specific for depression. They have been observed in a variety of other disorders including alcoholism (131, 132); borderline personality disorder, even in the absence of depression (133); and chronic pain syndromes (134). Furthermore, a delayed or blunted TSH response to TRH occurs in patients with anorexia nervosa (135,136). On the other hand, a blunted TRH test response is seen uncommonly in patients with schizophrenia (137,138). Because patients with mania tend to have a higher frequency of blunted responses (137,138), it has been suggested that this test may be of some clinical use in distinguishing patients with psychotic mania from those with schizophrenia. In this regard, earlier studies involving small samples suggested that the TRH test may distinguish unipolar from bipolar depression (139,140). Data from these studies indicated that the TSH response would be blunted in unipolar depression but augmented in bipolar depression. Subsequent studies (113,114) have failed to confirm these preliminary observations.

It has been suggested that TSH blunting may occur not only in the acute depressed state but also after recovery. In other words, it has been postulated that a blunted TRH test response is not only a state marker but also a trait marker for depression. Several studies (24,141–147) have shown that in a substantial proportion of patients, perhaps as many as one-half, a blunted TSH response persists even after remission from the depression. It has been concluded from these studies that a blunted TRH test response may be a trait marker for vulnerability to depression.

Because of its low frequency of occurrence, a blunted TRH test response probably has limited clinical use in the diagnosis of depression or in its differentiation from other psychiatric disorders. However, several studies have examined whether the TRH test may be useful in predicting either whether a depressed patient will respond to antidepressant treatment or whether, once they have responded, they are more likely to relapse after remission.

Although the data are inconclusive as to whether a blunted TRH test response predicts response to an antidepressant (148, 149), there is a consensus among several studies (146,149–151) that failure of normalization of a blunted TSH response after recovery from depression predicts early relapse for such patients. These observations may have clinical application. Krog-Meyer et al. (151) observed that the early relapse predicted by a blunted TRH test response could be prevented by long-term treatment with amitriptyline.

Several clinical correlates of a blunted TRH test have been reported, including chronicity of depression (152), associated anxiety disorder (153), and a history of violent suicidal behavior (154,155). Differences in diagnostic criteria for major depression may also affect the frequency of a blunted test (156).

In summary, there is convincing evidence that an abnormality of the TSH response to TRH occurs in a substantial minority of depressed patients. Although this test is of limited clinical use, it provides further evidence that abnormalities of the thyroid axis are associated with primary affective illness. Further studies in which both the techniques to administer the test and the definition of blunting are well standardized are required to elucidate the clinical correlates of this abnormality in depressed patients and its potential use in predicting response to treatment and subsequent relapse.

d. Pathophysiology

The etiological factors involved in a blunted TRH test response are poorly understood. However, several biological mechanisms have been postulated to explain this abnormality in patients with depression.

First, it has been suggested that an abnormal TSH response to TRH may reflect abnormalities of brain function. The hypothalamic-pituitary-thyroid axis, like other endocrine systems, provides a "window" for studying abnormalities of brain, particularly neurotransmitter, function (157). Various neurotransmitters (e.g., acetylcholine, serotonin, norepinephrine, and dopamine), as well as several neuropeptides (e.g., somatostatin and neurotensin), will affect the thyroid axis. Therefore, it is possible that abnormalities of these various neurochemicals in brain may lead to alterations in various measures of thyroid function including the TRH test (113,114). It is, of course, extremely difficult to infer exactly which neurochemical abnormality may result in an abnormal TRH test response because each of these neurotransmitters has complex interactions with each other and affects the thyroid axis at many levels (113,114). Several studies have attempted to evaluate the relationship between the TSH response to TRH and various measures of monoamine function. Although the TSH response to TRH is affected by norepinephrine, serotonin, and dopamine, studies that have examined the relationship between various measures of these monoamines and a blunted TRH test response have been largely inconclusive (158–162). With regard to the neuropeptides, somatostatin inhibits the TSH response to TRH.

However, most studies (163,164) have reported low cerebrospinal fluid somatostatin levels in depressed patients, which is not consistent with a blunted TSH response. Therefore, the role of somatostatin in this abnormality in patients with depression requires further study. Although neurotensin is also known to blunt the TSH response to TRH in animal studies (165), its potential role in affecting the thyroid axis in humans has not been studied.

Second, there are several lines of evidence that suggest that a blunted TRH test response may be due to chronic and excessive hypersecretion of TRH. Several studies (166–173) have examined the effects of chronic administration of exogenous TRH in healthy control subjects. The data from these studies show variable increases in circulating levels of peripheral thyroid hormones, particularly T_4, loss of the diurnal TSH rhythm, and blunting of the TSH response to TRH. These observations are similar to the various abnormalities of thyroid functions reported in depressed patients (Tables 6–1 and 6–7). Unfortunately, studies that have examined chronic administration of TRH in control subjects failed to carefully evaluate potential concomitant changes in mental state. Future studies should assess the relationship between changes in thyroid function and potential alterations in affective and cognitive state with chronic TRH administration in healthy control subjects.

Third, it is possible that a blunted TRH test response represents a form of subclinical hyperthyroidism that would be analogous to grade II subclinical hypothyroidism (57). It may be postulated that, at least in a subgroup of depressed patients, there is a relative increase in thyroid function that is associated with a blunting of the TRH test and increases in circulating thyroid hormone levels even though they remain within the normal range. This hypothesis would be consistent with the studies reviewed in Table 6–2, which suggest that depression is associated with relative increases in measures of T_4 and FT_4. It would also be consistent with the hypothesis (described above) that depression is a state of TRH hypersecretion. If this were the case, it would follow that the relative increases in thyroid function may be of central origin. In support of this hypothesis is the finding, in some studies, that a blunted TRH test response is related to increased levels of circulating T_4 (174,175). Furthermore, the TSH response to TRH has also been shown to be related to basal levels of circulating thyroid hormones in healthy control subjects (116). Although many studies in depressed patients do not show such a relationship (reviewed in 113,114), the association between relative increases in circulating T_4 and a blunted TRH test response in both depressed patients (174,175) and healthy control subjects (116) suggests that, in at least some patients, a blunted TRH test response may reflect a state of relative hyperactivity of the thyroid axis. This hypothesis is further supported by the recent observation by Kirkegaard et al. (176), using radiolabeled T_4, that there is an increased production of T_4 in depressed patients compared with healthy control subjects. On the other hand, a blunted TSH response has also been reported to be associated with low levels of T_4 and T_3 (113), indicating some disturbance of feedback inhibition in the regulation of the thyroid axis. Other abnormalities of thyroid function associated with a blunted TRH test response support such a hypothesis (114), although the specific inhibitor of thyroid axis regulation is unknown.

The last hypothesis to explain a blunted TRH test response is that this abnormality of the thyroid axis may reflect abnormalities of other endocrine systems. These may include other pituitary abnormalities or dysregulation of the hypothalamic-pituitary-adrenal axis. (For an extensive review, see Chapter 3.)

4. EFFECT OF SOMATIC TREATMENT ON THYROID FUNCTION TESTS

In addition to the various abnormalities of thyroid function tests reported in the depressed and remitted state, it has been shown that a wide variety of treatments proven effective in affective illness may have effects on the thyroid axis. In the sections that follow, we discuss the effect of each of these treatments on thyroid function.

4.1 Antidepressants

Both animal and human studies have shown that antidepressants, particularly tricyclics and electroconvulsive therapy (ECT) have consistent effects on thyroid function tests.

Earlier studies (177–179) involving less than 10 subjects each reported no effect of tricyclic antidepressants on thyroid function tests in depressed patients. However, these studies were limited by several methodological problems, including small sample sizes and failure to distinguish patients who respondedxto antidepressants from those who did not in assessing the effect of these drugs on thyroid hormone levels. Later studies (32,35,36) clearly suggested that response to tricyclic antidepressants is associated with decreases in T_4 and measures of FT_4 without a consistent effect on T_3 or TSH. The animal studies (180–183) support the clinical data. A variety of measures of thyroid function have been shown to decrease with chronic antidepressant treatment in several animal species (178–181).

Many of the clinical studies reviewed in Table 6–2 also support the notion that ECT is associated with substantial decrements in measures of T_4 without significantly affecting TSH levels (24–27,29,30). The animal studies using electroconvulsive shock are less conclusive (183–185). Many of these studies have evaluated the acute effects of electroconvulsive shock on the secretion of pituitary hormones including TSH (184). Studies in animals that have examined longer-term effects of electroconvulsive shock on thyroid function have been inconsistent, but have generally observed some evidence of decreased thyroid function reflected either as decreases in peripheral hormones or as increases in TSH (183,184).

In the only study to date that has evaluated the effect of monoamine oxidase inhibitors on thyroid function (31), we observed no effect of 4 weeks of phenelzine treatment on thyroid function tests in 16 depressed patients. As previously noted, the small sample size and resultant failure to distinguish patients who responded to treatment from those who did not in this study may have favored a negative result. Further studies in both animals and clinical populations are required to evaluate the effects of this class of monoamine oxidase inhibitor on peripheral thyroid hormone levels. In clinical samples, particular attention should be paid to the relationship between alterations in thyroid function and antidepressant response.

In summary, most studies to date suggest that treatment with a variety of antidepressants leads to substantial decrements in thyroid function tests. Because these decreases in thyroid function appear related to antidepressant response, it is likely that the effect of these drugs is due to a change in clinical state rather than a direct, intrinsic effect of the antidepressant on the thyroid axis.

4.2 Lithium

Soon after it was established that lithium was effective in the treatment of manic-depressive illness, its effects on the thyroid gland were observed (186). Since then, the effects of this compound on different aspects of thyroid function have been extensively examined in both animal and human studies.

Lithium has been shown to affect many stages in the production of thyroid hormones, including reduction in iodine uptake by the thyroid gland (187,188), inhibition of thyroid hormone production at various stages of synthesis (187,188), and blocking of the secretion of thyroid hormone (187,189–191). Studies suggest that lithium has its greatest inhibitory effect on the release of thyroid hormones, rather than on other stages of thyroid hormone production (189). In addition, lithium is a potent inhibitor of the conversion, by monodeiodination, of T_4 to T_3 (192). In addition to its direct effects on thyroid hormone production and release at the level of the thyroid gland, studies (193,194) suggest that lithium may have inhibitory effects on both TRH and TSH levels, indicating that it may diminish thyroid function by altering feedback mechanisms at several levels of the thyroid axis.

The effect of lithium on thyroid function tests has been extensively studied in both healthy volunteers and patients with affective illness. Data from healthy volunteers (195–199) have shown that up to 6 weeks of treatment with lithium leads to limited decreases in peripheral thyroid hormone levels with increases in basal or TRH-stimulated TSH levels. The data from studies examining short-term effects of lithium in patients with affective illness are consistent with those in healthy volunteers and confirm the thyrostatic effects of lithium (194,200–205). All these studies suggest that lithium treatment for up to 4–6 weeks is associated with decreases in measures of peripheral thyroid function with compensatory increases in TSH levels (194, 200–205). These studies (194–205) of acute lithium treatment in both healthy volunteers and clinical samples are summarized in Table 6–8. If changes in thyroid function are followed over a 3-month period, thyroid function tends to normalize as the increases in TSH levels restore normal circulating peripheral thyroid hormone levels (204).

Table 6–8. Acute effects of lithium on thyroid function

Study	Subjects	Controls	Measures	Result
Normal				
Halmi and Noyes 1972 (195)	6 male volunteers	—	T_4, baseline and 14 days	Decreased T_4
Kirkegaard et al. 1973 (196)	8 volunteers	—	T_3, baseline and 3 weeks	No change
Lauridsen et al. 1974 (197)	8 volunteers	—	T_4, T_3, T_3RU, TSH, basal and stimulated, baseline and 3 weeks	Increased TSH response to TRH
Child et al. 1977 (198)	4 volunteers	—	T_4, T_3, TSH and thyroid size, baseline and 6 weeks	Increased TSH and thyroid size
Perrild et al. 1984 (199)	16 volunteers	—	T_4, TSH basal and stimulated, iodine uptake and thyroid volume, baseline and 4 weeks	Decreased T_4, increased TSH, iodine uptake, thyroid volume
Clinical				
Sedvall et al. 1968 (200)	14 manic-depressive subjects on lithium 7–20 days	11 healthy volunteers	PBI, T_3RU iodine uptake	Decreased PBI, increased uptake
Cooper and Simpson 1969 (201)	25 manic-depressive subjects on lithium several weeks	139 psychiatric control subjects not on lithium	PBI, FT_4, iodine uptake	Decreased PBI and FT_4, increased uptake
Burrow et al. 1971 (202)	9 manic-depressive subjects	—	PBI and TSH before and after 4 weeks	Decreased PBI
Fyrö et al. 1973 (203)	43 manic-depressive subjects on lithium 2 weeks	17 healthy control subjects on lithium 2 weeks	PBI, T_3RU, iodine uptake	Decreased PBI, increased uptake
Emerson et al. 1973 (204)	27 manic-depressive subjects on lithium 1–3 months	27 healthy control subjects and 38 psychiatric control subjects not on lithium	T_4, TSH	Increased TSH, slight decrease in T_4
Rifkin et al. 1974 (205)	11 character disorder subjects	—	PBI, T_4 before and after 6 weeks	Decreased PBI and T_4
Bakker 1982 (194)	7 affective illness subjects	—	TSH stimulated, baseline and 6 weeks of lithium	Increased TSH response

Note. T_4 = thyroxine; T_3 = triiodothyronine; T_3RU = triiodothyronine resin uptake; TSH = thyroid-stimulating hormone; TRH = thyrotropin-releasing hormone; PBI = protein-bound iodine; FT_4 = free thyroxine.

Despite this normalization of thyroid function tests over several months of treatment, the acute effects of lithium on thyroid function are similar to those observed with other antidepressant treatments. Furthermore, Page et al. (206) reported that response to lithium treatment in patients with primary affective illness is directly related to decrements in thyroid function tests.

Although most patients tolerate long-term lithium treatment well and show minimal evidence of clinical thyroid dysfunction, it is well known that a substantial minority of patients on long-term lithium treatment will develop evidence of clinical hypothyroidism. Studies (68–71,194,204,207–227) that have examined the prevalence of hypothyroidism in patients on long-term lithium therapy are reviewed in Table 6–9. Although the reported prevalence varies considerably in the different studies (from none to 47%), this may be due to methodological issues such as the sample size used, the duration of lithium treatment at the time of thyroid hormone measurement, and the diagnostic types of patients included in the study. Collectively, these studies suggest that approximately 5%–10% of patients who receive long-term lithium treatment will develop evidence of clinical hypothyroidism.

It is unknown why some patients become hypothyroid whereas the majority are able to compensate for the effects of lithium on the thyroid axis. Two possible explanations have been suggested. First, it is possible that iodine and lithium act synergistically to produce hypothyroidism (228,229). Therefore, variability in iodine intake may be a risk factor for the development of hypothyroidism in lithium-treated patients.

Second, it has been suggested that the hypothyroidism associated with lithium treatment may be due to autoimmune phenomena. This second hypothesis is based on the observation from several cross-sectional studies that there is a high prevalence of positive thyroid antibody titers in lithium-treated patients, especially in those who develop hypothyroidism (210,211,218). Furthermore, some (230,231), but not all (232), studies suggest that an increased titer of thyroid antibodies develops with long-term lithium treatment. Unfortunately, these studies (230,231) have compared antibodies at two points during lithium treatment rather than before and after the initiation of lithium therapy. This methodological factor may account for the inconclusive results to date (230–232).

Although there is no doubt that lithium does affect immune function (230–232), the role of autoimmune thyroiditis in the etiology of lithium-induced hypothyroidism remains to be clarified. Furthermore, in most but not all cases, the discontinuation of lithium treatment will result in reversal of the hypothyroidism (194), which would not be expected if it was due to an autoimmune process. In those

Table 6–9.   Hypothyroidism with chronic lithium treatment

Study	N patients	Prevalence of hypothyroidism n	%
Hofman et al. 1970 (207)	119	0	0
Rogers and Whybrow 1971 (208)	19	0	0
Hullin et al. 1972 (209)	69	3	4.3
Lazarus and Bennie 1972 (210)	25	0	0
Tucker and Bell 1972 (211)	59	5	8.5
Emerson et al. 1973 (204)	255	6	2.1
Lindstedt et al. 1973 (212)	334	2	0.6
Villeneuve et al. 1974 (213)	149	22	14.7
Abuzzahab and Dahlam 1975 (214)	17	0	0
McLarty et al. 1975 (215)	17	2	11.7
Serry and Serry 1976 (216)	200	10	5
Williams and Gyory 1976 (217)	52	1	1.9
Lindstedt et al. 1977 (218)	53	8	15.1
Piziak et al. 1978 (219)	52	2	1.9
Transbol et al. 1978 (220)	86	20	23.3
Wasilewski et al. 1978 (221)	62	4	6.5
Botterman et al. 1979 (222)	88	0	0
Cho et al. 1979 (68)	195	7	3.6
Lazarus et al. 1981 (223)	73	1	1.4
Amdisen and Andersen 1982 (224)	237	10	4.2
Bakker 1982 (194)	13	0	0
Cowdry et al. 1983 (69)	43	12	27.9
Smigan et al. 1984 (225)	51	1	1.9
Maarbjerg et al. 1987 (226)	430	8	1.8
Wehr et al. 1988 (70)	70	33	47
Joffe et al. 1988 (71)	42	5	11.9
Yassa et al. 1988 (227)	116	9	7.8

patients in whom lithium cannot be discontinued, replacement therapy with L-T$_4$ is indicated. As previously discussed, patients with the rapid-cycling form of bipolar affective disorder may be particularly susceptible to lithium-induced hypothyroidism (Table 6–5).

There are practical implications of the varying effects of lithium on the thyroid axis. First, if patients develop clinical hypothyroidism, they require thyroid replacement therapy. However, the occurrence of this side effect does not indicate that lithium should be discontinued. Second, it follows from the data that cases of subclinical hypothyroidism on lithium therapy frequently occur. The approach to management is less certain than with clinical hypothyroidism. With very high levels of TSH, even in the presence of normal T$_4$ and T$_3$ levels, thyroid replacement appears warranted. With small increases in TSH, specific therapy is probably not indicated except in very treatment-resistant cases where an empirical trial of thyroid hormones, in addition to antidepressants or mood stabilizers, may be undertaken. In those cases in which thyroid hormones are not used, there should be regular monitoring of thyroid function tests, particularly T$_4$ and TSH, to detect the development of overt hypothyroidism. This monitoring is particularly pertinent in cases in which TSH elevation occurs in the presence of positive antithyroid antibodies (60).

The thyrostatic effects of lithium are well established. However, there is also preliminary evidence that hyperthyroidism may be occasionally associated with lithium treatment. Several clinical studies (233–243) have documented cases in which hyperthyroidism developed during lithium therapy. There is still no direct evidence that lithium, in fact, causes the overactivity of thyroid function, although it has been suggested that it may be due to lithium-induced immune dysfunction (233–243). Furthermore, exophthalmos not necessarily associated with thyroid hyperfunction has been reported in some patients on lithium treatment (244).

In conclusion, there is no doubt that lithium has widespread effects on thyroid function. Because of its predominantly thyrostatic effects, it has been used as a therapeutic agent in the treatment of hyperthyroidism. However, it has been found to be of limited use for various types of hyperthyroidism and is certainly not comparable in efficacy to standard antithyroid treatments (245).

4.3   Anticonvulsants

Several of the anticonvulsants, particularly carbamazepine and val-proic acid, have been shown to be effective in the acute and prophylactic treatment of patients with bipolar affective disorder. A number of studies have also shown that the anticonvulsants have effects on thyroid function. With regard to carbamazepine, a number of studies comparing epileptic patients receiving carbamazepine with healthy control subjects have reported substantially lower levels of T_4, FT_4, and T_3 but no significant alteration in TSH in the carbamazepine-treated group (246–248). Furthermore, T_4 and FT_4 have been found to decrease in studies examining changes in thyroid function in epileptic patients before and after taking carbamazepine (246–250). Cases of clinical hypothyroidism on carbamazepine have been very rarely reported (251). It has also been shown that carbamazepine causes a reduction in the TSH response to TRH in patients with epilepsy (252). Similar findings in epileptic patients have been observed for valproic acid (250,252), which has also been shown to be effective in the treatment of bipolar affective disorder, and for diphenylhydan-toin (253), although the utility of the latter drug in the treatment of affective illness remains uncertain.

We have extended the previous findings in epileptic patients to those with primary affective illness (28,254–257). We have observed that carbamazepine treatment is associated with a relative secondary hypothyroidism in that it causes substantial decrements in measures of T_4 and T_3 without affecting basal TSH levels. Moreover, it does cause a substantial reduction in the TRH-stimulated TSH response (28,254–257). We have further observed that response to carbamazepine in 50 patients with primary affective illness is associated with substantial decreases in measures of T_4 (28,254). The relationship between treatment response and decreases in thyroid function observed with carbamazepine (28,254) is consistent with the observed association between antidepressant response and changes in thyroid hormone levels with other antidepressant treatments in several studies to date (27,32,36). The effect of other anticonvulsants on thyroid function in affectively ill patients has not been systematically evaluated. It would be of particular interest to determine whether valproic acid has effects on thyroid function similar to those observed with carbamazepine in patients with primary affective disorder.

4.4 Sleep Deprivation

Total or partial sleep deprivation has been shown to be an effective antidepressant for patients with major depression in up to 60% of cases (258). Because this effect is usually transient, patients tend to relapse back into depression after a night of recovery sleep (258). Therefore, the antidepressant effect of sleep deprivation is of limited clinical use. Nonetheless, several studies have examined the effect of sleep deprivation on thyroid function in both healthy volunteers (259) and patients with major depression (260–264).

Palmblad et al. (259) observed increases in measures of both T_3 and T_4, as well as TSH, in 12 healthy male college students deprived of sleep for 48 hours. Because thyroid hormones are responsive to stress, it was suggested that this may be a nonspecific response to the stress of being kept awake for a prolonged period of time (259). All the studies (261–264) with depressed patients found a significant increase in TSH levels in both unipolar and bipolar depressed subjects. Although two of the studies (262,263) did not measure peripheral thyroid hormones, those that did (261,264) reported significant increases in measures of T_4 and T_3.

Despite this consensus about the effect of sleep deprivation on thyroid function, there is some disagreement about the relationship of changes in thyroid function to antidepressant response (261–263). Whereas Baumgartner and Meinhold (261) reported an association between changes in TSH and antidepressant response, the other three studies (260,263,264) did not find such a relationship. This lack of an association between changes in thyroid function and antidepressant response, together with similar changes in thyroid function with sleep deprivation in healthy volunteers (259), suggests that the changes observed may be a nonspecific stress response rather than due to changes in the mood state of the clinical samples. Although Kvist and Kirkegaard (260) did not specifically address the effect of sleep deprivation on thyroid function tests, they did report that absence of normalization of the TRH test with sleep deprivation predicted subsequent relapse.

5. THYROID HORMONE TREATMENT OF AFFECTIVE ILLNESS

5.1 Thyrotropin-Releasing Hormone (TRH)

TRH has effects on brain function that are independent of its effects on the thyroid axis (265). This peptide appears to have a wide range of effects on cerebral function including reversal of drug-induced sedation or anesthesia and stimulation of locomotor activity, as well as extensive effects on cardiorespiratory, gastrointestinal, and neurological functions (265–267). As a result of its widespread behavioral effects, in addition to its effects on thyroid function, it has been suggested that TRH may have antidepressant properties. Several studies (268–279) have evaluated the antidepressant effects of either intravenous or oral administration of TRH in depressed subjects (Table 6–10). The initial studies by Kastin et al. (268) and Prange et al. (269) reported that TRH administered intravenously as a single dose produced a transient antidepressant effect that was superior to placebo in a small number of patients. Subsequent studies (270–279) have reported no effect or a clinically insignificant therapeutic response to the administration of either oral or intravenous TRH administered for differing periods of time. It can, therefore, be concluded that TRH does not have a substantial antidepressant effect and that the behavioral changes noted in some patients may be more a nonspecific activating effect rather than a specific antidepressant response.

5.2 Thyroid-Stimulating Hormone (TSH)

Because TSH stimulates thyroid function, it has been postulated that it may have antidepressant activity. Only one study to date has assessed the effects of TSH on antidepressant response. Prange et al. (280) reported that a single dose of TSH 10 IU iv administered to depressed women the day before the initiation of a standard imipramine trial led to a much more rapid antidepressant response compared with saline. Although these data are intriguing, they require replication before one can conclude that TSH accelerates response to antidepressants.

5.3 Triiodothyronine (T$_3$)

T$_3$ has been used in two ways to promote response to antidepressants. First, four studies (280–283) have shown that the addition of up to 25

Table 6–10. Antidepressant effect of thyrotropin-releasing hormone (TRH)

Study	N patients	Design	Route of administration of TRH	Result
Kastin et al. 1972 (268)	5	Double-blind, placebo-controlled	500 μg iv for 3 days	Transient effect in 4 of 5 patients
Prange et al. 1972 (269)	10 8	Double-blind, placebo-controlled Single-blind	600 μg iv single dose 200–800 μg iv single dose	TRH superior to saline Improved
Coppen et al. 1974 (270)	10 12	Double-blind, placebo-controlled Double-blind, placebo-controlled	600 μg iv days 1 and 4 600 μg iv for 3 days	No effect No effect
Ehrsening et al. 1974 (271)	8	Double-blind, placebo-controlled	1,000 μg iv single dose	No effect
Hollister et al. 1974 (272)	31	Double-blind	600 μg iv on 3 occasions	No effect
Mountjoy et al. 1974 (273)	29	Double-blind, placebo-controlled	40 mg po for 7 days	No effect
van der Burgh et al. 1975 (274)	10	Double-blind	500 μg iv in 2 doses over 4 days	Minimal effect
Furlong et al. 1976 (275)	3	Double-blind	500 μg iv for 3 days	1 of 3 responded
Kieley et al. 1976 (276)	11	Double-blind, placebo-controlled	200–300 mg po for 30 days	No effect
van der Burgh et al. 1976 (277)	10	Double-blind, placebo-controlled	1,000 μg slow iv	Minimal effect
Vogel et al. 1977 (278)	15	Double-blind	500 μg iv for 3 days	No effect
Karlberg et al. 1978 (279)	12	Double-blind compared to amitriptyline	80 mg po TRH vs. 100 mg amitriptyline for 3 weeks	No significant difference

μg/day of T_3 will accelerate the response to imipramine or amitripty-line. This acceleration of antidepressant response has been observed to be more prominent in women than in men (280–283). The reasons for this sex difference are unclear. These studies were all done approx-imately 20 years ago and, therefore, require replication using current criteria for the diagnosis of depression and for the assessment of treat-ment response. It is of interest that more recent studies examining this phenomenon have not been published. It would be of considerable clinical and theoretical importance to firmly establish whether T_3 ac-celerates response to antidepressants. As there is considerable mor-bidity associated with the lag in onset of therapeutic response to the various classes of antidepressants, clarification of this question may have important clinical applications.

Several studies (284–293) have also examined the use of small amounts of T_3 to potentiate the response to tricyclic antidepressants in patients who are nonresponsive to treatment (Table 6–11). In both open and controlled studies using a variety of antidepressants, it has been consistently observed that approximately 55% of patients who are nonresponsive to tricyclic antidepressants will become responsive within 2–3 weeks after the addition of 25–50 μg of T_3 to their antide-pressant. This effect of T_3 does not appear to be related to sex or to clinical correlates such as the absence of anxiety or agitation.

A study by Gitlin et al. (292) failed to find a significant difference between T_3 and placebo in the potentiation of tricyclics. However, the authors used a 2-week crossover, double-blind design, which is ex-tremely problematic in the evaluation of antidepressant treatments. Furthermore, the 2-week active thyroid hormone treatment phase may have been inadequate to produce a response, as we (293) have observed that it may require up to 3 weeks to obtain an antide-pressant-potentiating effect with T_3. Although the antidepressant-augmentating effect of T_3 has been met with skepticism in the recent literature, the evidence from studies to date (see Table 6–11) strongly suggests that, at least for some, T_3 may convert patients who are non-responsive to antidepressant treatment to responsive patients. At the dose of T_3 used, there are limited side effects so that this strategy rep-resents a potentially safe, rapid, and effective means of managing pa-tients who fail to respond to standard tricyclic treatment. The use of

Table 6–11.   Triiodothyronine (T3) potentiation of tricyclic antidepressants

Study	N patients	Dose of T3 (μg)	Tricyclic	Design	Response
Earle 1970 (284)	25	25	Imipramine, amitriptyline	Open	14 of 25
Banki 1975 (285)	52	20–40	Mixed	Open	39 of 52
Banki 1977 (286)	33	20	Amitriptyline	Partially controlled	23 of 33
Ogura et al. 1974 (287)	44	20–30	Mixed	Open	29 of 44
Tsutsui et al. 1979 (288)	11	5–25	Mixed	Open	10 of 11
Goodwin et al. 1982 (289)	12	25–50	Mixed	Double-blind	8 of 12
Schwarcz et al. 1984 (290)	8	25–50	Desipramine	Open	4 of 8
Gitlin et al. 1987 (292)	16	25	Imipramine	Double-blind	No difference T3 vs. placebo
Thase et al. 1989 (291)	20	25	Imipramine	Open	5 of 20
Joffe and Singer 1990 (293)	38	37.5	Desipramine, imipramine	Double-blind	9 of 17 T3 vs. 4 of 21 T4

Note. T4 = thyroxine.

T_3 as compared with lithium augmentation in patients nonresponsive to tricyclics remains to be clarified. Nonetheless, there are preliminary data that suggest that patients who respond to these two different augmentation strategies may differ (294). In a recently completed double-blind, placebo-controlled study with 51 patients nonresponsive to tricyclics, we (R. T. Joffe, W. Singer, A. J. Levitt, unpublished data, December 1991) observed that T_3 and lithium had comparable efficacy in augmenting antidepressant response and both were more effective than placebo.

5.4 Thyroxine (T_4)

The initial studies (280–293) that used thyroid hormone to accelerate or potentiate antidepressant response used T_3. It was assumed that T_4 would have an effect similar to that of T_3 largely because it was thought that both would increase thyroid function, which was assumed to favor antidepressant response (5). Few studies, however, have specifically evaluated the efficacy of T_3 versus T_4 in the augmentation of antidepressant response. Targum (146) and collaborators found that 7 of 21 patients responded to augmentation with either T_3 or T_4. However, 5 of these 7 patients had evidence of subclinical hypothyroidism. Therefore, the use of either T_4 or T_3 may have been more as replacement treatment rather than as augmentation for the antidepressant therapy.

In the only study (293) to date that has systematically compared T_4 to T_3 augmentation of antidepressants in euthyroid depressed patients, T_3 was found to be much more effective than T_4. In this study, 38 patients with major depression who failed to respond to either desipramine or imipramine received a 3-week, double-blind trial of thyroid hormone augmentation. Four of 21 responded to T_4 versus 9 of 17 for T_3. There was a significant difference in the frequency of response between the two thyroid hormones ($P = .026$, Fisher Exact Test). Furthermore, mean changes in Hamilton depression scores were significantly greater ($P < .05$) in the T_3- versus the T_4-treated group.

There are several possible explanations for these findings. First, the substantially longer half-life of T_4 may mean that it takes much longer to observe an antidepressant-augmentating effect with T_4 (295). Even if this explanation were correct, it would still mean that T_3 was more clinically useful than T_4 because it would reduce the delay in observing the antidepressant-augmenting effect. However, as the intended alteration of thyroid function with each thyroid hormone was achieved early in the thyroid hormone trial (293), this explanation appears unlikely.

Second, the concurrent use of tricyclic antidepressants may inhibit the conversion of T_4 to T_3, which is required for the initiation of thyroid hormone action. If this were the case, levels of rT_3 would increase as this is the alternative pathway for metabolism of T_4 (295). This is also an unlikely explanation because rT_3 levels tend to decrease with antidepressant treatment (see Table 6–4).

Last, it is possible that T_4 and T_3 have differential effects on antidepressant augmentation. The difference in therapeutic effect of these hormones may be explained by their differential utilization in brain as compared with peripheral organs. In peripheral tissues such as liver and kidney, the T_3 that acts at the thyroid hormone receptor is derived from peripheral conversion of T_4 (100,295). In brain, however, approximately 80% of the T_3 in cortical neurons derives from the intracellular conversion of T_4 to T_3 (100). Hence, the major determinant of intracellular T_3 in peripheral organs is plasma T_3, whereas in brain, it is plasma T_4.

Although these data (100,295) are derived from animal studies, the physicochemical properties of thyroid hormones and their receptors in rats are similar to those in humans, and, therefore, these findings may apply across species. Based on these studies (100,295), we (37) have hypothesized that administration of T_3 by negative feedback on the thyroid axis lowers plasma T_4 levels and, therefore, makes less thyroid hormone available to the brain. Administration of T_4, however, increases plasma T_4 levels and therefore increases cerebral thyroid hormone levels. The resultant opposite effect of these two hormones on cerebral thyroid function may account for their differential antidepressant effects (37,293). If our hypothesis is correct, then it can also be suggested that T_3 potentiation of antidepressants acts by lowering cerebral thyroid hormone levels, which is consistent with the effect of other antidepressants (see Table 6–2). There are preliminary animal data to suggest that T_4 and T_3 may have differential effects on various aspects of brain function (296,297). Moreover, T_3 has been shown to reverse learned helplessness in rats (298).

Although preliminary data (293) suggest that T_4 is not as effective as T_3 in augmentation of antidepressants in patients with unipolar depression, there is also preliminary evidence that T_4 may be effective in the treatment of patients with bipolar affective disorder. Several case studies and an open trial (299) suggest that high doses of T_4, sufficient to induce a state of chemical hyperthyroidism, may decrease the frequency and severity of cycling in patients with bipolar affective disorder, particularly the rapid-cycling form. These initial findings suggest that high doses of T_4 are particularly useful when added to other mood-stabilizing agents such as lithium (300).

Although the data on the use of T_4 in unipolar versus bipolar patients appear to be conflicting, it is quite conceivable that T_4 may be effective in one group of affectively ill patients and not in others. Certainly, there are well-documented biological and clinical differences between unipolar and bipolar patients (96). Furthermore, there is also preliminary evidence that thyroid function differs in unipolar and bipolar subjects so that decreases in thyroid function favor recovery in the former group and increases in thyroid function favor recovery in the latter group (95). It is also important to note that the rapid-cycling group of bipolar patients, in which hypermetabolic T_4 may be particularly useful (299), are reported to have a high frequency of varying degrees of hypothyroidism, which may partially explain their response to thyroid hormone treatment (see Table 6–5).

6. CONCLUSIONS

We have summarized a vast literature on the relationship between primary affective illness and the thyroid axis. The initial assumption that there would be a direct and clear relationship between alterations of thyroid function and affective illness based on observations from clinical thyroid disorders has proved disappointingly incorrect. Nonetheless, although the literature is often conflicting, there are several consistent observations.

First, most patients with affective illness have normal thyroid function test responses. A significant minority do have varying degrees of hypothyroidism. This appears to be relevant to a small subgroup of patients with unipolar depression, but may be particularly pertinent to those bipolar patients with rapid-cycling illness. In this group of subjects, particularly those with subclinical forms of hypothyroidism, the efficacy of thyroid hormone treatment either as replacement or for augmentation of standard antidepressant or mood-stabilizing therapies appears promising.

Second, most studies concur that there are relative increases in measures of T_4, within the normal range, in patients who are depressed. This observation appears to hold whether depressed patients are compared with control subjects or thyroid function tests are compared before and after successful antidepressant treatment. It is uncertain whether these relative increases in T_4 are of etiological importance or secondary to the depression. There are opposing hypotheses in the literature to explain this phenomenon. Further studies are required to clarify the precise relationship between changes in T_4 levels and changes in clinical state. These issues could be resolved with careful prospective and longitudinal studies that carefully evaluate changes in thyroid function tests in relationship to changes in mental state.

Third, the various treatments used for patients with affective illness appear to have relatively consistent effects on thyroid function tests. The effects of lithium on thyroid function have been most extensively and best described. However, with some exceptions, other antidepressant and mood-stabilizing drugs appear to have effects similar to those of lithium, although treatment with these other agents has not been associated with the occurrence of clinical hypothyroidism.

Fourth, there is a definite place for the use of thyroid hormones, particularly T_3, in the treatment of affective disorders. At least in some depressed patients, T_3 may be valuable in converting patients who are nonresponsive to antidepressant treatment to responsive patients. There is also the intriguing possibility that this hormone may accelerate response to antidepressant treatment.

In conclusion, there is no doubt that thyroid hormones play an important part in the regulation of mood and are involved, to some extent, in the pathophysiology of mood disorders. Although there is an extensive literature, the precise relationship between alterations in thyroid functions and changes in mood has not been established. Future studies using more advanced and recently developed technologies will afford the opportunity to understand further how thyroid hormones affect brain function and whether they play a major role in the pathogenesis of mood disorders.

REFERENCES

1. Parry CH: Collections From the Unpublished Writings of the Late Caleb Hillier Parry, Vol 1. London, Underwoods, 1825
2. Clinical Society of London: Report of a committee nominated December 14, 1883 to investigate the subject of myxoedema. Transactions of the Clinical Society of London 21 (suppl), 1888
3. Asher R: Myxodematous madness. BMJ 2:555–562, 1949
4. Loosen PT: Hormones of the hypothalamic-pituitary-thyroid axis: a psychoneuroendocrine perspective. Pharmacopsychiatry 19:401–415, 1986
5. Bauer MS, Whybrow PC: Thyroid hormones and the central nervous system in affective illness: interactions that may have clinical significance. Integrative Psychiatry 6:75–100, 1988

6. Joffe RT: A perspective of the thyroid and depression. Can J Psychiatry 35:754–758, 1990

7. Board F, Wadeson R, Persky H: Depressive affect and endocrine functions. Archives of Neurology and Psychiatry 78:612–620, 1959

8. Dewhurst KE, Kabir DJ, Exley D, et al: Blood levels of thyrotropic hormone, protein-bound iodine, and cortisol in schizophrenia and affective states. Lancet 2:1160–1162, 1968

9. Whybrow PC, Coppen A, Prange AJ Jr, et al: Thyroid function and the response to liothyronine in depression. Arch Gen Psychiatry 26:242–245, 1972

10. Rybakowski J, Sowinski J: Free-thyroxine index and absolute free-thyroxine in affective disorders (letter). Lancet 1:889, 1973

11. Takahashi S, Kaondo H, Yoshimura M, et al: Thyrotropin responses to TRH in depressive illness: relationship to clinical subtypes after duration of depressive episode. Folia Psychiatrica Neurologica Japonica 28:255–265, 1974

12. Yamaguchi T, Nomura JA, Nishikubo M, et al: Studies on thyroid therapy and thyroid function in depressive patients. Folia Psychiatrica Neurologica Japonica 29:221–230, 1975

13. Kolakowska T, Swigar ME: Thyroid function in depression and alcohol abuse: a retrospective study. Arch Gen Psychiatry 34:984–988, 1977

14. Hatotani N, Nomura J, Yamaguchi T, et al: Clinical and experimental studies on the pathogenesis of depression. Psychoneuroendocrinology 2:115–130, 1977

15. Rinieris PM, Christodoulou CN, Souvatzoglou GA, et al: Thyroid function in primary depression. Acta Psychiatr Belg 78:248–255, 1978

16. Linnoila M, Lamberg BA, Rosberg G, et al: Thyroid hormones and TSH, prolactin and LH responses to repeated TRH and LRH injections in depressed patients. Acta Psychiatr Scand 59:536–544, 1979

17. Nordgren L, van Scheele VC: Nortriptyline and pituitary-thyroid function in affective disorder. Pharmacopsychiatry 40:61–65, 1981

18. Targum SD, Sullivan C, Burnes SM: Compensating pituitary-thyroid mechanisms in major depressive disorder. Psychiatry Res 6:85–96, 1982

19. Joffe RT, Blank DW, Post RM, et al: Decreased triiodothyronines in depression: a preliminary report. Biol Psychiatry 20:922–925, 1985

20. Orsulak BJ, Crowley G, Schlesser MA, et al: Free triiodothyronine (T_3) and thyroxine (T_4) in a group of unipolar depressed patients and normal subjects. Biol Psychiatry 20:1047–1054, 1985

21. Wahby V, Ibrahim G, Friedenthal S, et al: Serum concentrations of circulating thyroid hormones in a group of depressed men. Neuropsychobiology 22:8–10, 1989

22. Gibbons JL, Gibson JG, Maxwell AE, et al: An endocrine study of depressive illness. J Psychosom Res 5:32–41, 1960

23. Ferrari G: On some biochemical aspects of affective disorders. Revista Sperimentale Di Freniatriae: Medicina Legale Delle Alienazioni Mentali 93:1167–1175, 1973

24. Kirkegaard C, Norlem N, Lauridsen UB, et al: Protirelin stimulation test and thyroid function during treatment of depression. Arch Gen Psychiatry 32:1115–1118, 1975

25. Kirkegaard C, Norlem N, Lauridsen UB, et al: Prognostic value of thyrotropin releasing hormone stimulation test in endogenous depression. Acta Psychiatr Scand 52:170–177, 1975

26. Kirkegaard C, Bjorum N, Cohn N, et al: Studies on the influence of biogenic amines and psychoactive drugs on the prognostic value of the TRH stimulation test in endogenous depression. Psychoneuroendocrinology 2:131–136, 1977

27. Kirkegaard C, Faber J: Altered serum levels of thyroxine, triiodothyronines and diiodothyronines in endogenous depression. Acta Endocrinol (Copenh) 96:199–207, 1981

28. Roy-Byrne PP, Joffe RT, Uhde TW, et al: Effects of carbamazepine on thyroid function in affectively ill patients: clinical and theoretical implications. Arch Gen Psychiatry 41:1150–1153, 1984

29. Kirkegaard C, Faber J: Influence of free-thyroid hormone levels on the TSH response to TRH in endogenous depression. Psychoneuroendocrinology 11:491–497, 1986

30. Unden F, Ljunggren JG, Kjellman BF, et al: Twenty-four hour serum levels of T_4 and T_3 in relation to decreased TSH serum levels and decreased TSH response to TRH in affective disorders. Acta Psychiatr Scand 73:358–365, 1986

31. Joffe RT, Singer W: Effect of phenelzine on thyroid function in depressed patients. Biol Psychiatry 22:1033–1034, 1987

32. Baumgartner A, Graf KJ, Kurten I, et al: Repeated measurements of thyroxine, free-thyroxine, triiodothyronine and reverse triiodothyronine in patients with major depressive disorder and schizophrenia and in healthy subjects. Psychiatry Res 24:283–305, 1988

33. Muller B, Boning GJ: Changes in the pituitary-thyroid axis accompanying major affective disorders. Acta Psychiatr Scand 77:143–150, 1988

34. Brady KT, Anton RF: The thyroid axis and desipramine treatment in depression. Biol Psychiatry 25:703–709, 1989

35. Mason JW, Kennedy JL, Kosten TR, et al: Serum thyroxine levels in schizophrenic and affective disorder diagnostic subgroups. J Nerv Ment Dis 177:351–358, 1989

36. Joffe RT, Singer W: Effect of tricyclic antidepressants on thyroid hormone levels in depressed patients. Pharmacopsychiatry 23:67–69, 1990

37. Joffe RT, Roy-Byrne PP, Uhde TW, et al: Thyroid function and affective illness: a reappraisal. Biol Psychiatry 19:1685–1691, 1984

38. McLarty BG, Ratcliffe WA, Ratcliffe JG, et al: A study of thyroid function in psychiatric inpatients. Br J Psychiatry 133:211–218, 1978

39. Cohen RKL, Swigar ME: Thyroid function screening in psychiatric patients. JAMA 242:254–257, 1979

40. Levy RP, Jensen JB, Laus VG: Serum thyroid hormone abnormalities in psychiatric disease. Metabolism 30:1060–1064, 1981

41. Morley JE, Shafer RB: Thyroid function screening in new psychiatric admissions. Arch Intern Med 142:591–593, 1982

42. Spratt DI, Pont A, Miller MB, et al: Hyperthyroxinemia in patients with acute psychiatric disorders. Am J Med 73:41–48, 1982

43. Caplan RH, Pagliara AS, Wickus G, et al: Elevation of free-thyroxine index in psychiatric patients. J Psychiatr Res 17:267–274, 1982/83

44. Kramlinger KG, Gharib M, Swanson DW, et al: Normal serum thyroxine values in patients with acute psychiatric illness. Am J Med 76:799–801, 1984

45. Styra R, Joffe RT, Singer W: Transient hyperthyroxinemia in patients with primary affective disorder. Acta Psychiatr Scand 83:61–63, 1991

46. Chopra IJ, Solomon DH, Huang TS: Serum thyrotropin in hospitalized psychiatric patients: evidence for hyperthyrotropinemia as measured by an ultrasensitive thyrotropin assay. Metabolism 39:538–543, 1990

47. Joffe RT, Levitt AJ: Thyroid function and psychotic depression. Psychiatry Res 33:321–322, 1990

48. Joffe RT, Levitt AJ: Major depression and sub-clinical (Grade II) hypothyroidism. Psychoneuroendocrinology (in press)

49. Schimmel M, Utiger RD: Thyroidal and peripheral production of thyroid hormones. Ann Intern Med 87:760–765, 1977

50. Shulkin BL, Utiger RD: Reverse triiodothyronine does not alter pituitary-thyroid function in normal subjects. J Clin Endocrinol Metab 58:1184–1187, 1984

51. Kaplan MN, Yaskoski KA: Phenolic and tyrosyl ring deiodination of iodothyronines in rat brain homogenates. J Clin Invest 66:551–556, 1980

52. Nishikawa M, Inada M, Naito K, et al: 3,3',5'-triiodothyronine (reverse T_3) in human cerebrospinal fluid. J Clin Endocrinol Metab 53:1030–1034, 1981

53. Linnoila M, Lamberg BA, Potter WZ, et al: High reverse T_3 levels in manic and unipolar depressed women. Psychiatry Res 6:271–276, 1982

54. Linnoila M, Cowdry R, Lamberg BA, et al: CSF triiodothyronine (rT_3) levels in patients with affective disorders. Biol Psychiatry 18:1489–1492, 1983

55. Kjellman BF, Ljunggren JG, Beck-Friis J, et al: Reverse T_3 levels in affective disorders. Psychiatry Res 10:1–9, 1983

56. Wenzel KW, Meinhold D, Raffenberg N, et al: Classification of hypothyroidism in evaluating patients of radioiodine therapy by serum cholesterol T_3 uptake, total T_4, FT_4 index, total T_3, basal TSH and TRH test. Eur J Clin Invest 4:141–150, 1974

57. Evered DC, Ormston BJ, Smith PA: Grades of hypothyroidism. BMJ 1:657–659, 1973

58. Haggerty JJ Jr, Garbutt JC, Evans DL, et al: Subclinical hypothyroidism: a review of neuropsychiatric aspects. Int J Psychiatry Med 20:193–208, 1990

59. Tunbridge WMG, Brews M, French JM, et al: Natural history of autoimmune thyroiditis. BMJ 282:258–265, 1981
60. Cooper DS: Subclinical hypothyroidism (editorial). JAMA 258:246–247, 1987
61. Bigos ST, Ridgeway EC, Kourides IA, et al: A spectrum of pituitary alterations with mild and severe thyroid impairment. J Clin Endocrinol Metab 46:317–325, 1978
62. Cooper DS, Halpern R, Wood LC, et al: L-thyroxine therapy in subclinical hypothyroidism: a double-blind placebo-controlled trial. Ann Intern Med 101:18–24, 1984
63. Bell GM, Todd WTA, Forfar JC, et al: End-organ responses to thyroxine therapy in subclinical hypothyroidism. Clin Endocrinol 22:83–89, 1985
64. Gold MS, Pottash AC, Mueller EA, et al: Grades of thyroid failure in 100 depressed and anergic psychiatric inpatients. Am J Psychiatry 138:253–255, 1981
65. Gold MS, Pottash ALC, Extein I: Hypothyroidism and depression: evidence from complete thyroid function evaluation. JAMA 242:1919–1922, 1981
66. Goodnick PG, Extein IL, Gold MS: TRH test and the treatment of depression (New Research Abstract), in Proceedings of the 143rd Annual Meeting of the American Psychiatric Association, San Francisco, CA, May 1989. Washington, DC, American Psychiatric Association, 1989, p 126
67. Targum SD, Greenberg RD, Harmon RL, et al: Thyroid hormone and the TRH stimulation test in refractory depression. J Clin Psychiatry 45:345–347, 1984
68. Cho JT, Bone S, Donner DL, et al: The effect of lithium treatment on thyroid function in patients with primary affective disorder. Am J Psychiatry 136:115–117, 1979
69. Cowdry RW, Wehr TA, Zis AP, et al: Thyroid abnormalities associated with rapid-cycling bipolar illness. Arch Gen Psychiatry 40:414–420, 1983
70. Wehr TA, Sack DA, Rosenthal NE, et al: Rapid-cycling affective disorder: contributing factors and treatment responses in 51 patients. Am J Psychiatry 145:179–184, 1988
71. Joffe RT, Kutcher S, MacDonald C: Thyroid function and bipolar affective disorder. Psychiatry Res 25:117–121, 1988
72. Bauer MS, Whybrow PC, Winokur A: Rapid-cycling bipolar affective disorder, I: association with grade I hypothyroidism. Arch Gen Psychiatry 47:427–432, 1990
73. Gold MS, Pottash ALC, Extein I: "Symtomless" autoimmune thyroiditis in depression. Psychiatry Res 6:261–269, 1982
74. Nemeroff CB, Simon JS, Haggerty JJ Jr, et al: Antithyroid antibodies in depressed patients. Am J Psychiatry 142:840–843, 1985
75. Reus VI, Berlant J, Galante M, et al: Autoimmune thyroiditis in female depressives. Paper presented at the annual meeting of the Society of Biological Psychiatry, Washington, DC, May 1986

76. Joffe RT: Antithyroid antibodies in major depression. Acta Psychiatr Scand 76:598–599, 1987
77. Haggerty JJ Jr, Evans DL, Golden RN, et al: The presence of antithyroid antibodies in patients with affective and nonaffective psychiatric disorders. Biol Psychiatry 27:51–60, 1990
78. Tunbridge WMG, Evered DC, Hall R, et al: The spectrum of thyroid disease in a community: the Wickham survey. Clin Endocrinol 7:481–493, 1977
79. Vancauter E, Leclerc QR, Vanhaelst L, et al: Simultaneous study of cortisol and TSH daily variation in normal subjects and patients with hyperadrenal-corticism. J Clin Endocrinol Metab 39:645–652, 1974
80. Patel YC, Alford FP, Berger HG: The 24-hour plasma thyrotrophin profile. Clin Sci 43:71–77, 1972
81. Chan V, Jones A, Liendo-Ch P, et al: The relationship between circadian variations in circulating thyrotrophin, thyroid hormones and prolactin. Clin Endocrinol 9:337–349, 1978
82. Decostre P, Buhler U, Degroot LJ, et al: Diurnal rhythm in total serum thyroxine levels. Metabolism 20:782–791, 1971
83. Weeke A, Weeke J: Disturbed circadian variation of serum thyrotropin in patients with endogenous depression. Acta Psychiatr Scand 57:281–289, 1978
84. Weeke A, Weeke J: The 24-hour pattern of serum TSH in patients with endogenous depression. Acta Psychiatr Scand 62:69–74, 1980
85. Golstein J, Vancauter RE, Linkowski P, et al: Thyrotropin nyctohemeral pattern in primary depression: differences between unipolar and bipolar women. Life Sci 27:1695–1703, 1980
86. Kijne B, Aggernaes H, Fog-Moller F, et al: Circadian variation of serum thyrotropin in endogenous depression. Psychiatry Res 6:277–282, 1982
87. Kjellman BF, Beck-Friss J, Ljunggren JG, et al: 24-hour serum levels of TSH in affective disorders. Acta Psychiatr Scand 69:491–502, 1984
88. Winokur A, Utiger RD: TRH: regional distribution in the rat brain. Science 185:265–267, 1974
89. Lighton C, Bennett GW, Marsden CA: Increase in levels and ex vivo release of thyrotrophin-releasing hormone (TRH) in specific regions of the CNS of the rat by chronic treatment with antidepressants. Neuropharmacology 24:401–406, 1985
90. Yarbrough GG: On the neuropharmacology of thyrotropin-releasing hormone (TRH). Prog Neurobiol 12:291–312, 1979
91. Przegalinski E, Jaworska L: The effect of repeated administration of antidepressant drugs on the thyrotropin-releasing hormone (TRH) content of rat brain structures. Psychoneuroendocrinology 15:147–153, 1990
92. Kirkegaard C, Faber J, Hemmer L, et al: Increased levels of TRH in cerebrospinal fluid from patients with endogenous depression. Psychoneuroendocrinology 4:227–235, 1979

93. Banki CM, Bissette G, Arato M, et al: Elevation of immunoreactive CSF TRH in depressed patients. Am J Psychiatry 145:1526–1531, 1988

94. Biggins JA, Parry BK, McDermott JR, et al: Postmortem levels of thyrotropin-releasing hormone and neurotensin in the amygdala in Alzheimer's disease, schizophrenia and depression. J Neurol Sci 58:117–122, 1983

95. Bech B, Kirkegaard C, Bock E, et al: Hormones, electrolytes and cerebrospinal fluid proteins in manic-melancholic patients. Neuropsychobiology 4:99–112, 1978

96. Schildkraut JJ, Orsulak PJ, Schatzberg A, et al: Toward a biochemical classification of depressive disorders, I: differences in MHPG and other catecholamine metabolites in clinically defined subtypes of depression. Arch Gen Psychiatry 35:1427–1435, 1978

97. Oppenheimer JH: Thyroid hormone action at the cellular level. Science 203:971–979, 1979

98. Dratman MB, Crutchfield FL: Synaptosomal 125-I-triiodothyronine after intravenous 125-I-thyroxine. Am J Physiol 235:E638–E647, 1978

99. Dratman MB, Futaesku Y, Crutchfield FL, et al: Iodine-125-labelled triiodothyronine in rat brain: evidence for localization in discreet neural systems. Science 215:309–312, 1982

100. Crantz FR, Silver JE, Larsen PR: An analysis of the sources and quantity of 3,5,3-triiodothyronine specifically bound to nuclear receptors in rat cerebral cortex and cerebellum. Endocrinology 110:367–375, 1982

101. Dratman MB, Crutchfield FL: Normally high levels of T_3 generated from T_4 in brain markedly increased by hypothyroidism: contrasting the minimum responses in other tissues. Endocrinology 106:223, 1980

102. Dratman MB, Crutchfield FL: Contrasting effects of hyperthyroidism on formation of label 3,3,5-triiodothyronine (T_3) in rat brain and liver after IV 125-I-thyroxine (T_4). Program of the 56th Annual American Thyroid Association, San Diego, CA, September 1980

103. Jennings A, Crutchfield FL, Dratman MB: Effect of hyper- and hypothyroidism on triiodothyronine production in perfused rat liver (abstract). Clin Res 28:261a, 1980

104. Kaplan MM, Utiger RD: Iodothyronine metabolism in liver and kidney homogenates from hyperthyroid and hypothyroid rat. Endocrinology 103:156–161, 1978

105. Leonard JL, Kaplan MM, Visser TJ, et al: Cerebral cortex responds rapidly to thyroid hormones. Science 214:571–573, 1981

106. Surks MI, Oppenheimer JH: Concentration of L-thyroxine and L-triiodothyronine specifically bound to nuclear receptors in rat liver and kidney: quantitative evidence favoring a major role of T_3 in thyroid hormone action. J Clin Invest 60:555–562, 1977

107. Whybrow PC, Prange AJ Jr.: A hypothesis of thyroid-catecholamine-receptor interaction. Arch Gen Psychiatry 38:106–113, 1981

108. Tucker DM, Penland JG, Beckwith BE, et al: Thyroid function in normals: influences on the electroencephalogram and cognitive performance. Psychophysiology 21:72–78, 1984

109. Wadden TA, Mason G, Foster GD, et al: Effects of a very low calorie diet on weight, thyroid hormones and mood. Int J Obes 14:249–258, 1990

110. Haggerty JJ, Evans DL, Prange AJ Jr: Organic brain syndrome associated with marginal hypothyroidism. Am J Psychiatry 143:785–786, 1986

111. Nystrom E, Caidahl K, Fager G, et al: A double-blind cross-over twelve month study of L-thyroxine treatment of women with "subclinical" hypothyroidism. Clin Endocrinol 29:63–76, 1988

112. Sternbach H, Gerner RH, Gwirtsman HE: The thyrotropin releasing hormone stimulation test: a review. J Clin Psychiatry 43:4–6, 1982

113. Loosen PT, Prange AJ Jr.: Serum thyrotropin response to thyrotropin-releasing hormone in psychiatric patients: a review. Am J Psychiatry 139:405–416, 1982

114. Loosen PT: TRH-induced TSH response in psychiatric patients: a possible neuroendocrine marker. Psychoneuroendocrinology 10:237–260, 1985

115. Ingbar SH, Woeber KA: The thyroid gland, in Textbook of Endocrinology. Edited by William RH. Philadelphia, PA, WB Saunders, 1981, pp 117–248

116. Sawin TT, Hershman JM: Clinical use of thyrotropin-releasing hormone. Pharmacology and Therapeutic Currents 1:351–366, 1976

117. Burger HG, Patel YC: TSH and TRH: their physiological regulation and the clinical application of TRH, in Clinical Neuroendocrinology. Edited by Martini L, Besser GN. New York, Academic Press, 1977, pp 69–131

118. Anderson MS, Bowers CJ, Kastin HA, et al: Synthetic TRH: a potent stimulator of thyrotropin secretion in man. N Engl J Med 285:1279–1283, 1981

119. Amsterdam JD, Winokur A, Lucki A, et al: A neuroendocrine test battery in bipolar patients and healthy subjects. Arch Gen Psychiatry 40:515–521, 1983

120. Winokur A, Amsterdam J, Caroff S, et al: Variability of hormonal responses to a series of neuroendocrine challenges in depressed patients. Am J Psychiatry 139:39–44, 1982

121. Snyder PJ, Utiger RD: Response to thyrotropin releasing hormone (TRH) in normal man. J Clin Endocrinol Metab 34:380–385, 1972

122. Haigler ED Jr, Pittman JA Jr, Hershman JM, et al: Direct evaluation of pituitary thyrotropin reserve utilizing synthetic thyrotropin-releasing hormone. J Clin Endocrinol Metab 33:573–581, 1971

123. Portany GK, O'Brian JT, Bush J, et al: The effect of starvation on the concentration and binding of thyroxine and triiodothyronine in serum and on the response to TRH. J Clin Endocrinol Metab 39:191–194, 1974

124. Wenzel KW, Meinhold H, Herpich M, et al: TRH-Stimulationstest mit alters- und geschlechtsabhängigem TSH-Anstieg bei Normalpersonen. Klin Wochenschr 52:722–727, 1974

125. Smals AGH, Kloppenberg PWC, Lequin RL, et al: The pituitary-thyroid axis in Klinefelter's syndrome. Acta Endocrinol 84:72–90, 1977

126. Kaptein EM, Kletzky OA, Spencer CA, et al: Effects of prolonged dopamine infusion on anterior pituitary function in normal males. J Clin Endocrinol Metab 51:488–491, 1980

127. Kaptein EM, Spencer CA, Kamiel MB: Prolonged dopamine administration and thyroid economy in normal and critically ill subjects. J Clin Endocrinol Metab 51:387–393, 1980

128. Berger AG, Weissel M, Berger M: Starvation induces a partial failure of tri-iodothyronine to inhibit the thyrotropin response to thyrotropin-releasing hormone. J Clin Endocrinol Metab 51:1064–1067, 1980

129. Nemeroff CB, Bissette G, Manberg PJ: Neurotensin-induced hypothermia: evidence for an interaction with dopaminergic systems and the hypotha-lamic-pituitary-thyroid axis. Brain Res 195:68–86, 1980

130. Vale W, Brazea UP, Rivier C, et al: Inhibitory hypophysiotropic activity of hypothalamic somatostostatin. Federation Proceedings 32:211–218, 1973

131. Loosen PT, Prange AJ Jr, Wilson IC: TRH (protirelin) in depressed alcoholic men: behavioral changes and endocrine responses. Arch Gen Psychiatry 36:540–547, 1979

132. Loosen PT, Wilson IC, Dew BW, et al: TRH in abstinent alcoholic men. Am J Psychiatry 140:1145–1149, 1983

133. Garbutt JC, Loosen PT, Tipermas A, et al: The TRH test in borderline per-sonality disorder. Psychiatry Res 9:107–113, 1983

134. Krishnan AR, France RD: TRH stimulation test in chronic pain. Paper pre-sented at the 138th annual meeting of the American Psychiatric Association, Los Angeles, CA, May 1984

135. Mayai K, Toshihide Y, Azukizawa M, et al: Serum thyroid hormones and thy-rotropin in anorexia nervosa. J Clin Endocrinol Metab 40:344–348, 1975

136. Wakeling A, DeSourza VA, Gore MBR, et al: Amenorrhea, body weight and serum hormone concentrations with particular reference to prolactin and thyroid hormones in anorexia nervosa. Psychol Med 9:265–272, 1979

137. Extein I, Pottash ALC, Gold MS, et al: Using the protirelin test to distinguish mania from schizophrenia. Arch Gen Psychiatry 39:77–81, 1982

138. Kirike N, Izumiya Y, Nishiwaka S, et al: TRH test and DST in schizoaffective mania, mania and schizophrenia. Biol Psychiatry 24:415–422, 1988

139. Gold MS, Pottash ALC, Ryan N, et al: TRH-induced TSH response in unipo-lar and secondary depression: possible utility in clinical assessment and dif-ferential diagnosis. Psychoneuroendocrinology 5:147–155, 1980

140. Gold PW, Goodwin FK, Wehr T, et al: Pituitary thyrotropin response to thy-rotropin-releasing hormone in affective illness: relationship to spinal fluid amine metabolites. Am J Psychiatry 134:1028–1031, 1977

141. Coppen A, Montgomery S, Peet M, et al: Thyrotropin-releasing hormone in the treatment of depression. Lancet 2:433–434, 1974

142. Maeda K, Kato Y, Ohgo S, et al: Growth hormone and prolactin release after the injection of thyrotropin-releasing hormone in patients with depression. J Clin Endocrinol Metab 40:501–505, 1975

143. Newson PT, Prange AJ Jr, Wilson IC, et al: Thyroid stimulating hormone response after thyrotropin releasing hormone in depressed, schizophrenic and normal women. Psychoneuroendocrinology 2:137–148, 1977

144. Kirkegaard C, Carroll BJ: Dissociation of TSH and adrenocortical disturbances in endogenous depression. Psychiatry Res 3:253–264, 1980

145. Papakostas V, Fink M, Lee J, et al: Neuroendocrine measures in psychiatric patients: course and outcome to treatment. Psychiatry Res 4:55–65, 1981

146. Targum SD: The application of serial neuroendocrine challenge studies in the management of depressive disorder. Biol Psychiatry 18:3–19, 1983

147. Kathol RG, Sherman BM, Winokur G, et al: Dexamethasone suppression, protirelin stimulation and insulin infusion in subtypes of recovered depressive patients. Psychiatry Res 9:99–106, 1983

148. Larsen JK, Bjorum N, Kirkegaard C, et al: Dexamethasone suppression test, TRH test and Newcastle II depression rating in the diagnosis of depressive disorders. Acta Psychiatr Scand 71:499–505, 1985

149. Langer G, Aschauer H, Koinig G, et al: The TSH-response to TRH: a possible predictive outcome to antidepressant and neuroleptic treatment. Prog Neuropsychopharmacol Biol Psychiatry 7:335–342, 1983

150. Kirkegaard C: The thyrotropin response to thyrotropin-releasing hormone in endogenous depression. Psychoneuroendocrinology 6:189–212, 1981

151. Krog-Meyer J, Kirkegaard C, Kijne B, et al: Prediction of relapse with a TRH test and prophylactic amitriptyline in 39 patients with endogenous depression. Am J Psychiatry 141:945–948, 1984

152. Takahashi CS, Kondo H, Yoshimura M, et al: Thyrotropin responses to TRH in depressive illness: relation to clinical subtypes and prolonged duration of depressive episode. Folia Psychiatrica Neurologica Japonica 28:355–365, 1974

153. Gillette GM, Garbutt JC, Quade DE: TSH response to TRH in depression with and without panic attacks. Am J Psychiatry 146:743–748, 1989

154. Linkowski P, Van Wettere JP, Kerkhofs M, et al: Violent suicidal behaviour and the thyrotropin-releasing hormone–thyroid stimulating hormone test: a clinical outcome study. Neruopsychobiology 12:19–22, 1984

155. Linkowski P, Van Witter JP, Kerkhofs M, et al: Thyrotropin response to thyreostimulin in affectively ill patients: relationships to suicidal behavior. Br J Psychiatry 143:401–405, 1983

156. Arana GW, Zarzar MN, Baker E: The effect of diagnostic methodology on the sensitivity of the TRH stimulation test for depression: a literature review. Biol Psychiatry 28:733–737, 1990

157. Carroll BJ: Neuroendocrine functions in psychiatric disorders, in Psychopharmacology: A Generation of Progress. Edited by Lipton MA, DeMascio A, Killam KF. New York, Raven Press, 1978, pp 487–497

158. Roy A, Karoum F, Linnoila M, et al: Thyrotropin releasing hormone test in unipolar depressed patients and controls: relationship to clinical and biologic variables. Acta Psychiatr Scand 77:151–159, 1988
159. Morley J: Neuroendocrine control of thyrotropin secretion. Endocr Rev 2:396–436, 1981
160. Sternbach AJ, Kirstein L, Pottash ALC, et al: The TRH test and urinary MHPG in unipolar depression. J Affective Disord 5:233–237, 1983
161. Davis KL, Hollister LE, Mathe AA: Neuroendocrine and neurochemical measurements in depression. Am J Psychiatry 138:1555–1561, 1981
162. Gwirtsman H: TSH and MHPG levels of depressed patients. Am J Psychiatry 139:967, 1982
163. Gerner RH, Yamada T: Altered neuropeptide concentration in cerebrospinal fluid of psychiatric patients. Brain Res 238:298–302, 1982
164. Rubinow DR, Gold PW, Post RM, et al: CSF somatostatin in affective illness. Arch Gen Psychiatry 40:409–412, 1983
165. Nemeroff CB, Evans DL: Thyrotropin-releasing hormone (TRH), the thyroid axis and affective disorder. Ann N Y Acad Sci 553:304–310, 1988
166. Frey HMM, Haug E: Effect of prolonged oral administration of TRH on plasma levels of thyrotropin and prolactin in normal individuals and in patients with primary hypothyroidism. Acta Endocrinol 85:744–752, 1977
167. Staub JJ, Girard J, Mueller-Brand J, et al: Blunting of TSH response after repeated oral administration of TRH in normal and hypothyroid subjects. J Clin Endocrinol Metab 46:260–266, 1978
168. Spencer CA, Greenstadt MA, Wheeler WS, et al: The influence of long-term low dose thyrotropin-releasing hormone infusions on serum thyrotropin and prolactin concentrations in man. J Clin Endocrinol Metab 51:771–775, 1980
169. Pavasuthipaisit K, Norman RL, Ellenwood WE, et al: Different prolactin, thyrotropin and thyroxine responses after prolonged, intermittent or continuous infusions of thyrotropin-releasing hormone in rhesus monkeys. J Clin Endocrinol Metab 56:541–548, 1983
170. Winokur A, Caroff SN, Amsterdam JD, et al: Administration of thyrotropin-releasing hormone at weekly intervals results in a diminished thyrotropin response. Biol Psychiatry 19:695–702, 1984
171. Iglesia SR, Llobra M, Montoya E: Sequential changes in the pituitary-thyroid axis after chronic TRH administration: effects on euthyroid and thyroxine treated female rats. Acta Endocrinol 109:237–242, 1985
172. Kaplan MM, Taft JA, Reichlin S, et al: Sustained rises in serum thyrotropin, thyroxine and triiodothyronine during long-term continuous thyrotropin-releasing hormone treatment in patients with amyotrophic lateral sclerosis. J Clin Endocrinol Metab 63:808–814, 1986
173. Hartnell JM, Pekary AE, Hershman JM: Comparison of the effects of pulsatile and continuous TRH infusion on TSH release in men. Metabolism 36:878–882, 1987

174. Loosen PT, Kistler K, Prange AJ Jr: The use of TRH induced TSH responses as an independent variable. Am J Psychiatry 140:700–703, 1983
175. Calloway SP, Dolan RJ, Fonagy P, et al: Endocrine changes and clinical profiles in depression, II: the thyrotropin-releasing hormone test. Psychol Med 14:759–765, 1984
176. Kirkegaard DC, Korner A, Faber J: Increased production of thyroxine and inappropriately elevated serum thyrotropin levels in endogenous depression. Biol Psychiatry 27:472–476, 1990
177. Leichter SB, Kirstein L, Martin ND: Thyroid function and growth hormone secretion in amitriptyline-treated depression. Am J Psychiatry 134:1270–1272, 1977
178. Gregoire F, Brauman H, DeBuch R, et al: Hormone release in depressed patients before and after recovery. Psychoneuroendocrinology 2:303–312, 1977
179. Linnoila M, Gold P, Potter WZ, et al: Tricyclic antidepressants do not alter the thyroid hormone levels in patients suffering from a major affective disorder. Psychiatry Res 4:357–360, 1981
180. Fischetti B: Pharmacological influences on thyroid activities. Arch Ital Sci Farmacol 12:33–109, 1962
181. Prange A, Wilson I, Knox A, et al: Thyroid-imipramine clinical and chemical interaction: evidence for a receptor defect in depression. J Psychiatr Res 9:196–205, 1972
182. Morley JE, Brammer GR, Shop B, et al: Neurotransmitter controls of hypothalamic-pituitary-thyroid function in rats. Eur J Pharmacol 70:263–271, 1981
183. Atterwill CK, Catto LC, Heal DJ, et al: The effects of desipramine (DMI) and electroconvulsive shock (ECS) on the function of the hypothalamo-pituitary-thyroid axis in the rat. Psychoneuroendocrinology 40:339–346, 1989
184. Aperia B, Bergman H, Englbrektson K, et al: Effects of electroconvulsive therapy on neuropsychological function and circulating levels of ACTH cortisol, prolactin and TSH in patients with major depressive illness. Acta Psychiatr Scand 72:536–541, 1985
185. Duque C, Franco-Vicario JM, Franco-Vicario R, et al: Changes in T_3, T_4 and TSH rat plasma levels following electroconvulsive shock. Br J Pharmacology 80:566–570, 1983
186. Schou M, Amdisen A, Jansen SE: Occurrence of goiter during lithium treatment. BMJ 3:710–713, 1968
187. Burrow GN, Burke WR, Himmelhoch JM, et al: Effect of lithium on thyroid function. J Clin Endocrinol Metab 32:647–652, 1971
188. Mannisto PT: Thyroid iodine metabolism in vitro, II: effect of lithium ion. Annals of Medical and Experimental Biology 51:42–45, 1973
189. Berens SC, Wolff J: The endocrine effects of lithium, in Lithium Research and Therapy. Edited by Johnson FN. New York, Academic Press, 1975, pp 443–472

190. Bagchi N, Brown TR, Mack RE: Effects of chronic lithium treatment on hypothalamic-pituitary regulation of thyroid function. Horm Metab Res 14:92–93, 1982

191. Sedvall G, Jonsson B, Pettersson U: Evidence of altered thyroid function in man during treatment with lithium carbonate. Acta Psychiatr Scand 207:59–67, 1969

192. Voss C, Schober HC, Hartman N: Einfluss von Lithium auf die in vitro Dejodierung von L-Thyroxine in der Rattenleber. Acta Biologica Medica Germanica 36:1061–1065, 1977

193. Bagchi N, Brown TR, Mack RE: Effect of chronic lithium treatment on hypothalamic-pituitary regulation of thyroid function. Horm Metab Res 14:92–93, 1982

194. Bakker K: The influence of lithium carbonate on the hypothalamic-pituitary-thyroid axis. Agressologie 23:89–93, 1982

195. Halmi KA, Noyes R Jr: Effects of lithium on thyroid function. Biol Psychiatry 5:211–215, 1972

196. Kirkegaard C, Lauridsen UB, Nerup J: Lithium and the thyroid (letter). Lancet 2:1210, 1973

197. Lauridsen UB, Kirkegaard C, Nerup J: Lithium and the pituitary-thyroid axis in normal subjects. J Clin Endocrinol Metab 39:383–385, 1974

198. Child C, Nolan G, Jubiz W: Changes in serum thyroxine, triiodothyronine and thyrotropin induced by lithium in normal subjects and in rats. Clin Pharmacol Ther 20:715–719, 1977

199. Perrild H, Hegdus L, Arnung K: Sex related goiterogenic effect of lithium carbonate in healthy young subjects. Acta Endocrinol 106:203–208, 1984

200. Sedvall G, Jonsson B, Pettersson U, et al: Effects of lithium salts on plasma protein bound iodine and uptake of I in thyroid gland of man and rat. Life Sci 7:1257–1264, 1968

201. Cooper TB, Simpson GM: Preliminary report of a longitudinal study on the effects of lithium on iodine metabolism. Current Therapeutic Research 11:603–608, 1969

202. Burrow GN, Burke WR, Himmelhoch JM, et al: Effect of lithium on thyroid function. J Clin Endocrinol Metab 32:647–652, 1971

203. Fyrx B, Petterson U, Sedvall G: Time course for the effect of lithium on thyroid function in men and women. Acta Psychiatr Scand 49:230–236, 1973

204. Emerson CH, Dyson WL, Utiger RD: Serum thyrotropin and thyroxine concentrations in patients receiving lithium carbonate. J Clin Endocrinol Metab 36:338–346, 1973

205. Rifkin A, Quitkin F, Blumberg AG, et al: The effect of lithium on thyroid functioning: a controlled study. J Psychiatr Res 10:115–120, 1974

206. Page C, Benaim S, Lappin F: A long-term retrospective follow-up study of patients treated with prophylactic lithium carbonate. Br J psychiatry 150:175–179, 1987

207. Hofman G, Hofer R, Jolei I: The prophylaktische Wirkung von Lithium-Salzen und Schildrusenhormone auf Manifestatione des manis-depressiven Karakenheitsgschehens und der Legierrungs-Psychosen: klinische und experimentelle Ergebnisse. International Pharmacopsychiatry 5:221–226, 1970

208. Rogers MP, Whybrow PC: Clinical hypothyroidism occurring during lithium treatment: two case histories and a review of thyroid function in 19 patients. Am J Psychiatry 128:50–55, 1971

209. Hullin RP, McDonald DR, Allsopp MNE: Prophylactic lithium in recurrent affective disorders. Lancet 1:1044–1046, 1972

210. Lazarus JH, Bennie EH: Effect of lithium on thyroid function in man. Acta Endocrinol 70:266–272, 1972

211. Tucker WI, Bell GO: Effectiveness of lithium carbonate in the prevention of manic and depressive disorders. Med Clin North Am 56:681–686, 1972

212. Lindstedt G, Lundberg PA, Tofft M: Serum thyrotropin and hypothyroidism during lithium therapy. Clin Chim Acta 48:127–133, 1973

213. Villeneuve A, Gautier J, Jos A, et al: The effect of lithium on thyroid in man. International Journal of Clinical Pharmacology 9:75–80, 1974

214. Abuzzahab FS, Dahlam HC: Long-term effects of lithium carbonate on serum protein bound iodine in affective disorders. Progr Neuropsychopharmacol Biol Psychiatry 2:269–277, 1975

215. McLarty DG, O'Boyle JH, Spencer CA, et al: Effect of lithium on hypothalamic-pituitary-thyroid function in patients with affective disorders. BMJ 3:623–626, 1975

216. Serry M, Serry D: Lithium carbonate and hypothyroidism. Med J Aust 79:505–508, 1976

217. Williams WO, Gyory AZ: Aspects of the use of lithium for the non-psychiatrist. Aust N Z J Med 6:233–242, 1976

218. Lindstedt G, Nilsson LA, Walinder J, et al: On the prevalence, diagnosis and management of lithium induced hypothyroidism in psychiatric patients. Br J Psychiatry 130:452–458, 1977

219. Piziak VK, Sellman JE, Othmer E: Lithium and hypothyroidism. J Clin Psychiatry 39:709–711, 1978

220. Transbol I, Christiansen C, Baastrupp C: Endocrine effects of lithium, I: hypothyroidism, its prevalence in long-term treated patients. Acta Endocrinol 87:759–767, 1978

221. Wasilewski VB, Steinbock H, Kohl R, et al: Thyroid function in prophylactic therapy with lithium. Arzniemittelforschung 28:1297–1298, 1978

222. Botterman P, Greil W, Steinbock H, et al: Thyroid function in patients with episodic affective disorders in the course of lithium therapy. Acta Endocrinol 225 (suppl):36, 1979

223. Lazarus JH, John R, Bennie EH, et al: Lithium therapy and thyroid function: a long-term study. Psychol Med 11:85–92, 1981

224. Amdisen A, Andersen CJ: Lithium treatment and thyroid function: a survey of 237 patients in long-term lithium treatment. Pharmacopsychiatry 15:149–155, 1982

225. Smigan L, Wahlin A, Jacobsson L, et al: Lithium therapy and thyroid function tests: a prospective study. Neuropsychobiology 11:39–43, 1984

226. Maarbjerg K, Vestergaard P, Schou M: Changes in serum thyroxine (T4) and serum thyroid stimulating hormone (TSH) during prolonged lithium treatment. Acta Psychiatr Scand 75:217–221, 1987

227. Yassa R, Saunders A, Nastas EC, et al: Lithium-induced thyroid disorders: a prevalence study. J Clin Psychiatry 49:14–16, 1988

228. Braverman LE, Woeber KA, Ingbar SH: Induction of myxedema by iodide in patients euthyroid after the radioiodine or surgical treatment of diffuse goiter. N Engl J Med 281:816–821, 1969

229. Braverman LE, Ingbar SH, Vagenakis AG, et al: Enhanced susceptibility to iodide myxedema in patients with Hashimoto's disease. J Clin Endocrinol Metab 32:515–521, 1971

230. Calabrese JR, Gulledge AD, Hahn K, et al: Autoimmune thyroiditis in manic depressive patients treated with lithium. Am J Psychiatry 142:1318–1321, 1985

231. Lazarus JH, McGregor AM, Ludgat UM, et al: Effective lithium carbonate therapy on thyroid immune status in manic depressive patients: a prospective study. J Affective Disord 11:155–160, 1986

232. Leroy MC, Villeneuve A, Lajeunesse C: Lithium, thyroid function and antithyroid antibodies. Prog Neuropsychopharmacol Biol Psychiatry 12:483–490, 1988

233. Franklin LM: Thyrotoxicosis developing during lithium treatment: case report (letter). N Z Med J 79:782, 1974

234. Cubitt T: Lithium and thyrotoxicosis. Lancet 1:1247–1248, 1976

235. Rosser R: Thyrotoxicosis and lithium. Br J Psychiatry 128:61–66, 1976

236. Brownlie BEW, Chambers ST, Saddler WA, et al: Lithium associated thyroid disease: a report of 14 cases of hypothyroidism and 4 cases of thyrotoxicosis. Aust N Z J Med 6:223–229, 1976

237. Bafaqee HH, Myers DH: Lithium and thyrotoxicosis (letter). Lancet 1:1409, 1976

238. Chauhdry MA, Bebbington PE: Lithium therapy and ophthalmic Grave's disease. Br J Psychiatry 130:420, 1977

239. Merry J: Lithium and thyrotoxicosis (letter). BMJ 3:765, 1977

240. Pallisgaard G, Frederickson PK: Thyrotoxicosis in a patient treated with lithium carbonate for mental disease. Acta Medica Scandinavica 204:141–143, 1978

241. Reus VI, Gold P, Post R: Lithium-induced thyrotoxicosis. Am J Psychiatry 136:724–725, 1979

242. Rabin PL, Evans DC: Exophthalamos and elevated thyroxine levels in association with lithium therapy. J Clin Psychiatry 42:398–400, 1981

243. Valenta LJ, Elias AN, Weber DJ: Hyperthyroidism and propylthiouracil-induced agranulocytosis during chronic lithium carbonate therapy. Am J Psychiatry 138:1605–1607, 1981

244. Segal RL, Rosenblatt S, Eliasoph I: Endocrine exophthalamos during lithium therapy in manic depressive illness. N Engl J Med 289:136–138, 1973

245. Kristensen O, Harrestrup H, Andersen H, et al: Lithium carbonate and the treatment of thyrotoxicosis: a control trial. Lancet 1:603–605, 1976

246. Rootwelt K, Ganes T, Johannessen SI: Effects of carbamazepine, phenytoin and phenobarbitone on serum levels of thyroid hormones and thyrotropin in humans. Scand J Clin Lab Invest 38:731–736, 1978

247. Leiwendahl K, Majuri H, Helenius T: Thyroid function tests in patients on long-term treatment with various anticonvulsant drugs. Clin Endocrinol 8:185–191, 1978

248. Strandjord RE, Aanderud S, Myking OL, et al: Influence of carbamazepine on serum thyroxine and triiodothyronine in patients with epilepsy. Acta Neurol Scand 63:111–121, 1981

249. Luhdorf K, Christiansen P, Hansen JM, et al: The influence of phenytoin and carbamazepine on endocrine function: preliminary results, in Epilepsy: The 8th International Symposium. Edited by Penry JK. New York, Raven Press, 1977, pp 209–213

250. Bentsen KD, Gram L, Veje A: Serum thyroid hormones and blood folic acid during monotherapy with carbamazepine or valproate. Acta Neurol Scand 67:235–241, 1983

251. Aanderud S, Strandjord RE: Hypothyroidism induced by anti-epileptic therapy. Acta Neurol Scand 61:330–332, 1980

252. Fichsel H, Knopfle G: Effect of anticonvulsants on thyroid hormones. Epilepsia 19:323–335, 1978

253. Smith PJ, Surks MI: Multiple effects of 5,5'-diphenylhydantoin on the thyroid hormone system. Endocr Rev 5:514–524, 1984

254. Post RM, Kramlinger KG, Joffe RT, et al: Thyroid indices in the course of affective illness. Am J Psychiatry (in press)

255. Joffe RT, Gold PW, Uhde TW, et al: The effects of carbamazepine on the thyrotropin response to thyrotropin releasing hormone. Psychiatry Res 12:161–166, 1984

256. Joffe RT, Post RM, Eil C: Carbamazepine does not interact with thyroid hormone receptors in human skin fibroblasts. Neuropharmacology 23:1301–1303, 1984

257. Blank D, Joffe RT: Effect of carbamazepine on thyroid hormone in vitro. Clin Chim Acta 143:173–176, 1984

258. Joffe RT, Brown P: Clinical and biological correlates of sleep deprivation in depression. Can J Psychiatry 29:530–536, 1984

259. Palmblad J, Akerstedt T, Froberg J, et al: Thyroid and adrenomedullary reactions during sleep deprivation. Acta Endocrinol 90:233–239, 1979

260. Kvist J, Kirkegaard C: Effect of repeated sleep deprivation on clinical symptoms and the TRH test in endogenous depression. Acta Psychiatr Scand 62:494–502, 1980

261. Baumgartner A, Meinhold H: Sleep deprivation and thyroid hormone concentrations. Psychiatry Res 19:241–242, 1986

262. Kasper S, Sack DA, Wehr TA, et al: Nocturnal TSH and prolactin secretion during sleep deprivation and prediction of antidepressant response in patients with major depression. Biol Psychiatry 24:631–641, 1988

263. Sack DA, James SP, Rosenthal NE, et al: Deficient nocturnal surge of TSH secretion during sleep and sleep deprivation in rapid-cycling bipolar illness. Psychiatry Res 23:179–191, 1988

264. Kaschka WP, Flugle D, Negle-Antsberger J, et al: Total sleep deprivation and thyroid function in depression. Psychiatry Res 29:231–234, 1989

265. Griffiths EC: TRH: endocrine and central effects. Psychoneuroendocrinology 10:225–235, 1985

266. Prange AJ Jr, Nemeroff CB, Lipton MA, et al: Peptides and the central nervous system, in Handbook of Psychopharmacology, Vol 13. Edited by Iversen LL, Iversen SD, Snyder SH. New York, Plenum, 1978, pp 1–107

267. Griffiths ED: Thyrotropin-releasing hormone: endocrine and central effects. Psychoneuroendocrinology 3:225–235, 1985

268. Kastin AJ, Ehrensing RH, Schalch DS, et al: Improvement in mental depression with decreased thyrotropin response after administration of thyrotropin releasing hormone. Lancet 2:740–742, 1972

269. Prange AJ Jr, Wilson IC, Lara PP, et al: Effects of thyrotropin-releasing hormone in depression. Lancet 2:999–1001, 1972

270. Coppen A, Montgomery S, Peet M, et al: Thyrotropin-releasing hormone in the treatment of depression. Lancet 1:433–435, 1974

271. Ehrensing RH, Kastin AJ, Schalch DS, et al: Affective state and thyrotropin and prolactin responses after repeated injections of thyrotropin-releasing hormone in depressed patients. Am J Psychiatry 131:714–718, 1974

272. Hollister LE, Berger P, Ogle FL, et al: Protirelin (TRH) in depression. Arch Gen Psychiatry 31:468–470, 1974

273. Mountjoy CQ, Price JS, Weller M, et al: A double-blind cross-over sequential trial of oral thyrotropin-releasing hormone in depression. Lancet 2:958–960, 1970

274. Van Den Burgh W, Van Praag HM, Bos ERH, et al: Thyrotropin releasing hormone (TRH) as a possible quick acting but short lasting antidepressant. Psychol Med 5:404–412, 1975

275. Furlong FW, Brown GM, Beeching MF: Thyrotropin-releasing hormone: differential antidepressant and endocrinological effects. Am J Psychiatry 133:1187–1190, 1976

276. Kiely WF, Adrian AD, Lee JH, et al: Therapeutic failure of oral thyrotropin-releasing hormone in depression. Psychosom Med 38:233–241, 1976

277. Van Den Burgh W, Van Praag HM, Bos ERH, et al: TRH by slow, continuous infusion: an antidepressant? Psychol Med 6:393–397, 1976
278. Vogle HP, Benkert O, Illig R, et al: Psychoendocrinological and therapeutic effects of TRH in depression. Acta Psychiatr Scand 56:223–232, 1977
279. Karlberg BE, Kjellman BF, Kagedel B: Treatment of endogenous depression with oral thyrotropin-releasing hormone and amitriptyline. Acta Psychiatr Scand 58:389–400, 1978
280. Prange AJ Jr, Wilson IC, Raybon AM, et al: Enhancement of the imipramine antidepressant activity by thyroid hormone. Am J Psychiatry 126:457–469, 1969
281. Wilson IC, Prange AJ Jr, McClane TK, et al: Thyroid hormone enhancement of imipramine in nonretarded depression. N Engl J Med 282:1063–1067, 1970
282. Wheathley D: Potentiation of amitriptyline by thyroid hormone. Arch Gen Psychiatry 26:229–233, 1972
283. Coppen A, Whybrow PC, Noguera R, et al: Comparative antidepressant value of L-tryptophan and imipramine with and without attempted potentiation by liothyronine. Arch Gen Psychiatry 26:234–241, 1972
284. Earle BV: Thyroid hormone and tricyclic antidepressants in resistant depression. Am J Psychiatry 126:1667–1669, 1970
285. Banki CM: Triiodothyronine in the treatment of depression. Orvieti Hetilia 116:2543–2547, 1975
286. Banki C: Cerebrospinal fluid amine metabolites after combined amitriptyline-triiodothyronine treatment of depressed women. Eur J Clin Pharmacol 11:311–315, 1977
287. Ogura C, Okuma T, Uchida Y, et al: Combined thyroid (triiodothyronine)-tricyclic antidepressant treatment in depressed states. Folia Psychiatrica Neurologica Japonica 28:179–186, 1974
288. Tsutsui S, Yamazaki Y, Nanba T, et al: Combined therapy of T3 and antidepressants in depression. J Int Med Res 7:138–146, 1979
289. Goodwin FK, Prange AJ Jr, Post RM, et al: Potentiation of antidepressant effects by L-triiodothyronine in tricyclic nonresponders. Am J Psychiatry 139:34–38, 1982
290. Schwarcz G, Halaris A, Baxter L, et al: Normal thyroid function in desipramine nonresponders compared to responders by the addition of L-triiodothyronine. Am J Psychiatry 141:1614–1616, 1984
291. Thase ME, Kupfer DJ, Jarrett DB: Treatment of imipramine-resistant recurrent depression, I: an open clinical trial of adjunctive L-triiodothyronine. J Clin Psychiatry 50:385–388, 1989
292. Gitlin MJ, Winer H, Fairbanks L, et al: Failure of T3 to potentiate tricyclic antidepressant response. J Affective Disord 13:267–272, 1987
293. Joffe RT, Singer W: A comparison of triiodothyronine and thyroxine in the potentiation of tricyclic antidepressants. Psychiatry Res 32:241–252, 1990

294. Joffe RT: Triiodothyronine (T_3) and lithium potentiation of tricyclic antidepressants. Am J Psychiatry 145:1317–1318, 1988
295. Larsen PR: Thyroid-pituitary interaction. N Engl J Med 306:23–32, 1982
296. Joffe RT, Post RM, Sulser F, et al: Altered thyroid function and cortical beta-adrenergic receptors in rat brain: lack of effect of carbamazepine. Neuropharmacology 27:171–174, 1988
297. Mason GA, Walker CH, Prange AJ Jr: Depolarization-dependent ^{45}Ca uptake by synaptosomes of rat cerebral cortex is enhanced by L-triiodothyronine. Neuropsychopharmacology 3:291–295, 1990
298. Martin P, Brochet D, Soubrie P, et al: Triiodothyronine-induced reversal of learned helplessness in rats. Biol Psychiatry 20:1023–1025, 1985
299. Stancer HC, Persad E: Treatment of intractable rapid-cycling manic-depressive disorder with levothyroxine. Arch Gen Psychiatry 39:311–312, 1982
300. Bauer MS, Whybrow PC: Rapid-cycling bipolar affective disorder, II: treatment of refractory rapid cycling with high-dose levothyroxine: a preliminary study. Arch Gen Psychiatry 47:435–440, 1990

Chapter 7

The Thyroid
and Anxiety Disorders

Murray B. Stein, M.D.
Thomas W. Uhde, M.D.

CONTENTS

1. INTRODUCTION

Clinicians have long been aware of the considerable psychiatric morbidity that may occur in patients with thyroid disorders. In fact, early descriptions of the hyperthyroid state (1,2) prominently featured the changes in mental state associated with these syndromes; these have variously been referred to as agitation, anxiety, restlessness, or nervousness. Although it is not our intent here to rigorously detail the psychiatric manifestations of clinical thyroid disorders (for a discussion, see Chapter 5), we do wish to allude to several studies that have specifically focused on the occurrence of anxiety syndromes in patients with thyroid disorders. In this chapter, we also review the abnormalities in thyroid axis function that have been examined in patients with specific anxiety disorders.

2. ANXIETY DISORDERS IN PATIENTS WITH CLINICAL THYROID DISEASE

Although the occurrence of anxiety as a symptom of hyperthyroidism, in particular, is well recognized (3–6), surprisingly few studies have examined the prevalence of diagnosable anxiety disorders in patients with thyroid dysfunction. In one study, Kathol and Delahunt (7) observed that depressive and anxiety disorders were extremely common in patients with hyperthyroidism seen in a general endocrinology clinic. The authors were able to prospectively follow 29 consecutively evaluated patients, and found that 23 of these individuals met criteria for generalized anxiety and/or panic disorder. In 21 of these 23, they found that the anxiety resolved completely with antithyroid therapy alone (8). This study would suggest that anxiety disorders are far from rare in clinical endocrinology practice and that the thyroid dysfunction may be directly responsible for the occurrence of the anxious symptomatology.

Several clinicians have also reported the occurrence of panic attacks with or without agoraphobia in patients with hyperthyroidism (9–12). Despite these observations, a more recent article (13) on the medical evaluation of patients with panic attacks suggested that routine thyroid hormone screening was not indicated in these individuals. This suggestion seems to have been based on the observation that patients with panic disorder in psychiatric clinics almost uniformly have normal thyroid indices. Nonetheless, the available evidence would clearly indicate that, particularly in a primary care practice or when psychiatrists serve as the first line of referral from nonmedical sources, it would be imprudent not to rule out thyroid disease in patients presenting with anxiety disorders (14,15). (For a more complete discussion, see Chapter 5.)

3. HYPOTHALAMIC-PITUITARY-THYROID (HPT) AXIS IN ANXIETY DISORDERS

In contrast to the limited data addressing the prevalence of anxiety disorders in patients with thyroid disease, a number of studies in the past 5 years have begun to examine the hypothalamic-pituitary-thyroid (HPT) axis in patients with anxiety disorders. The stimulus to these studies has been twofold: *1)* to ascertain whether the high rate of anxiety in patients with thyroid disease corresponds with a high rate of thyroid abnormalities in patients with primary anxiety disorders and *2)* to determine whether the anxiety disorders, which exhibit considerable comorbidity with depression, also exhibit similar HPT axis abnormalities found in major affective disorders (see Chapter 6). In the remainder of this chapter, we review the studies that have examined the HPT axis in each of the anxiety disorders. We examine the findings in the context of each of the two major hypotheses outlined above.

4. THE THYROID AND PANIC DISORDER

In marked contrast to the paucity of thyroid studies in generalized anxiety disorder (GAD), a number of studies have examined HPT axis function in patients with panic disorder.

In the first of several retrospective studies, Lindeman et al. (16) found that 10.8% of patients with panic attacks reported a history of thyroid disease (this included hypothyroidism or hyperthyroidism), compared to less than 1% reported by the general population. In another study, Orenstein et al. (17) found that women with panic disorder and histories of depression had elevated personal and family histories of thyroid disease, but women with panic disorder alone (i.e., no history of depression) did not. These studies, limited by their retrospective nature, fail to determine whether patients with panic disorder have a higher rate of overt thyroid dysfunction than nonpsychiatric control subjects or individuals with other psychiatric disorders (e.g., depression). In the following five sections, we review current knowledge of HPT function in panic disorder. Data from studies investigating thyroid indices, antithyroid antibodies, thyroid-stimulating hormone (TSH) responsivity to thyrotropin-releasing hormone (TRH), and pulse wave arrival time (QK_d intervals) in panic patients versus healthy control subjects are presented. In addition, preliminary information is provided on the treatment effects of triiodothyronine (T_3) in tricyclic-nonresponsive panic disorder patients.

4.1 Thyroid Indices

The most conventional strategy for examining the prevalence of thyroid dysfunction in patients with panic disorder is to assess peripheral thyroid indices (18–24). Such studies have two goals. The first is to determine the true rate of abnormal (i.e., hypo- or hyperthyroidism) thyroid indices. To achieve this aim, subjects should not be pre-screened by another health practitioner to rule out overt thyroid disease. This is obviously a difficult criterion to meet, as there is likely to be considerable heterogeneity in referral sources and the degree to which these referral sources have conducted prior thyroid tests. Consequently, previous reports using this strategy tend to underestimate the true rate of thyroid dysfunction in panic disorder.

The second research goal is to determine if, in the absence of overt thyroid disease, panic disorder patients typically exhibit more subtle alterations in thyroid hormonal levels. To achieve this aim, two criteria must be met: *1)* patients who exhibit overt thyroid disease (on the basis of clinical and laboratory examinations) would be a priori excluded and *2)* a control group would be needed for comparison. Most studies have managed to meet the first criterion and have excluded subjects with clinically evident thyroid disease. Meeting the second criterion has, however, proved more elusive, and most studies have determined the "normality" of their findings in patients with panic disorder by comparing only to published laboratory norms, rather than to healthy control subjects. We (24) recently investigated thyroid indices in 26 patients with panic disorder and compared the findings with those of a group of 26 age- and sex-matched healthy control subjects. We found no significant differences in T_3, thyroxine (T_4), free thyroxine (FT_4), or TSH between the two groups, in keeping with the consensus from other studies (18–23). These studies (15,18–23) suggest that abnormalities in peripheral indices of thyroid function are not a requisite biological correlate of panic disorder (see Table 7–1).

4.2 Antithyroid Antibodies

The presence of antithyroid antibodies is a marker for several varieties of autoimmune thyroiditis, including Hashimoto's thyroiditis. It is believed that the presence of thyroid autoantibodies may precede the development of overt thyroid dysfunction, making their detection of some prognostic significance (25). In recent years, it has been recognized that some patients with depression exhibit the presence of antithyroid antibodies (26–28), with reported rates varying from 9% to 20%. Most recently, Haggerty et al. (29) determined the frequency of antithyroglobulin and antimicrosomal antibodies in 173 consecutively admitted psychiatric inpatients and found that the rate of positive antithyroid antibody titers in patients with affective disorders (9%) did not differ from that of patients with nonaffective disorders

Table 7–1.   Studies of thyroid hormone levels in patients with panic disorder

Study	n subjects	Control group	Findings
Pariser et al. 1979 (19)	17	Laboratory norms	Normal
Fishman et al. 1985 (20)	82	Laboratory norms	22% of subjects had undetectable TSH levels, T_3 and T_4 were normal
Matuzas et al. 1987 (22)	55	Laboratory norms	4 patients had an elevation in T_3, T_4, or FT_4 index
Yeragani et al. 1987 (21)	46	Matched healthy subjects	No differences versus control subjects
Lesser et al. 1987 (23)	165	Laboratory norms	Less than 1% of subjects had evidence of current thyroid dysfunction
Stein and Uhde 1988 (15)	26	Age- and sex-matched healthy control subjects	No differences versus control subjects
Munjack and Palmer 1988 (18)	41	Healthy subjects	No differences versus control subjects

Note. TSH = thyroid-stimulating hormone; T_3 = triiodothyronine; T_4 = thyroxine; FT_4 = free thyroxine.

(10%). They did find, however, that patients with bipolar disorder (mixed or depressed type) had an exceptionally high rate of antithyroid antibodies (approximately 29%). These observations are paralleled by the recent findings of Bauer et al. (30) of high rates of grade I hypothyroidism (i.e., elevated thyrotropin [TSH] responses to protirelin [TRH]) in rapid-cycling bipolar patients, possibly indicative of early or subclinical thyroid dysfunction in the same way that antithyroid antibodies are believed to be.

Clinicians have long been aware of the tremendous overlap between anxious and depressive syndromes, and it is generally acknowledged that approximately one-third of depressed patients experience panic attacks while depressed. Examining the data from a longitudinal perspective, there is also a consensus that approximately two-thirds of patients with panic disorder experience major depressive episode(s) at some point during the course of their illness (31–34). In this light, given the high degree of comorbidity between anxiety and depression, it is reasonable to wonder if patients with anxiety disorders might exhibit elevated rates of antithyroid antibodies, similar to those reported in some studies of depressed patients.

To our knowledge, only one study has examined this issue in an anxious population. This is a study we conducted wherein we compared the rate of positive antithyroid titers in 38 patients with panic disorder to that of 38 matched healthy control subjects. Contrary to reports in depression, the proportion of patients with panic disorder (11%) who had positive antithyroid antibodies did not differ significantly from the control subjects (5%).

Two women with panic disorder who had antithyroid antibodies at the time of initial evaluation continued under our care, giving us the opportunity to obtain a longitudinal perspective on this issue. We were able to document their titers serially over time, as shown in Figure 7–1. In both cases, their titers of antithyroid antibodies became undetectable within a 6-month timeframe. The course of their anxiety disorder did not, however, closely parallel the course of their antibody titers. Furthermore, neither of these women showed clinical or biochemical evidence of the development of hypothyroidism during this period of observation.

In addition to indicating that autoimmune thyroiditis is unlikely to be playing a role in most patients with panic disorder, our observations underscore the need for longitudinal monitoring of antithyroid titers in future studies of psychiatric patients. The cross-sectional detection of antithyroid antibodies may be of little clinical significance, particularly as these titers may wax and wane, and, as in the case of the two patients we presented, may normalize altogether. On the other hand, antithyroid antibodies that persist at high titers may be of considerable importance in some psychiatric syndromes (perhaps, as suggested above, bipolar illness), but this remains to be confirmed from prospective studies.

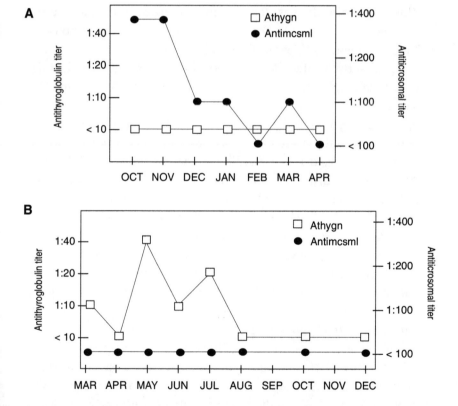

Figure 7–1. Two women with panic disorder and elevated antithyroid hormones were followed for up to 8 consecutive months. In both cases, elevated titers of antimicrosomal (Antimcsml) (*Panel A:* 29-year-old woman) or antithyroglobulin (Anthygn) (*Panel B:* 41-year-old woman) antibodies became undetectable within several months.

4.3   Thyroid-Stimulating Hormone (TSH) Response to Thyrotropin-Releasing Hormone (TRH)

Although the static indices of thyroid status do not point toward the existence of thyroid abnormalities in patients with panic disorder, more intricate assessment of the HPT axis in these patients has been attempted using the TRH-stimulation test. As reviewed in Chapter 4, the pituitary thyrotrophs respond to TRH stimulation by releasing TSH, which can then be measured in blood. This test provides an indication of the functional status of the HPT axis and has been widely studied in patients with affective disorders (see Chapter 6) with the oft-replicated finding that approximately one-third of depressed patients exhibit a reduced TSH response to TRH administration. Because panic disorder has close phenomenological and biological ties to major depression (31–35), examination of the TSH response to TRH in patients with panic disorder is of interest.

The first two studies of TSH responsivity to TRH in panic disorder both found high rates of "blunting." Roy-Byrne et al. (36) found that 4 of 12 patients (33%) had TSH responses less than 7 μU/ml, similar to the 8 of 20 patients (40%) in the study by Hamlin and Pottash (37). Subsequent to this, Castellani et al. (38) found that 3 of 9 (33%) patients with panic disorder had blunted TSH responses to TRH (i.e., Δ_{max} TSH $< 7\,\mu U/ml$). Therefore, these three studies, albeit conducted in fairly small patient samples, seemed to indicate that reduced TSH responses to TRH were found in approximately the same proportion of patients with panic disorder as of patients with depression.

A report (39) of 46 patients with major depression used an interesting approach whereby the investigators subdivided the depressed patients into those with and those without panic attacks during the current depressive episode. They found that the 14 depressed patients with panic attacks had a significantly higher ($P < .05$) prevalence (50%) of low TSH responses to TRH (i.e., ΔTSH $< 7.0\,\mu U/ml$ at 30 minutes after TRH injection) than the 32 depressed patients without panic attacks (22%). Similarly, mean TSH responses were significantly lower ($P < .05$) in the group of patients with panic attacks. In this study, the TSH responses in the depressed patients without panic attacks did not differ significantly from those of healthy control subjects. This set of findings implied that diminished TSH responsivity to TRH might actually be more a feature of panic than of depression.

To shed additional light on this topic, we (40) sought to reexamine the dynamic status of the HPT axis in panic disorder by conducting a study of neuroendocrine responses to TRH in a larger, completely new sample of panic disorder patients and healthy control subjects. We compared 26 patients with panic disorder, none of whom met simultaneous criteria for major depression, with 22 healthy volunteers. There were no differences observed in hormonal responses to TRH between groups, either in terms of the prevalence of blunted responses or in the comparison of mean responses. However, higher Beck Depression Inventory scores, even within this relatively nondysphoric group of patients, were negatively correlated with Δ_{max} TSH responses ($r_s = -.60$, $P < .002$) (Figure 7–2).

These findings of normal TSH responses to TRH in panic disorder, which have recently been replicated elsewhere in another sample of 26 patients with panic disorder (41), raise an intriguing possibility. Taken together, our observation and those of Gillette et al. (39) may

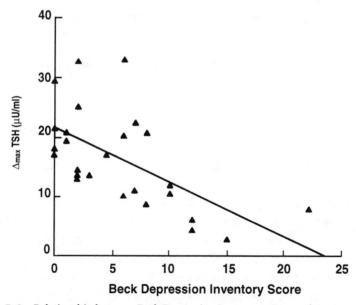

Figure 7–2. Relationship between Beck Depression Inventory score and Δ_{max} thyroid-stimulating hormone (TSH) in patients with panic disorder ($r_s = -.60$, $P < .002$). Panic disorder patients with the highest ratings of depression had the most blunted TSH responses to thyrotropin-releasing hormone.

indicate that it is the combined or interactive influence of both panic and depression that yield the highest rates of TSH hyposensitivity to TRH. This hypothesis remains to be tested in studies that take into account the various ways in which affective illness and anxiety may be expressed (e.g., major depression with panic attacks, panic disorder with dysthymia, and "atypical depression").

We wish to point out another interesting facet of our study (40) that has implications toward the use of TRH testing in psychiatry. We used an immunoradiometric assay with a sensitivity of 1 µU/ml (IRMA, Serono Diagnostics, Norwell, MA), and found that basal TSH levels (i.e., before TRH administration) correlated positively with the Δ_{max} TSH values obtained after TRH stimulation (panic disorder patients, $r = .55$, $P < .005$; healthy control subjects, $r = .85$, $P < .0001$) (Figure 7–3). These observations suggest, as recognized by other investigators (42,43), that, with a TSH assay with good detection limits at the low end of the scale, basal TSH values may in certain clinical circumstances supplant the more expensive and time-consuming TRH test. The generalizability of these observations to psychiatric research remains to be determined, but appears promising.

4.4 Measurement of End-Organ Thyroid Hormone Response

It can be seen from the preceding studies that there is not much evidence to support a major role for thyroid dysfunction in the pathogenesis of panic disorder. It must be remembered, however, that each of the aforementioned studies relies on the assessment of thyroid function through the measurement of peripheral thyroid hormonal levels (including TSH). It remains possible, but heretofore untested, that patients with panic disorder might exhibit abnormal end-organ responsivity to apparently normal thyroid hormonal levels. We entertained the notion that patients with panic disorder might actually demonstrate supersensitivity to thyroid hormones at a receptor level and sought a way to indirectly test this hypothesis in vivo.

The metabolic and other physiological effects of thyroid hormones are well established (see Chapters 1, 2, and 3). It is possible to use one or more of these physiological effects of thyroid hormones as indicators of functional thyroid hormone effect at the tissue level. Examples include the use of basal metabolic rate (reduced in hypothyroidism), ankle reflex relaxation time (known to be reduced in hypothyroidism), serum carotene (elevated in hypothyroidism), and sex hormone–binding globulin (elevated in hyperthyroidism) (44). Each of these is seen to be altered, albeit nonspecifically, in patients with thyroid disease. Another similar measure that has received renewed attention is the use of the pulse wave arrival time (QK_d interval) as a means to assess thyroid function. The QK_d *interval* refers to the timing of the Korotkoff arterial sounds at diastolic pressure with reference to the QRS complex of the electrocardiogram. This interval is seen to in-

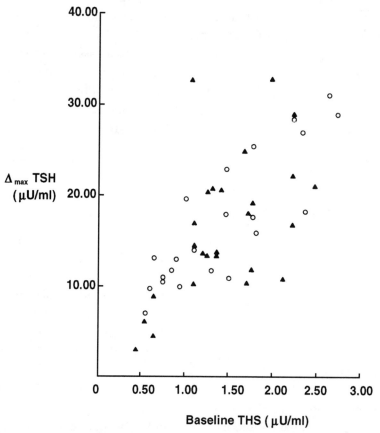

Figure 7–3. Baseline levels of thyroid-stimulating hormone (TSH) significantly correlate with Δ_{max} TSH responses to thyrotropin-releasing hormone in both panic disorder patients (*blackened triangles;* $r = .55$, $P < .005$) and healthy control subjects (*open circles;* $r = .85$, $P < .0001$).

crease in hypothyroidism and to decrease in hyperthyroidism. It has been used to demonstrate the existence of reduced thyroid hormonal function in patients with "thyroid hormone resistance" syndromes (45,46).

In our study (47), we hypothesized that patients with panic disorder would have decreased QK_d intervals, consistent with functional hyperthyroidism as a result of tissue supersensitivity to thyroid hormones. We compared the QK_d interval at rest in 15 patients with panic disorder with that of 20 healthy control subjects. We found no significant differences between the patients with panic disorder (230 ± 50 milliseconds) and the control subjects (224 ± 29 milliseconds) while drug free, suggesting that these patients have normal tissue-level responsivity to thyroid hormones (Figure 7–4).

Recently, one group of investigators has used basal metabolic rate measurements to suggest that some depressed patients may exhibit abnormalities in thyroid hormone responsivity (48). Thus although probably not directly relevant to our understanding of panic disorder, the further use of these techniques to study thyroid hormone function may be germane to the elucidation of the genesis and maintenance of other psychiatric syndromes such as depressive disorders.

4.5 Triiodothyronine (T_3) Potentiation of Treatment for Panic Disorder

The use of thyroid hormones as an adjunct in the pharmacotherapy of treatment-refractory depression has gained considerable attention. Several reports (49–51) have provided evidence that the supplemental administration of thyroid hormones may lead to additional improvement or even complete remission in a proportion of depressed patients who have responded only partially to cyclic antidepressants, although there are also reports (52,53) pointing to the lack of efficacy of this approach.

Patients with panic disorder generally respond well to tricyclic antidepressants (54,55), but a subset of patients clearly continue to experience residual symptoms. In view of the fact that many treatments that are effective in depression are also effective in panic disorder, we elected to conduct a study of the adjunctive use of T_3 in patients with panic disorder who were poorly responsive or nonresponsive to tricyclic antidepressants. In this study (56), T_3 was administered on a single-blind basis to eight consecutive patients partially responsive to imipramine ($n = 7$) or nortriptyline ($n = 1$). T_3 was administered at a starting dose of 10–25 µg each morning and adjusted upward on a weekly basis, taking into account clinical response and side effects.

The mean duration of treatment with T_3 was 3.4 ± 1.2 weeks (range 2–5) and the mean maximal dose of T_3 was 25 ± 5 µg/day (range 20–30). The addition of T_3 failed to produce significant

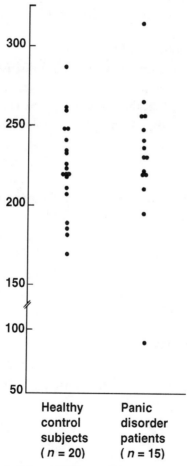

Figure 7–4. Pulse wave arrival time (QK_d interval) in patients with panic disorder and healthy control subjects. There is no difference in the mean QK_d interval in panic disorder patients (230 ± 50 milliseconds) compared with healthy control subjects (224 ± 29 milliseconds).

changes on any of the anxiety rating scales used in the study. On an individual basis, three patients experienced no change in their clinical status, four actually worsened, and only one patient appeared to benefit. The latter patient had a history of recurrent depressive episodes in addition to panic disorder with agoraphobia. Overall, this pilot study, although limited by the small sample size, suggests that T_3 potentiation is unlikely to be of widespread benefit to the majority of patients with panic disorder who respond poorly to tricyclic antidepressants.

5. THE THYROID AND OTHER ANXIETY DISORDERS

5.1 Generalized Anxiety Disorder (GAD)

Clinical studies of patients with thyroid diseases suggest that GAD may be the most common of the anxiety syndromes seen in these individuals. Nonetheless, the relationship between thyroid dysfunction and GAD has largely gone unexplored. Only one study (18) of thyroid hormone levels in patients with GAD ($n = 52$) has been performed, and this found no consistent evidence of abnormalities. To the best of our knowledge, other indices of HPT axis functioning have not been explored in GAD. This is unfortunate, because GAD is a chronic, persistent, and pervasive syndrome, in which it would be reasonable to speculate that HPT axis abnormalities might exist (as in depression). It is unclear why there is such a dearth of information on this subject, but it is our impression that the problem may lie, at least in part, in the difficulty most researchers experience in accumulating large numbers of "pure" GAD subjects for their studies.

5.2 Obsessive-Compulsive Disorder

Only a single study has examined the thyroid in obsessive-compulsive disorder. In this study, Joffe and Swinson (57) failed to find abnormalities in peripheral thyroid indices in patients with obsessive-compulsive disorder.

5.3 Social Phobia

A single study (23) has examined the HPT axis in patients with social phobia. No differences were found between patients with social phobia and age- and sex-matched control subjects in plasma T_3, T_4, FT_4, or TSH levels, or in the proportion of subjects with positive antithyroid antibodies. Furthermore, there was not convincing evidence of a higher rate of blunted TSH responses to TRH in the patients with social phobia, although it was thought that this deserved replication in a larger sample size.

5.4 Posttraumatic Stress Disorder (PTSD)

In a recent study of patients with posttraumatic stress disorder (PTSD), Kosten et al. (58) found that 3 of 11 (27%) male veterans with PTSD had blunted (i.e., Δ_{max} TSH < 7 μU/ml) TSH responses to TRH, a proportion not different than that of 28 male control subjects, but significantly less ($P < .05$) than the proportion of veterans with major depressive disorder (12 of 18 [67%]). Although the depressed veterans showed a significant increase ($P < .05$) in Δ_{max} TSH during repeat TRH-testing at discharge, this was not seen in the veterans with PTSD. These data would appear to provide some support for a neurobiological distinction between major depressive disorder and PTSD. In the only other study of TRH-responsivity in PTSD, Kauffman et al. (59) found that 4 of 8 (50%) patients with PTSD had blunted TSH responses. Clearly, the small sample sizes in which these studies were conducted make it impossible at this juncture to draw definitive conclusions about HPT axis functioning in PTSD.

6. EFFECTS OF TREATMENT ON THE HYPOTHALAMIC-PITUITARY-THYROID (HPT) AXIS

Although the aforementioned studies of thyroid function in anxiety disorders have generally failed to provide strong evidence for the involvement of overt or subclinical thyroid dysfunction in these syndromes, there remains a rationale for studying the effects of treatment on these parameters. In depression, several investigators (see Chapter 6) have reported changes in thyroid function associated with successful pharmacotherapy. For example, Joffe and Singer (60) reported that serum T_4 declined during treatment of 28 depressed patients with tricyclic antidepressants and that patients who responded had significantly greater decrements ($P < .05$) in T_4 than did nonresponsive patients. These findings contradict those of an earlier study (61) in which imipramine treatment was not accompanied by changes in peripheral thyroid hormones. Nonetheless, these studies emphasize that although clinical thyroid "disease" may not be a regular manifestation of affective illness, it remains entirely possible that some of the treatments we employ may result in changes in thyroid function that play a role in therapy. For example, even a nonpharmacological antidepressant, sleep deprivation, has been reported to result in changes in TSH responsivity to TRH (62) and peripheral thyroid indices (63). These changes, particularly those involving the anterior pituitary release of TSH and growth hormone (64), may provide a window into the neurotransmitter systems that mediate these changes, and, ultimately, the biological mechanisms that mediate clinical improvement.

We have conducted what we believe to be the only study of thyroid function in patients with panic disorder before and after treatment (65). Fourteen patients with panic disorder had basal peripheral thyroid indices and TSH responses to 500 µg TRH measured before and during chronic imipramine treatment. The mean imipramine dose at the time of TRH-testing was 107 ± 43 mg (range 50–175 mg) daily, and patients had been treated for a mean of 22 ± 9 weeks. During imipramine treatment, there were no significant changes noted in serum T_3, T_4, FT_4, or thyroid-binding globulin. However, patients exhibited significant increases in the TSH response to TRH ($P < .05$) (Figure 7–5) and in the prolactin response to TRH ($P < .02$) (Figure 7–6) during imipramine pharmacotherapy.

In this study, all 14 patients studied responded to imipramine. Consequently, we were unable to determine if the changes observed were confined to patients who showed clinical improvement; this remains a question to be answered through further study. Furthermore, we wish to emphasize that peripheral and central neuroendocrine events are often dissociated, making us extremely cautious about inferring what may be occurring in the brain on the basis of plasma hormonal measurements. With these caveats in mind, it is nonetheless possible that inhibition of dopaminergic tone, which could account for the enhanced prolactin and TSH responses to TRH, may be an important ingredient in the therapeutic response to imipramine in panic disorder.

7. CONCLUSIONS

It is clear from the material reviewed above that the study of the HPT axis in anxiety disorders is at a much more primitive stage of development than

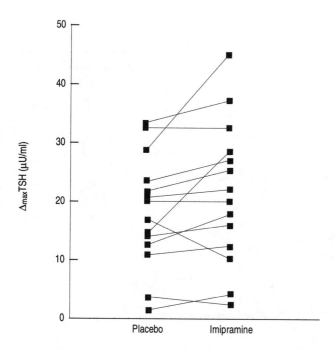

Figure 7–5. Increase in thyroid-stimulating hormone (TSH) response to thyrotropin-releasing hormone (TRH) during imipramine therapy in panic disorder patients ($n = 14$). The Δ_{max} TSH response to TRH significantly increased from a mean pretreatment change score of 18.2 ± 9.44 to 21.8 ± 12.1 after imipramine pharmacotherapy ($P < .05$, two-tailed Wilcoxon signed rank test).

is the case for the affective disorders. Few detailed dynamic studies of HPT axis in anxiety disorders have been undertaken. However, current knowledge suggests that alterations in thyroid function are unlikely to play a major role in the pathogenesis of panic disorder; it may be too early to generalize this opinion to the other anxiety disorders. Although there should be little argument that overt thyroid dysfunction (either hypo- or hyperthyroidism) may present with prominent symptoms of generalized anxiety or panic and should be conceptualized as an organic anxiety disorder (DSM-III-R), there is at present no reason to believe that thyroid dysfunction is a component of the primary anxiety disorders.

The apparent lack of thyroid abnormalities associated with panic disorder seems to differ from what is reported in the literature on major depression. At least a subgroup of patients with major depression seem to exhibit HPT axis dysfunction; at present, the most compelling evidence would

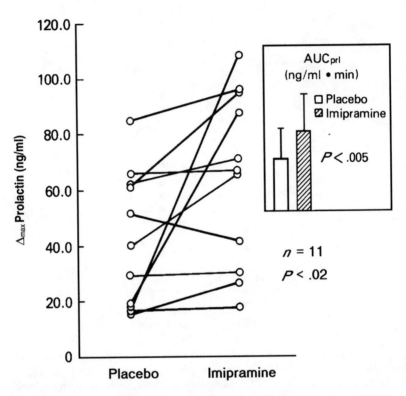

Figure 7–6. Increase in prolactin response to thyrotropin-releasing hormone (TRH) during imipramine therapy in panic disorder patients ($n = 11$, $P < .02$). The prolactin response to TRH (AUCprl, ng/ml • min) was significantly higher ($P < .005$) after imipramine treatment (2048 ± 984) compared with the placebo-treatment response profile (1367 ± 806).

seem to exist for patients with bipolar disorder or refractory (e.g., rapid-cycling) affective illness. This does not seem to be the case for panic disorder, and hence, on a theoretical note, this may mark an area of biological discontinuity between panic disorder and major depression.

This is not to say, however, that the thyroid gland is irrelevant to our understanding of the anxiety disorders. Certainly, the mere fact that anxiety is such a prominent feature of diseases such as Graves' disease suggests that we may benefit from the further study of these illnesses. In addition, there may be relatively rare clinical circumstances in which aberrations in thyroid function may play a role that is as yet unrecognized. An interesting candidate for such a scenario would be the changes in panic attack frequency that may occur around the time of pregnancy. Some patients with panic disorder exhibit a remission during pregnancy (66) or a worsening (or onset) in the postpartum period (67). This pattern is consistent with the course of postpartum thyroiditis, which often wanes during pregnancy and may recur following delivery. Therefore, a role for thyroid dysfunction in these clinical syndromes is deserving of further study.

REFERENCES

1. Graves RJ: Clinical lectures. London Medicine and Surgery Journal 7:516, 1835
2. Wartofsky L, Ingbar SH: Diseases of the thyroid, in Harrison's Principles of Internal Medicine, 12th Edition. Edited by Wilson JD, Braunwald E, Petersdorf RG, et al. New York, McGraw-Hill, 1991, pp 1692–1712
3. Whybrow PC, Prange AJ, Treadway CR: Mental changes accompanying thyroid gland dysfunction. Arch Gen Psychiatry 20:48–62, 1969
4. Dunlap GH, Moersch FP: Psychic manifestations associated with hyperthyroidism. Am J Psychiatry 91:1215–1236, 1935
5. MacCrimmon DJ, Wallace JE, Goldberg WM, et al: Emotional disturbance and cognitive deficits in hyperthyroidism. Psychosom Med 41:331–340, 1979
6. Rockey PH, Griep RJ: Behavioral dysfunction in hyperthyroidism. Arch Intern Med 140:1194–1197, 1980
7. Kathol RG, Delahunt JW: The relationship of anxiety and depression to symptoms of hyperthyroidism using operational criteria. Gen Hosp Psychiatry 8:23–28, 1986
8. Kathol RG, Turner R, Delahunt J: Depression and anxiety associated with hyperthyroidism: response to antithyroid therapy. Psychosomatics 27:501–505, 1986
9. Ficcara BJ, Nelson RA: Phobia as a symptom in hyperthyroidism. Am J Psychiatry 103:831–832, 1947
10. Katerndahl DA, Van de Creek L: Hyperthyroidism and panic attacks. Psychosomatics 24:491–496, 1983
11. Weller MPI: Agoraphobia and hyperthyroidism. Br J Psychiatry 144:553–554, 1984
12. Turner TH: Agoraphobia and hyperthyroidism. Br J Psychiatry 145:215–216, 1985
13. Raj A, Sheehan DV: Medical evaluation of panic attacks. J Clin Psychiatry 48:309–313, 1987
14. Stein MB: Panic disorder and medical illness. Psychosomatics 27:833–840, 1986

15. Stein MB, Uhde TW: Routine screening of thyroid indices in patients with panic attacks (letter). J Clin Psychiatry 49:204, 1988
16. Lindeman CG, Zitrin CM, Klein DF: Thyroid dysfunction in phobic patients. Psychosomatics 25:603–606, 1984
17. Orenstein H, Peskind A, Raskind MA: Thyroid disorders in female psychiatric patients with panic disorder or agoraphobia. Am J Psychiatry 145:1428–1430, 1988
18. Munjack DJ, Palmer R: Thyroid hormones in panic disorder, panic disorder with agoraphobia, and generalized anxiety disorder. J Clin Psychiatry 49:229–231, 1988
19. Pariser SF, Jones BA, Pinta ER, et al: Panic attacks: diagnostic evaluations of 17 patients. Am J Psychiatry 136:105–106, 1979
20. Fishman SM, Sheehan DV, Carr DB: Thyroid indices in panic disorder. J Clin Psychiatry 46:432–433, 1985
21. Yeragani VK, Rainey JM, Pohl R, et al: Thyroid hormone levels in panic disorder. Can J Psychiatry 32:467–469, 1987
22. Matuzas W, Al-Sadir J, Uhlenhuth EH, et al: Mitral valve prolapse and thyroid abnormalities in patients with panic attacks. Am J Psychiatry 144:493–496, 1987
23. Lesser IM, Rubin RT, Lydiard RB, et al: Past and current thyroid function in subjects with panic disorder. J Clin Psychiatry 48:473–476, 1987
24. Stein MB, Uhde TW: Thyroid indices in panic disorder. Am J Psychiatry 145:745–747, 1988
25. Turnbridge WMG, Brewis M, French JM, et al: Natural history of autoimmune thyroiditis. BMJ 282:258–262, 1981
26. Gold MS, Pottash ALC, Extein I: "Symptomless" autoimmune thyroiditis in depression. Psychiatry Res 6:261–269, 1982
27. Nemeroff CB, Simon JS, Haggerty JJ Jr, et al: Antithyroid antibodies in depressed patients. Am J Psychiatry 142:840–843, 1985
28. Joffe RT: Antithyroid antibodies in major depression. Acta Psychiatr Scand 76:598–599, 1987
29. Haggerty JJ Jr, Evans DL, Golden RN, et al: The presence of antithyroid antibodies in patients with affective and nonaffective psychiatric disorders. Biol Psychiatry 27:51–60, 1990
30. Bauer MS, Whybrow PC, Winokur A: Rapid cycling bipolar disorder, I: association with grade I hypothyroidism. Arch Gen Psychiatry 47:427–432, 1990
31. Uhde TW, Boulenger JP, Roy-Byrne PP, et al: Longitudinal course of panic disorder: clinical and biological considerations. Prog Neuropsychopharmacol Biol Psychiatry 9:39–51, 1985
32. Breier A, Charney DS, Heninger GR: Major depression in patients with agoraphobia and panic disorder. Arch Gen Psychiatry 41:1129–1135, 1984
33. Stein MB, Uhde TW: Panic disorder and major depression: a tale of two syndromes. Psychiatr Clin North Am 11:441–461, 1988

34. Stein MB, Tancer ME, Uhde TW: Major depression in patients with panic disorder: factors associated with course and recurrence. J Affective Disord 19:287–296, 1990

35. Heninger GR: A biologic perspective on comorbidity of major depressive disorder and panic disorder, in Comorbidity of Mood and Anxiety Disorders. Edited by Maser JD, Cloninger CR. Washington, DC, American Psychiatric Press, 1990, pp 381–401

36. Roy-Byrne PP, Uhde TW, Rubinow DR, et al: Reduced TRH and prolactin responses to TRH in patients with panic disorder. Am J Psychiatry 143:503–507, 1986

37. Hamlin CL, Pottash ALC: Evaluation of anxiety disorders, in Diagnostic and Laboratory Testing in Psychiatry. Edited by Gold MS, Pottash ALC. New York, Plenum, 1986, pp 215–233

38. Castellani S, Quillen MA, Vaughan DA, et al: TSH and catecholamine response to TRH in panic disorder. Biol Psychiatry 24:87–90, 1988

39. Gillette GM, Garbutt JC, Quade DE: TSH response to TRH in depression with and without panic attacks. Am J Psychiatry 146:743–748, 1989

40. Stein MB, Uhde TW: Endocrine, cardiovascular, and behavioral effects of intravenous TRH in patients with panic disorder. Arch Gen Psychiatry 48:148–156, 1991

41. Eriksson E, Westberg P, Modigh K: Panic disorder, I: GH response to clonidine, TSH response to TRH, and dexamethasone suppression test in patients and controls. Neuroendocrinology Letters 12:313, 1990

42. Seth J, Kellett HA, Cladwell G, et al: A sensitive immunoradiometric assay for serum thyroid stimulating hormone: a replacement for the thyrotropin releasing hormone test? BMJ 289:1334–1336, 1984

43. Baumgartner A, Hahnenkamp L, Meinhold H: Effects of age and diagnosis on thyrotropin response to thyrotropin-releasing hormone in psychiatric patients. Psychiatry Res 17:285–294, 1986

44. Moore WT, Eastman RC: Thyroid disease, in Diagnostic Endocrinology. Edited by Moore WT, Eastman RC. Philadelphia, PA, BC Decker, 1990, pp 127–148

45. Refetoff S: Syndromes of thyroid hormone resistance. Am J Physiol 243:E88–E98, 1982

46. Usala SJ, Tennyson GE, Bale AE, et al: A base mutation of the c-erbA beta thyroid hormone receptor in a kindred with generalized thyroid hormone resistance. J Clin Invest 85:93–100, 1990

47. Stein MB, Muir-Nash J, Uhde TW: The QK_d interval in panic disorder: an assessment of end-organ thyroid hormone responsivity. Biol Psychiatry 29:1209–1214, 1991

48. Gewirtz GR, Malaspina D, Hatterer JA, et al: Occult thyroid dysfunction in patients with refractory depression. Am J Psychiatry 145:1012–1014, 1988

49. Goodwin FK, Prange AJ Jr, Post RM, et al: Potentiation of antidepressant effects of L-triiodothyronine in tricyclic nonresponders. Am J Psychiatry 139:34–38, 1982

50. Targum SD, Greenburg RD, Harmon RL, et al: Thyroid hormone and the TRH stimulation test in refractory depression. J Clin Psychiatry 45:345–346, 1984

51. Joffe RT, Singer W: A comparison of triiodothyronine and thyroxine in the potentiation of tricyclic antidepressants. Psychiatry Res 32:241–252, 1990

52. Gitlin MJ, Weiner H, Fairbanks L: Failure of T3 to potentiate tricyclic anti-depressant response. J Affective Disord 38:106–113, 1987

53. Thase ME, Kupfer DJ, Jarrett DB: Treatment of imipramine-resistant recurrent depression, I: an open clinical trial of adjunctive L-triiodothyronine. J Clin Psychiatry 50:385–388, 1989

54. Lydiard RB, Ballenger JC: Antidepressants in panic disorder and agoraphobia. J Affective Disord 13:153–168, 1987

55. Uhde TW, Stein MB: The biology and pharmacological treatment of panic disorder, in Panic and Phobias II: Treatments and Variables Affecting Outcome. Edited by Hand I, Wittchen H-U. Berlin, Springer-Verlag, 1988, pp 18–35

56. Stein MB, Uhde TW: Triiodothyronine potentiation of tricyclic antidepressant treatment in patients with panic disorder. Biol Psychiatry 28:1061–1064, 1990

57. Joffe RT, Swinson RP: Thyroid function in obsessive-compulsive disorder. Psychiatr J Univ Ottawa 13:215–216, 1988

58. Kosten TR, Wahby V, Giller E Jr, et al: The dexamethasone suppression test and thyrotropin-releasing hormone stimulation test in posttraumatic stress disorder. Biol Psychiatry 28:657–664, 1990

59. Kauffman CD, Reist C, Djenderedjian A, et al: Biological markers of affective disorders and posttraumatic stress disorder: a pilot study with desipramine. J Clin Psychiatry 48:366–367, 1987

60. Joffe RT, Singer W: The effect of tricyclic antidepressants on basal thyroid hormone levels in depressed patients. Pharmacopsychiatry 23:67–69, 1990

61. Linnoila M, Gold P, Potter WZ, et al: Tricyclic antidepressants do not alter thyroid hormone levels in patients suffering from a major affective disorder. Psychiatry Res 4:357–360, 1981

62. Kasper S, Sack DA, Wehr TA, et al: Nocturnal TSH and prolactin secretion during sleep deprivation and prediction of antidepressant response in patients with major depression. Biol Psychiatry 24:631–641, 1988

63. Baumgartner A, Graf K-J, Kurten I, et al: Neuroendocrinological investigations during sleep deprivation in depression, I: early morning levels of thyrotropin, TH, cortisol, prolactin, LH, FSH, estradiol, and testosterone. Biol Psychiatry 28:556–568, 1990

64. Uhde TW, Tancer ME, Rubinow DR, et al: Evidence for hypothalamo-growth hormone dysfunction in panic disorder: profile of growth hormone (GH) responses to clonidine, yohimbine, caffeine, glucose, GRF and TRH in panic disorder patients versus healthy volunteers. Neuropsychopharmacology 6:101–118, 1992
65. Stein MB, Uhde TW: Thyrotropin and prolactin responses to TRH prior to and during chronic imipramine treatment in patients with panic disorder. Psychoneuroendocrinology 15:381–389, 1990
66. George DT, Ladenheim JA, Nutt DJ, et al: Effect of pregnancy on panic attacks. Am J Psychiatry 144:1078–1079, 1987
67. Metz A, Sichel DA, Goff DC: Postpartum panic disorder. J Clin Psychiatry 49:278–279, 1988

Chapter 8

Interrelationships Between the Hypothalamic-Pituitary-Thyroid Axis and Alcoholism

James C. Garbutt, M.D.
Peter T. Loosen, M.D.
Arthur J. Prange, Jr., M.D.

CONTENTS

1. INTRODUCTION

Alcoholism is a common and serious illness that may affect as many as 25% of American men and 4% of American women at some time in their lives

(1). Alcoholism has been referred to as the *modern syphilis* because its clinical presentation can mimic many other illnesses and, accordingly, it is frequently misdiagnosed. One estimate has suggested that as many as 20%–40% of all inpatient hospital admissions in the United States are alcohol related (2). A disease as prevalent and destructive as alcoholism needs to be understood at many levels (i.e., genetic, neurobiological, medical, behavioral, and social) to lead to effective prevention and treatment.

In this chapter, we focus on only two aspects of alcoholism: its effects on the hypothalamic-pituitary-thyroid (HPT) axis and a possible role of the HPT axis in the pathogenesis of the illness. We examine abnormalities that have been reported in HPT axis function in various stages of alcoholism, and we focus on the clinical relevance of such findings when they are known.

Before a review of findings in the HPT axis, however, a brief discussion of its physiology may be useful (see also, Chapters 1 and 4) (3). The principal hormones of the HPT axis are thyroxine (T_4) and triiodothyronine (T_3), the latter much more potent than the former. Although both T_4 and T_3 are released from the thyroid gland, about 80% of circulating T_3 is derived from deiodination of T_4 in the liver and other tissues. Because the major site of deiodination is the liver, dysfunction of this organ is likely to alter thyroid hormone dynamics. Thyroid hormones are strongly bound to the serum proteins, thyroxine-binding globulin (TBG), albumin, and thyroid-binding prealbumin. More than 99% of T_4 and T_3 are bound to these proteins, with the remaining free fractions having biological activity. Alterations in levels of these proteins (as occurs with liver pathology), changes in estrogen levels, and other factors can affect total T_4 and T_3 levels, as well as free thyroxine (FT_4) and free triiodothyronine (FT_3) levels.

The release of T_4 and T_3 from the thyroid gland is primarily controlled by the anterior pituitary hormone thyroid-stimulating hormone (TSH) (or thyrotropin). After being released from thyrotroph cells in the pituitary gland, TSH stimulates both the synthesis and release of thyroid hormones. The control of TSH release in turn is mediated principally by thyrotropin-releasing hormone (TRH), which is released into the hypothalamic-pituitary-portal vascular system from hypothalamic neurons that originate in the paraventricular nucleus. TRH also stimulates the release of prolactin from pituitary lactotroph cells. Homeostatic control within the HPT axis is provided principally by negative feedback inhibition by T_4 and T_3 at the thyrotroph cell, leading to diminished synthesis and release of TSH. Thyroid hormones have recently been shown to selectively reduce TRH biosynthesis in the hypothalamus, which may provide yet another means of regulation (4). Furthermore, many neurotransmitters and non-HPT axis hormones affect TRH and TSH release (5,6).

Because ethanol can affect many neurotransmitter systems in brain and, over time, can produce cell damage in several organ systems, it is not surprising that the interaction between ethanol and the HPT axis is indeed a complicated one. One of the major methods that has been used to assess the HPT axis in subjects with alcoholism is the TRH test. Until recently, this test was the most sensitive method to ascertain subtle changes in HPT axis function and was used to help in the diagnosis of hypothyroidism and hyperthyroidism. Advances in TSH assay sensitivity and specificity now allow measurement of basal TSH to provide much of the information that was formerly available only through the TRH test. However, the TRH test remains the most direct method to determine pituitary responsiveness to TRH and thereby provides information about the central nervous system inputs to the HPT axis that basal TSH likely does not. A methodological problem with the interpretation of TRH test findings is that different research groups have used different doses of TRH and different definitions of an abnormal response. As we review individual studies, we will use the definition of a blunted TSH response employed by their authors.

2. ACUTE EFFECTS OF ETHANOL

The acute effects of ethanol on HPT axis function in nonalcoholic subjects have been investigated to determine whether ethanol exhibits pharmacological effects at any level of the axis. Identification of such effects on the HPT axis in healthy subjects might help identify potential sites of pathological change in the HPT axis in alcoholic patients. Leppaluoto et al. (7) administered 1.5 g/kg of ethanol to healthy volunteers over 3 hours and found no effects on basal TSH levels measured during or 12 hours after ethanol administration. The TSH response to 200 µg TRH given 1 hour after ethanol was not different from the response after placebo. The prolactin response to TRH was not assessed.

Ylikahri et al. (8) also gave 1.5 g/kg of ethanol to volunteers over 3 hours, assessing thyroid hormone levels at intervals over the next 17 hours. In this study, a TRH test was given 4 and 14 hours after the beginning of the drinking session. Analyses compared hormone values after ethanol to hormone values obtained at identical time points after drinking water. Thyroid hormone levels were not altered by ethanol, nor were basal or TRH-induced TSH levels different between the two conditions. In fact, the only difference observed was a marked reduction in prolactin response to TRH 14 hours after drinking had begun, during the "hangover" period.

Van Thiel et al. (9) administered ethanol daily for 3 days to healthy subjects and then performed a TRH challenge test 12 hours after subjects had stopped drinking. Hormone values between ethanol and placebo conditions were compared. No differences in T_4 or T_3 levels or in the TSH response to TRH were observed after ethanol; prolactin responses were not measured.

The above data indicate that ethanol does not acutely affect the HPT axis at either the thyroidal or pituitary level. Whether acute ethanol exerts any central effect on TRH activity in brain in humans is unknown because there is no accurate way to measure this. The reduction in prolactin response to TRH several hours after cessation of drinking is of interest and has been interpreted as possibly secondary to an ethanol-induced increase in dopaminergic tone (8,10).

3. ETHANOL WITHDRAWAL

Withdrawal from ethanol can produce major physiological changes, their severity being determined by duration and extent of prior ethanol use, presence of prior withdrawal reactions from ethanol, nutritional status, and medical status. Major manifestations of moderate to severe ethanol withdrawal include tachycardia, tremor, diaphoresis, and increased temperature. The origin of these symptoms has been attributed, in part, to increased sympathetic tone with both peripheral and central components. The similarity between these withdrawal features and hyperthyroidism is apparent, though overt hyperthyroidism has not been shown to be a consequence of ethanol withdrawal.

HPT axis studies performed during ethanol withdrawal have focused on assessment of thyroid hormones and the TSH response to TRH. Of the studies cited in Table 8–1 (11–17), only two have reported differences in thyroid hormone levels compared with those in control subjects. We (11) found that alcoholic subjects in the acute withdrawal phase had elevations in the free thyroxine index (FT_4I) when compared with control subjects. However, the FT_4I values in the alcoholic subjects were within the normal range. In contrast, Geurts et al. (12) reported a decrease in total T_4 and T_3 accompanied by a reduction in TBG and a normal measured FT_4 level in alcoholic subjects, compared with those in control subjects, when thyroid measures were taken within 24 hours after the subjects had stopped drinking. This group reported an increase in T_4, T_3, and TBG levels in the alcoholic subjects when their thyroid hormone values immediately after stopping drinking were compared with their values taken 2 weeks after stopping drinking.

Anton et al. (18) have also recently reported that FT_4 and total T_4 increased as alcoholic subjects progressed from the acute intoxicated phase to abstinence. Furthermore, the degree of increase was positively related to the extent of ethanol intake prior to detoxification. T_4 levels were again reduced in alcoholic subjects who relapsed, suggesting that ethanol pro-

Table 8–1. Hypothalamic-pituitary-thyroid axis findings in alcoholic men during acute ethanol withdrawal

Study	T_4	T_3	rT_3	TSH	Δ_{max}TSH	Other
Loosen et al. 1979 (11)	+	0	NA	0	−	50% (6 of 12) blunted response; T_4 decreased with abstinence; basal prolactin reduced.
Geurts et al. 1981 (12)	−	−	0	0	0	T_4 and T_3 increased with abstinence; thyroid-binding globulin low at entry.
Valimaki et al. 1984 (13)	0	0	0	0	−	36% (9 of 25) blunted response. T_4 decreased with abstinence.
Rojdmark et al. 1984 (14)	0	0	NA	0	−	Prolactin response reduced, TSH and prolactin response increased by dopamine blockade.
Dackis et al 1984 (15)	0	0	NA	0	−	33% (5 of 15) blunted response, men and women.
Banki et al. 1984 (17)	NA	NA	NA	NA	−	77% (7 of 9) blunted response, women only.
Muller et al.	NA	NA	NA	NA	−	31% (11 of 35) blunted response, men and women.

Note. T_4 = thyroxine; T_3 = triiodothyronine; rT_3 = reverse triiodothyronine; TSH = thyroid-stimulating hormone; + = increased; − = decreased; 0 = no change; NA = not assessed.

duced suppression of T_4. Conversely, we (11) and Valimaki et al. (13) reported that FT_4I values decreased as alcoholic subjects progressed from the acute withdrawal state to the postwithdrawal state. We (11) did not find any changes in T_3 levels during withdrawal, although Valimaki et al. (13) did report a slight decrease in the free triiodothyronine index (FT_3I) after withdrawal. Rojdmark et al. (14) and Dackis et al. (15) did not find changes in either T_4 or T_3 levels over the course of withdrawal.

In summary, the data suggest that slight and transient increases or decreases in T_4 can occur during ethanol withdrawal and that these changes are of a smaller magnitude than those observed in overt thyroid disease. No clinical significance is presently attributed to these changes.

Regarding the TSH response to TRH during ethanol withdrawal, Table 8–1 shows that of the seven studies reviewed all but one reported a blunted TSH response to TRH. In all, 96 patients were tested, and 38 (39%) showed a blunted response.

Examination of the pathophysiology of this phenomenon has focused on thyroid hormones and dopamine. Given that there may be slight increases in T_4 during ethanol withdrawal (11,13) and given that thyroid hormones are potent inhibitors of TSH, one explanation for a reduced TSH response in withdrawal could be an increase in T_4 (or T_3). However, studying alcoholic patients in withdrawal, we (11) compared FT_4I levels between those with and those without a blunted TSH response; we observed no difference. Nevertheless, because it is the change in thyroid hormone levels within an individual that determines TSH response to TRH, it would be premature to conclude that relative increases in thyroid hormones are not responsible for at least some of the reduction in TSH response observed during ethanol withdrawal. It is also possible that small alterations in the free fractions of thyroid hormones may contribute to TSH blunting.

Increased dopamine input to the pituitary has been suggested by two groups (11,14) as a possible explanation for low TSH responses in ethanol withdrawal. Dopamine is known to inhibit TSH release in addition to its well-described inhibition of prolactin release (19). In support of overactive dopamine function, we (11) reported that basal prolactin was significantly reduced in alcoholic subjects in withdrawal when compared with either subjects in postwithdrawal or control subjects. A more definitive test of the hypothesis was carried out by Rojdmark et al. (14), who gave the dopamine receptor blocker metoclopramide to alcoholic subjects during acute withdrawal. Starting with the finding that the TSH and prolactin responses to TRH are reduced in alcoholic subjects in withdrawal, they found that metoclopramide produced partial normalization of both responses. These data strongly implicate increased dopamine activity as contributing to a reduced TSH response in ethanol withdrawal. They resonate with the findings of Ylikahri et al. (8) that in healthy subjects the prolactin response is reduced during the "withdrawal" from an acute dose of ethanol.

4. ABSTINENT ALCOHOLIC PATIENTS

4.1 Without Liver Disease

The long-term consequences of alcoholism on the HPT axis, other than in withdrawal syndromes, have been examined in alcoholic subjects with and without liver disease. In this section, we focus on studies that have excluded alcoholic subjects with significant liver disease, including cirrhosis. *Abstinence*, as used here, refers to at least a 1-week period without ethanol intake at the time of study; in fact, most studies have allowed a 3- to 4-week alcohol-free interval prior to study.

The early reports of Goldberg (20,21) that a large percentage of alcoholic patients were hypothyroid as determined by low values of protein-bound iodine, a deficient thyroidal response to TSH, and a prolonged ankle reflex time have not been confirmed (22,23). Table 8–2 shows the HPT axis findings in abstinent alcoholic subjects based on modern assessment methods (12,15,16,24–30). As can be seen, no evidence for either hypothyroidism or hyperthyroidism is present. Most studies have not found alterations in T_4 or T_3 levels, though two groups did find lower T_3 levels in alcoholic subjects compared with control subjects (24,25). Basal TSH was reported as substantially lower than normal by our groups (24,26), but not by three other groups (12,15,25).

A more consistent finding is a blunted TSH response to TRH, which has been reported in seven of nine studies that involved TRH testing. An eighth study (27) did not report significantly lower average TSH responses to TRH but did find a higher rate of blunted TSH responses in alcoholic subjects. A total of 163 alcoholic patients were studied in these eight projects; 43 (26%) were reported as having a blunted TSH response. However, methodological issues such as the use of different doses of TRH and the lack of control subjects in some studies make a precise estimate of prevalence uncertain. Nevertheless, it is clear that a blunted TSH response is often present in abstinent alcoholic patients.

The clinical significance of the blunted TSH response in abstinent alcoholic subjects is not known. It does not indicate any common form of thyroid disease. Although a reduction in TSH response might suggest marginal hyperthyroidism, supporting data (e.g., increased thyroid hormone production) are lacking. Pharmacokinetic differences in TRH metabolism between alcoholic and nonalcoholic subjects could explain the difference in TSH response. However, we (31) did not find this to be the case in a preliminary study. Moreover, most groups have reported normal prolactin responses in abstinent alco-

Table 8–2. Hypothalamic-pituitary-thyroid axis findings in abstinent alcoholic men without liver disease

Study	T_4	T_3	rT_3	TSH	Δ_{max} TSH	Other
Geurts et al. 1981 (12).	0	0	0	0	NA	TRH test not done
Loosen et al. 1983 (24)	0	–	+	–	–	31% (9 of 29) blunted response, prolactin response normal.
Dackis et al. 1984 (15)	–	0	NA	0	–	12% (4 of 32) blunted response, men and women.
Radouco-Thomas et al. 1984 (29)	NA	NA	NA	NA	–	44% (4 of 9) blunted response.
Casacchia et al. 1985 (28)	NA	NA	NA	NA	–	29% (2 of 7) blunted response, prolactin response normal.
Agner et al. 1986 (25)	0	–	–	0	0	Prolactin response normal.
Muller et al. 1989 (16)	NA	NA	NA	NA	–	41% (7 of 17) blunted response, men and women.
Marchesi et al. 1989 (30)	NA	NA	NA	NA	–	60% (9 of 15) blunted response, prolactin response decreased.
Willenbring et al. 1990 (27)	0	NA	NA	NA	0	15% (8 of 54) blunted response.
Garbutt et al. 1991 (26)	0	0	0	–	–	Dose-response design, prolactin response normal.

Note. T_4 = thyroxine; T_3 = triiodothyronine; rT_3 = reverse triiodothyronine; TSH = thyroid-stimulating hormone; + = increased; – = decreased; 0 = no change; NA = not assessed.

holic subjects, indicating an adequate lactotroph response to TRH and therefore an adequate amount of TRH reaching the pituitary. The finding of normal basal prolactin and normal TRH-stimulated prolactin also militates against excess dopamine input to the pituitary in abstinent alcoholic subjects.

Many other explanations for a blunted TSH response are possible, including reduced thyrotroph TRH receptors and excess activity of other TSH-inhibitory substances such as somatotropin release–inhibiting factor. Downregulation of thyrotroph TRH receptors could be caused by increases in the amount of TRH reaching the pituitary. However, Roy et al. (32) found that alcoholic patients do not differ from control subjects in levels of cerebrospinal fluid TRH. Of course, TRH levels in cerebrospinal fluid may not reflect TRH transmission to the pituitary. These authors did not compare TRH levels to TRH test findings.

4.2   With Liver Disease

Well known to clinicians (and a major public health problem) is ethanol-induced liver disease. Alcoholic liver disease is a progressive process leading to cellular destruction, fibrosis, and loss of function, as seen in cirrhosis. Cirrhosis and less severe forms of liver injury are associated with changes in protein synthesis and with alterations in the metabolism of many substances, including thyroid and steroid hormones. Therefore, it is not surprising that alcoholic subjects with cirrhosis or other forms of liver dysfunction exhibit a different profile of HPT axis changes than do abstinent alcoholic subjects without liver disease. Table 8–3 summarizes the findings (9,25,33–39).

With regard to thyroid hormones the data are quite uniform. For the most part, T_4 levels are not changed, whereas T_3 levels are decreased. Despite the decrease in T_3 levels, overt hypothyroidism is not present. The reductions in T_3 appear to derive from decreased conversion of T_4 to T_3, which in turn is thought to be secondary to liver cell damage and loss of deiodinating capacity. In support of this hypothesis, Israel et al. (33) observed a strong inverse correlation between an index of liver disease and serum T_3 levels. Furthermore, they reported that increases in T_3 levels over the course of hospitalization were associated with clinical improvement. In support of this finding, Hepner and Chopra (34) found that lower serum T_3 levels were associated with an increased risk of death. This suggests that the assessment of T_3 in alcoholic patients with cirrhosis may be used to gauge prognosis and to complement other indices of severity.

It is of interest that Orrego et al. (40) reported that the administration of propylthiouracil, an inhibitor of the conversion of T_4 to T_3, increases survival in alcoholic patients with liver disease. Although the underlying mechanism is not clear, it has been suggested that the effect is to decrease oxygen demand in hepatocytes by decreasing thyroid hormone levels, which in turn renders the cells less likely to experience hypoxic injury. Alcoholic liver disease is the only alcohol-related pathological change known to us in which a drug affecting thyroid hormone economy has been shown to be clinically efficacious. Hegedus et al. (41) reported that alcoholic patients with or without cirrhosis exhibit reductions in thyroid gland volume, as as-

Table 8–3. Hypothalamic-pituitary-thyroid axis findings in abstinent alcoholic men with liver disease

Study	T_4	T_3	rT_3	TSH	Δ_{max} TSH	Other
Chopra et al. 1974 (37)	−	−	NA	+	0	Physiological measures indicated subjects were euthyroid.
Nomura et al. 1975 (35)	0	−	NA	+	NA	Decreased conversion of T_4 to T_3.
Green et al. 1977 (36)	0	−	NA	+	+/−	60% (9 of 15) abnormal TSH response to TRH.
Van Thiel et al. 1979 (9)	−	−	NA	+	0	Free T_3 levels low and free T_4 levels high.
Israel et al. 1979 (33)	0	−	NA	NA	NA	T_3 levels inversely correlated with severity of liver disease.
Hepner and Chopra 1979 (34)	0	−	+	NA	NA	Low T_3 and high rT_3 levels predictive of bad outcome.
Monza et al. 1981 (38)	0	NA	NA	+	0	Prolactin response to TRH increased.
Hasselbalch et al. 1981 (39)	NA	NA	NA	0	0	Prolactin response to TRH increased.
Agner et al. 1986 (25)	0	−	NA	0	0	Thyroxine-binding globulin increased.

Note. T_4 = thyroxine; T_3 = triiodothyronine; rT_3 = reverse triiodothyronine; TSH = thyroid-stimulating hormone; + = increased; − = decreased; 0 = no change; NA = not assessed.

sessed by ultrasonic examination, and an increase in thyroid gland fibrosis at autopsy when compared with control subjects. Patients with nonalcoholic liver disease did not exhibit a reduction in thyroid gland volume. These data raise the question of a direct toxic effect of chronic ethanol ingestion on the thyroid gland. The clinical significance of this would appear doubtful, however, given that chronic alcoholism does not lead to overt hypothyroidism.

Another fairly consistent finding in alcoholic subjects with liver disease is an elevation in basal TSH levels, generally not accompanied by changes in the TSH response to TRH. Notably absent in this group is an increased prevalence of a blunted TSH response. The clinical significance of an increased basal TSH is not apparent. The lack of an increase in TSH response to TRH suggests that subclinical hypothyroidism is not present. The underlying reason(s) for the increased TSH is unknown; it could be related to decreased TSH clearance, increased estrogen levels (which potentiate TSH release), alterations in intrapituitary conversion of T_4 to T_3, or other factors.

5. SUBJECTS AT HIGH RISK FOR ALCOHOLISM

An important contribution to alcoholism research is the demonstration that genetic factors are among the determinants of the illness (42). Identification of the phenotypic expression of the underlying genetic risk has emerged as an important research direction to complement search for the alcoholic gene(s). A reduced TSH response to TRH has been preliminarily tested as a marker for alcoholism because, as noted above, it has been found in long-abstinent alcoholic subjects in the absence of thyroid or liver disease. Tests of a reduced TSH response to TRH as a putative marker have been carried out by comparing the prevalence of blunting in two groups: nonalcoholic offspring from alcoholic families (family history positive [FHP]) and nonalcoholic offspring from nonalcoholic families (family history negative [FHN]). This strategy requires that high-risk subjects be young enough not to have expressed alcoholic behavior, with its attendant consequences for neurobiological function.

Using this high-risk strategy, Radouco-Thomas et al. (29) found that 3 of 10 FHP subjects exhibited a blunted TSH response compared to 1 of 26 FHN subjects. All subjects were between 20 and 25 years old. In a study of very young subjects (ages 8–17 years), Moss et al. (43) reported that FHP boys exhibited a higher basal TSH and a higher peak TSH response after TRH administration compared with FHN boys. Girls, when compared by family history, did not differ in basal or TRH-stimulated TSH levels. In a comparison of 10 FHP and 10 FHN men (ages 18–25 years), Monteiro et al. (44) found no differences in basal T_4, basal TSH, or TSH responses. In our own work to date (45), we have found that 10 of 20 FHP subjects (ages 18–30 years) exhibited a blunted TSH response, defined as Δ_{max} TSH < 7 µU/ml, compared to 2 of 13 FHN subjects, a statistically significant difference ($P < .01$). No differences in mean T_4 or T_3 levels, basal TSH, or Δ_{max} TSH were found between the two groups.

The data summarized above indicate that alterations in the TSH response to TRH may be present in subjects at high risk for alcoholism, though the alterations are variable in sign and extent. A problem with risk-marker research is determining when one should accept negative findings as truly negative and not as a Type II error. Because only a portion of alcoholic subjects exhibit the marker and only a portion of their offspring are at risk for alcoholism, calculating what number of offspring would need to be studied to conclusively prove or disprove the marker hypothesis is complicated. We estimate the number to be on the order of 50 matched pairs. In any case, existing data suggest that this marker would not be a useful clinical test for risk for future alcoholism. Its sensitivity is low, and, given that other psychiatric and medical conditions are associated with a blunted TSH response, its specificity is poor. However, identification of an abnormality in TSH response to TRH in the offspring of alcoholic subjects would add to our understanding of the pathophysiology of the illness and could aid in the clarification of subtypes.

6. THYROTROPIN-RELEASING HORMONE (TRH) AND THE BEHAVIORAL EFFECTS OF ETHANOL

Shortly after the discovery of TRH as the hypothalamic releasing factor controlling TSH release, it was found that TRH is widely distributed throughout the central nervous system. The actions of TRH in these non-hypothalamic regions have been found to be diverse and not directly, if at all, related to endocrine function. One of the early observations regarding the central nervous system actions of TRH was that, in animals, TRH was a potent antagonist of the depressant effects (i.e., motor impairment, hypnosis, and hypothermia) of barbiturates (46) and ethanol (47,48). Interestingly, it was subsequently shown, again in an animal model, that TRH enhanced the anticonflict (anxiolytic) effects of ethanol, barbiturates, and benzodiazepines (49).

Several studies have examined interactions between TRH and sedating substances, including ethanol, in humans. Linnoila et al. (50) reported that TRH 10 µg/kg boy weight increased the sense of intoxication and potentiated several measures of impairment following ethanol 1.5 g/kg body weight in healthy volunteers. These findings were the opposite of what would be predicted from the animal data. Recently, Knutsen et al. (51) reported that five doses of TRH 20 mg po given before ethanol 1.0 g/kg body weight did antagonize a number of the impairing effects of ethanol. For instance, the rate of ethanol-induced errors in a choice-reaction task and ethanol-induced motor impairment was reduced by TRH. Interestingly, TRH produced a mild increase in subjective rating of relaxation in combination with ethanol.

We (52) have tested the effects of administering an acute injection of TRH, total dose of 500 µg, on ethanol-induced (0.8 g/kg) behaviors in healthy volunteers. In this paradigm we observed a mild antagonistic effect for TRH on ethanol-induced behaviors. In a preliminary study (53), we found that TRH 500 µg did counteract the sedative effect of chlordiazepoxide in humans, suggesting that TRH may indeed modulate the actions of sedative-hypnotics, such as ethanol, in humans.

In summary, data from animal research reveal TRH as a potent modulator of the behavioral effects of ethanol. TRH decreases the depressant effects of ethanol and probably enhances its anxiolytic actions. We believe that this combination of effects is unique; most agents that counteract the depressant effects of ethanol also counteract its anxiolytic effects. Results of attempts to extend these observations to humans have been mixed, but because of the lack of a good method to activate TRH systems in brain in humans, the failure to find effects must be considered preliminary. Therefore, whereas the hypothesis that TRH is involved in the neurobiological mechanisms underlying the pathological use of ethanol is attractive, it is not clear whether TRH systems play any role in the neurobiology of ethanol preference or tolerance. In our view, investigation in this area may offer the greatest likelihood of establishing an important link between a component of the HPT axis and alcoholism.

7. CONCLUSIONS

Examination of the relationships between the HPT axis and alcoholism has revealed findings with clinical and theoretical implications. Acute administration of ethanol does not produce changes in thyroid hormone levels or in the TSH response to TRH (7–9). Neuroendocrine evidence of an increase in dopaminergic input to the pituitary during the postdrinking period has been suggested by the finding of a reduction in prolactin response (8).

With chronic alcohol abuse, as occurs in alcoholic patients, perturbations in the HPT axis have been observed. The reported changes do not include the development of overt hypothyroidism, despite early reports by Goldberg (20,21) that a large portion of alcoholic individuals were hypothyroid. Similarly, the reported changes present no evidence for overt hyperthyroidism. Instead, subtle changes have been found in the HPT axis in various stages of alcoholism. These can be arranged within three groups of findings.

First, alcoholic patients undergoing withdrawal frequently exhibit a blunting in their TSH response to TRH compared with postwithdrawal values or control values. Some data indicate that this is related to dopaminergic inhibition of TSH (11,14). At present, this finding is of no known clinical value.

Second, a portion of alcoholic subjects who have been abstinent for long periods exhibit a blunted TSH response compared with control subjects. The pathophysiological basis of the blunted TSH response observed during abstinence is not known, though overt hyperthyroidism clearly is not the cause. The clinical significance of a blunted TSH response is not known. The TRH test is not recommended as a diagnostic measure because it has both low sensitivity and specificity in alcoholic patients. Present data also do not suggest that the TSH response to TRH will be able to provide robust discrimination between individuals who will and those who will not become alcoholic, though this area requires more study.

Finally, alcoholic patients with liver disease commonly have low T_3 levels; the extent of T_3 reduction and the failure to increase T_3 levels with recovery are indicative of a poor prognosis. The latter finding may be useful to clinicians managing patients with alcoholic liver disease. In a related way, pharmacological inhibition of the conversion of T_4 to T_3 is associated with increased survival (40), presumably by reducing metabolic demand on the liver. This latter observation may lead to improved strategies to manage and possibly prevent serious alcohol-related liver disease.

Perhaps the most intriguing aspect of the relationship between the HPT axis and alcoholism, and one that does not directly involve the neuroendocrine axis, is the possibility that the brain actions of TRH are connected to the neurobiology of alcoholism at a fundamental level. TRH, or its analogues, may have therapeutic value by counteracting craving or by preventing the transition from moderate to excessive ethanol use. This notion, although admittedly speculative, is supported by the finding that TRH has anxiolytic properties in animals (49) and may have similar actions in humans (51).

REFERENCES

1. Robins LN, Helzer JE, Weissman MW, et al: Lifetime prevalence of specific psychiatric disorders in three sites. Arch Gen Psychiatry 41:949–958, 1984
2. Burke TR: The economic impact of alcohol abuse and alcoholism. Public Health Rep 103:564–568, 1988
3. Ingbar SH: The thyroid gland, in Textbook of Endocrinology. Edited by Wilson JD, Foster DW. Philadelphia, PA, WB Saunders, 1985, pp 682–815
4. Segerson TP, Kauer J, Wolfe HC, et al: Thyroid hormone regulates TRH biosynthesis in the paraventricular nucleus of the rat hypothalamus. Science 238:78–80, 1987
5. Morley JE: Neuroendocrine control of thyrotropin secretion. Endocr Rev 2:396–436, 1981
6. Jacobowitz DM: Multifactorial control of pituitary hormone secretion: the "wheels" of the brain. Synapse 2:186–192, 1988
7. Leppaluoto J, Rapeli M, Varis R, et al: Secretion of anterior pituitary hormones in man: effects of ethyl alcohol. Acta Physiol Scand 95:400–406, 1975
8. Ylikahri RH, Huttunen MO, Harkonen M, et al: Acute effects of alcohol on anterior pituitary secretion of the tropic hormones. J Clin Endocrinol Metab 46:715–720, 1978
9. Van Thiel DH, Smith WI Jr, Wight C, et al: Elevated basal and abnormal thyrotropin-releasing hormone-induced thyroid-stimulating hormone secretion in chronic alcoholic men with liver disease. Alcohol Clin Exper Res 3:302–308, 1979
10. Liljquist S, Ahlenius S, Engel J: The effect of chronic ethanol treatment on behavior and central monoamines in the rat. Arch Pharmacol 300:205–212, 1977

11. Loosen PT, Prange AJ Jr, Wilson IC: TRH (Protirelin) in depressed alcoholic men. Arch Gen Psychiatry 36:540–547, 1979
12. Geurts J, Demeester-Mirkine N, Glinoer D, et al: Alterations in circulating thyroid hormones and thyroxine binding globulin in chronic alcoholism. Clin Endocrinol 14:113–118, 1981
13. Valimaki M, Pelkonen R, Harkonen M, et al: Hormonal changes in noncirrhotic male alcoholics during ethanol withdrawal. Alcohol Alcohol 19:235–242, 1984
14. Rojdmark S, Adner N, Andersson DEH, et al: Prolactin and thyrotropin responses to thyrotropin-releasing hormone and metoclopramide in men with chronic alcoholism. J Clin Endocrinol Metab 59:595–600, 1984
15. Dackis CA, Bailey J, Pottash ALC, et al: Specificity of the DST and TRH test for major depression in alcoholics. Am J Psychiatry 141:680–683, 1984
16. Muller N, Hoehe M, Klein HE, et al. : Endocrinological studies in alcoholics during withdrawal and after abstinence. Psychoneuroendocrinology 14:113–123, 1989
17. Banki CM, Arato M, Papp Z: Thyroid stimulation test in healthy subjects and psychiatric patients. Acta Psychiatr Scand 70:295–303, 1984
18. Anton R, Thevos A, Brady KT: Acute effects of alcohol consumption on the thyroid (abstract 419). Presented at the Fifth Congress of the International Society for Biomedical Research on Alcoholism, Toronto, Ontario, Canada, June 1990
19. Burrow GN, May PB, Spaulding SW, et al: TRH and dopamine interactions affecting pituitary hormone secretion. J Clin Endocrinol Metab 45:65–72, 1977
20. Goldberg M: The occurrence and treatment of hypothyroidism among alcoholics. Journal of Clinical Endocrinology 20:609–621, 1960
21. Goldberg M: Thyroid function in chronic alcoholism. Lancet 2:746–749, 1962
22. Selzer ML, VanHouten WH: Normal thyroid function in chronic alcoholism. J Clin Endocrinol Metab 24:380–383, 1964
23. Augustine JR: Laboratory studies in acute alcoholics. Can Med Assoc J 96:1367–1370, 1967
24. Loosen PT, Wilson IC, Dew BW, et al: Thyrotropin-releasing hormone (TRH) in abstinent alcoholic men. Am J Psychiatry 140:1145–1149, 1983
25. Agner T, Hagen C, Andersen BN, et al: Pituitary-thyroid function and thyrotropin, prolactin and growth hormone responses to TRH in patients with chronic alcoholism. Acta Medica Scandinavica 220:57–62, 1986
26. Garbutt JC, Mayo JP, Gillette GM, et al: Dose-response studies with thyrotropin-releasing hormone (TRH) in abstinent male alcoholics: evidence for selective thyrotroph dysfunction. J Stud Alcohol 52:275–280, 1991
27. Willenbring ML, Anton RF, Spring WD Jr, et al: Thyrotropin and prolactin response to thyrotropin-releasing hormone in depressed and nondepressed alcoholic men. Biol Psychiatry 27:31–38, 1990

28. Casacchia M, Rossi A, Stratta P: Thyrotropin-releasing hormone test in re-cently abstinent alcoholics. Psychiatry Res 16:249–251, 1985
29. Radouco-Thomas S, Garcin F, Murthy MRV, et al: Biological markers in major psychoses and alcoholism: phenotypic and genotypic markers. J Psy-chiatr Res 18:513–539, 1984
30. Marchesi C, Campanini T, Govi A, et al: Abnormal thyroid stimulating hor-mone, prolactin and growth hormone responses to thyrotropin-releasing hormone in abstinent alcoholic men with cerebral atrophy. Psychiatry Res 28:89–96, 1989
31. Loosen PT, Youngblood W, Dew B: Plasma levels of exogenous TRH in nor-mal subjects and two patients with TSH blunting. Psychopharmacol Bull 19:325–327, 1983
32. Roy A, Bissette G, Nemeroff CB, et al: Cerebrospinal fluid thyrotropin-re-leasing hormone concentrations in alcoholics and normal controls. Biol Psy-chiatry 28:767–772, 1990
33. Israel Y, Walfish PG, Orrego H, et al: Thyroid hormones in alcoholic liver disease. Gastroenterology 76:116–122, 1979
34. Hepner GW, Chopra IJ: Serum thyroid hormone levels in patients with liver disease. Arch Intern Med 139:1117–1120, 1979
35. Nomura S, Pittman CS, Chambers JB Jr, et al: Reduced peripheral conversion of thyroxine to triiodothyronine in patients with hepatic cirrhosis. J Clin Invest 56:643–652, 1975
36. Green JRB, Snitcher EJ, Mowat NAG, et al: Thyroid function and thyroid regulation in euthyroid men with chronic liver disease: evidence of multiple abnormalities. Clin Endocrinol 7:453–461, 1977
37. Chopra IJ, Soloman DH, Chopra U, et al: Alterations in circulating thyroid hormones and thyrotropin in hepatic cirrhosis: evidence for euthyroidism despite subnormal serum triiodothyronine. J Clin Endocrinol Metab 39:501–511, 1974
38. Monza GC, Lampertico M, Ferrari A, et al: Prolactin and thyrotropin se-cretion in alcoholic liver cirrhosis: study of the variations induced by TRH, metoclopramide and cimetidine. J Nucl Med Allied Sci 25:71–78, 1981
39. Hasselbalch HC, Bech K, Eskildsen PC: Serum prolactin and thyrotropin re-sponses to thyrotropin-releasing hormone in men with alcoholic cirrhosis. Acta Medica Scandinavica 209:37–40, 1981
40. Orrego H, Blake JE, Blendis LM, et al: Long-term treatment of alcoholic liver disease with propylthiouracil. N Engl J Med 317:1421–1427, 1987
41. Hegedus L, Rasmussen N, Ravn V, et al: Independent effects of liver disease and chronic alcoholism on thyroid function: the possibility of a toxic effect of alcohol on the thyroid gland. Metabolism 37:229–233, 1988
42. Cloninger CR: Neurogenetic adaptive mechanisms in alcoholism. Science 236:410–416, 1987

43. Moss HB, Guthrie S, Linnoila M: Enhanced thyrotropin response to thyrotropin-releasing hormone in boys at risk for alcoholism. Arch Gen Psychiatry 43:1137–1142, 1986

44. Monteiro MG, Irwin M, Hauger RL, et al: TSH response to TRH and family history of alcoholism. Biol Psychiatry 27:905–910, 1990

45. Garbutt JC, Miller L, Karnitschnig J, et al: Thyrotropin response to thyrotropin-releasing hormone in young men at high or low risk for alcoholism (abstract 356). Fifth Congress of the International Society for Biomedical Research on Alcoholism, Toronto, Ontario, Canada, June 1990

46. Prange AJ Jr, Breese GR, Cott JM, et al: Thyrotropin-releasing hormone: antagonism of pentobarbital in rodents. Life Sci 14:447–455, 1974

47. Breese GR, Cott JM, Cooper BR, et al: Antagonism of ethanol narcosis by thyrotropin-releasing hormone. Life Sci 14:1053–1063, 1974

48. Cott JM, Breese GR, Cooper BR, et al: Investigations into the mechanism of reduction of ethanol sleep by thyrotropin-releasing hormone (TRH). J Pharmacol Exp Ther 196:594–604, 1976

49. Witkin JM, Sickle J, Barrett JE: Potentiation of the behavioral effects of pentobarbital, chlordiazepoxide and ethanol by thyrotropin-releasing hormone. Peptides 5:809–813, 1984

50. Linnoila M, Mattila MJ, Karhunen P, et al: Failure of TRH and ORG 2766 hexapeptide to counteract alcoholic inebriation in man. Eur J Clin Pharmacol 21:27–32, 1981

51. Knutsen H, Dolva LO, Skrede S, et al: Thyrotropin-releasing hormone antagonism of ethanol inebriation. Alcohol Clin Exper Res 13:365–370, 1989

52. Garbutt JC, Hicks RE, Clayton C, et al: Behavioral and endocrine interactions between thyrotropin-releasing hormone and ethanol in normal human subjects. Alcoholism: Clinical and Experimental Research 15:1045–1049, 1991

53. Garbutt JC, Gillette GM, Hicks RE: TRH effect on chlordiazepoxide sedation. Biol Psychiatry 25:983–985, 1988

Chapter 9

The Thyroid
and Eating Disorders

Allan S. Kaplan, M.D.
D. Blake Woodside, M.D.

CONTENTS

1. INTRODUCTION

For almost two centuries, the thyroid gland has been known to play a role in psychiatric illness (1). The role of the thyroid gland in maintaining metabolic homeostasis has also been historically well described. There is an emerging literature regarding the neurobiology of appetitive behaviors suggesting that there is a disturbance in this metabolic homeostasis that may have pathophysiological significance in illnesses such as anorexia nervosa and bulimia nervosa.

Studying the role of thyroid hormone in eating disorders would seem to be clearly indicated for a number of reasons. First, a number of parameters of thyroid function are disturbed in anorexia nervosa and bulimia nervosa, and an understanding of the nature of these disturbances may lead to an understanding of pathophysiology and pathogenesis. Second, thyroid hormone is one of several drugs used by patients with eating disorders to control weight by altering metabolic rate and inducing a disturbance in metabolism. Finally, thyroid function is known to be disturbed in affective disorder and many patients with eating disorders have a comorbid affective disorder.

An understanding of the nature of the thyroid disturbance in affectively disordered anorexic and bulimic patients may help to elucidate the complex relationship between thyroid function, mood, and eating. In this chapter, we first review the effects of caloric deprivation on circulating levels of thyroid hormone and on the hypothalamic-pituitary-thyroid (HPT) axis. We then review thyroid function in anorexia nervosa and bulimia nervosa and conclude with a cautionary note about the risk of thyroid hormone abuse in patients with eating disorders.

2. NUTRITIONAL DEPRIVATION

2.1 Peripheral Thyroid Hormone Levels

Caloric restriction results in a characteristic picture of thyroid hormone serum levels, consisting of decreased levels of triiodothyronine (T_3), low average or decreased levels of thyroxine (T_4), and increased levels of reverse triiodothyronine (rT_3) (for a comprehensive review of the effects of nutrition on thyroid function, see Chapter 6 and 2). Investigation has revealed that this picture is caused by a number of factors. First, the deiodinase responsible for the bulk of T_3 production (type I) is highly sensitive to starvation, responding to this stimulus with decreased activity. Second, increases in serum rT_3—once thought to be the result of increased production—are now known to be related to decreased degradation of rT_3, related to the same decreases in type I deiodinase activity. It is also known that these changes are transient and return to more normal values after a short time, even in the face of continued caloric restriction. Further, it is known that this transient rise is highly dependent on dietary composition, with small amounts of carbohydrate blocking this transient rise due to a carbohydrate-specific induction of the type I deiodinase. T_4 concentrations are comparatively unaffected by short-term caloric restriction and do not begin to fall until there is either a decrease in thyroid-binding globulin (TBG) and transthyretin (TTR) concentrations or until there is a dietary iodide deficiency. Binding protein concentrations are also known to be sensitive to more chronic caloric deprivation, especially to carbohydrate deprivation. T_3 and T_4 concentrations may also be related to circulating levels of substances such as carotenes, with hypercarotenemia being associated with lowered T_3 and T_4 levels (3).

2.2 Hypothalamic-Pituitary-Thyroid (HPT) Axis

Although decreases in serum T_3 and T_4 normally result in increases in thyroid-stimulating hormone (TSH) (or thyrotropin), the situation in caloric deprivation is somewhat different. Serum TSH levels are not usually increased and the TSH response to thyrotropin-releasing hormone (TRH) is often blunted or delayed rather than augmented in starvation. Although this pattern is intuitively understandable from the point of view of a starved organism, the precise reason for the observed effect is unknown. It is possible that this effect is due to pituitary intracellular T_3 concentrations being maintained by conversion from T_4 by the type II deiodinase; T_4 concentrations are relatively unaffected by starvation in the short term.

As we discuss in the next section, thyroid function has been extensively studied in anorexia nervosa, and, for the most part, the pattern of thyroid indices seen in anorexia nervosa seems to be a physiological adaptation to starvation. Similar abnormalities have been reported in healthy control subjects experimentally starved over a 3-week period. These subjects demonstrated lowered basal TSH levels and blunted TSH response to TRH compared with prefasting baseline levels (4,5). Similar findings have been reported in a previous study (6) in which five of nine healthy male subjects who initially had a normal TSH response to TRH demonstrated blunted responses following a 36-hour fast. These studies demonstrate the importance of nutritional state and, specifically, level of caloric intake at the time of testing of the HPT axis.

3. ANOREXIA NERVOSA

3.1 Peripheral Thyroid Hormone Levels

There is now general agreement that low circulating levels of thyroid hormone are present in anorexia nervosa. However, there are differences noted between circulating levels of T_3 and T_4. Circulating levels of T_4 are routinely reported to be within the lower part of the normal range, with values consistently reported as lower than those for control groups (7–11). By contrast, circulating levels of T_3 are usually reported to be below the normal range with elevated levels of rT_3 (7, 9–17). It is hypothesized that the elevated levels of rT_3 that are observed are related to a shift from rT_3-T_3 conversion to T_4-rT_3 conversion as an energy conservation mechanism, rT_3 being less biologically active (18,19). The combination of low-normal T_4, low T_3, elevated rT_3, and normal TSH has been referred to as the "euthyroid sick" syndrome (20) and is often associated with conditions in which there is rapid weight loss. One group (21) has suggested that the occurrence of hypothyroid-like symptoms in anorexia nervosa is related to peripheral tissue being preferentially sensitive to T_3, with T_4 having an effect more on the pituitary.

T_3 resin uptake is usually normal in response to acute starvation (22), suggesting normal levels of TBG. T_3 resin levels would be expected to fall only when starvation was severe enough either to cause reduced TBG levels or a dietary iodide deficiency. Serum TBG may be low in anorexia nervosa (16) as it is lowered in states of profound starvation associated with hypoalbuminemia (2).

3.2 Hypothalamic-Pituitary-Thyroid (HPT) Axis

TSH levels are typically reported in the low-normal range in anorexia nervosa (9,10,13,22–24), as distinct from the case in hypothyroidism.

TSH responses to TRH have been variably reported as normal (10, 24), delayed (12,15,25,26), or blunted (14). It is noteworthy that Kiyohara et al. (27) observed that patients with the most abnormal TSH responses were those with the most severe eating disorder symptoms. As is the case with other indices of thyroid function, variable recovery of normal responses has been reported with weight restoration.

Although it has occasionally been suggested that nonrecovery of normal TSH response to TRH implies the existence of a primary hypothalamic disturbance in a subgroup of anorexia nervosa patients, no long-term follow-up studies have been performed. The existence of a possibly delayed return to normal of such endocrinologic markers should be viewed in the light of other endocrinologic manifestations of starvation that are known to take a variable time to recover, such as normal menstrual function, which can take many months or years to return to normal after weight restoration has occurred. The reasons for these delays are unknown but may relate to a primary, as yet unidentified, hypothalamic disorder or to the long-term effects of chaotic eating and starvation even after the acute effects resolve.

3.3 Weight Restoration

Most studies have shown that weight restoration and, more importantly, caloric intake lead to either partial or complete normalization of thyroid indices. The return of normal degradation of rT_3 after carbohydrate ingestion has been commented on above, as has the return of more normal TSH responses to TRH. These changes are largely sensitive to caloric intake and nutrient composition, rather than to weight, per se. However, thyroid hormone levels do not correlate well with weight, caloric intake, nor with rate of weight gain, and a proportion of patients will show abnormal indices and TSH responses after recovery. Kiyohara et al. (27) investigated this issue in 25 patients with anorexia nervosa who had abnormal TSH responses to TRH during starvation. After weight recovery, 13 of 25 patients demonstrated a persistence of abnormal responses. Of importance, the 12 patients who had normalized TSH responses had recovered from all symptoms of the eating disorder, whereas it is implied in this study that the patients with persistently abnormal responses did not.

In summary, the changes associated with acute caloric deprivation include a transient rise in rT_3, a decrease in T_3, and no change in serum TSH or T_4. With more prolonged starvation, TBG and TTR levels will eventually fall, causing an associated decrease in T_4. TSH responses to TRH will become blunted or delayed early on in this process and seem to return to normal after weight restoration in most cases.

A few studies have examined the relationship between dietary composition, metabolic rate, and weight gain during the refeeding process in anorexia nervosa. Forbes et al. (28) noted that there was no difference in the rate of weight gain in high- or low-protein diets. Walker et al. (29) demonstrated that patients presenting at a lower weight require fewer calories to gain a kilogram, possibly because of increases in metabolic rate associated with a less emaciated weight. Finally, Stordy et al. (30) noted that previously obese anorexic patients gained weight more rapidly on the same caloric intake than did anorexic patients with no history of obesity, suggesting that the previously obese were more efficient at utilizing the calories provided.

In the light of other studies examining basal metabolic rate in bulimia nervosa (31), it is unfortunate that this study did not delineate which patients may have had bulimic features. Although it is most likely that the abnormalities noted to occur in thyroid function in anorexia nervosa are epiphenomena of starvation and/or weight loss and adaptations to this state, an etiological role for an abnormality of peripheral or central thyroid metabolism has not been adequately investigated and cannot yet be completely ruled out. Further research is needed to clarify the relationship between metabolic rate and caloric requirements for weight gain in anorexia nervosa.

4. BULIMIA NERVOSA

Studying thyroid function in patients with bulimia nervosa who are apparently at a normal weight may reveal abnormalities that are not necessarily explained solely by weight loss or starvation. Such abnormalities could provide evidence for a trait disturbance in neuroendocrine function. However, it is noteworthy that most bulimic patients, although at a normal weight as defined by average body weight for age and height, have lost weight from a premorbidly heavier state (32). Biologically, these patients may be in a starvation state similar to patients underweight with anorexia nervosa or as a result of experimentally induced starvation. Such a notion is supported by evidence from several studies (14,33) that demonstrated that compared with control subjects, a majority of patients with bulimia nervosa had elevated plasma β-hydroxybutyric acid and free fatty acids, as well as lower levels of T_3 and glucose and a decreased noradrenaline response to an orthostatic challenge. These are metabolic signs of starvation and occur in bulimic patients at a normal weight similar to emaciated anorexic patients and unlike control subjects at normal weight. In addition, some studies (34,35) have reported enlarged cerebral ventricles in patients with bulimia nervosa, possibly reflecting the effects of chronic malnutrition or fluctuations in weight affecting brain function.

Chaotic eating associated with abnormal patterns of nutrient intake independent of weight could also indirectly alter central nervous system neurotransmission and disturb the HPT axis. In summary, an assessment of thyroid function, specifically the HPT axis in bulimia nervosa, may help more accurately determine the nature of the disturbance present and whether such a disturbance is state related (i.e., secondary to the nutritional and metabolic effects of disordered eating) or a trait disturbance (i.e., a primary neuroendocrinologic abnormality that has pathophysiological or pathogenetic significance).

4.1 Peripheral Thyroid Hormone Levels

A number of studies have examined basal levels of thyroid hormone in bulimia nervosa. These studies have generally not assessed the nutritional status of the patients at the time of testing. The results are therefore difficult to interpret in terms of their pathophysiological significance.

In an early study, Mitchell and Bantle (36) found that five of six normal-weight bulimic subjects had normal T_4 and T_3 concentrations and normal T_3 resin uptake. The authors felt that generally normal levels of thyroid hormone in bulimic subjects compared with anorexic subjects reflected the fact that bulimic patients were more stable nutritionally than anorexic patients and there was less of a need for decreased peripheral conversion of T_4 to T_3 as an adaptation to starvation. However, these findings do not agree with those by other investigators (14,33) who found that levels of T_3 in normal-weight bulimic patients were significantly lower compared with both control groups and anorexic subjects. These authors interpret this finding in combination with their findings of lowered levels of glucose, decreased elevation of noradrenaline in response to an orthostatic challenge, and significantly increased levels of free fatty acids and β-hydroxybutyric acid as indicative of starvation and evidence of intermittent inadequate energy supply in bulimia nervosa patients (14).

In a study (36) of 168 patients with bulimia nervosa at normal weight, 16 were found to have abnormal thyroid function, the most common abnormality being a decreased T_4 index, the product of the T_3 resin uptake and serum T_4. Of these 16 patients, 2 had documented preexisting thyroid dysfunction, whereas only 1 of the remaining 14 patients showed evidence of thyroid dysfunction on further investigation. A possible explanation for thyroid abnormalities found in the remaining patients may relate to the fact that 11% of these 168 patients were under 90% of ideal body weight. It was not stated whether the thyroid abnormalities occurred at greater frequency in this underweight group of patients.

A more recent study assessed the level of thyroid hormone in bulimia nervosa. Kiyohara et al. (27) measured levels of serum T_4, T_3, and rT_3 in 17 patients with bulimia nervosa who were within ±10% of ideal body weight for at least 2 years before the study. The mean T_4 concentration in the patient group was slightly but significantly lower ($P < .01$) than in the control group. The mean T_3 concentration in the bulimia nervosa patients was significantly lower ($P < .001$) than in the control subjects, whereas the mean basal serum rT_3 concentration of the patients was not significantly different from that of the control subjects. There was no significant correlation between basal serum T_4 or T_3 levels and percent decrease from ideal body weight. The authors of this study considered the possibility that changes in thyroid levels reflected either caloric restriction, malnutrition, or weight change. However, they concluded that because of the normal levels of rT_3 in these subjects, it was likely that factors other than weight loss or malnutrition could result in alterations in thyroid functioning in bulimia nervosa.

In a group of 40 patients with bulimia nervosa and between 90% and 110% of ideal body weight, Kaplan (37) found that all but 1 patient had normal levels of T_3 resin uptake and serum T_4. Normal levels of T_4, T_3, and rT_3 were also reported in a study of metabolic abnormalities in bulimia nervosa (31). However, these investigators found substantially lower levels of baseline serum TSH in bulimic subjects compared with control subjects, a finding that is difficult to interpret in the context of normal thyroid indices.

In a study (38) that analyzed the relationship between depression and starvation in bulimia nervosa, lower levels of serum T_3 along with lowered body weight, elevated levels of β-hydroxybutyric acid, and elevated levels of cortisol accounted for a significant amount of the variance ($P < .05$) in the depression score of the Beck Depression Inventory in a group of bulimic patients. These same investigators also found that in a group of healthy subjects experimentally placed on 1,000 kcal/day diet for 6 weeks who lost an average of 1 kg/week, average global mood ratings during the last 3 weeks of the study correlated significantly ($r = -.52; P < .01$) with carbohydrate content of the diet and with the ratio of tryptophan to large neutral amino acid. It has been suggested that low-carbohydrate intake results in a reduction of this ratio and less tryptophan available for brain synthesis of serotonin (39), with possible deterioration of mood as a result. These investigators concluded that the low-carbohydrate diet frequently followed by anorexic and bulimic patients could account in part for the accompanying mood disturbances found in these patients.

In another study (40), investigators examined thyroid function in 23 bulimic patients studied longitudinally while actively bingeing and purging and after at least 30 days of voluntary abstinence from these behaviors. All measures of thyroid functioning, including serum T_3, T_4, TSH, and TBG were within normal limits in patients studied while actively bingeing and purging. After at least 30 days of abstinence, there was a significant decrease ($P < .001$) in serum T_3 and serum T_4 compared with the symptomatic state. There were no significant changes in TSH and TBG. These investigators hypothesized that the fall in T_3 may be due to the fact that bulimic patients were consuming a calorically deficient diet low in carbohydrate in order to defend a weight set point that was artificially low for them. Another possible explanation for these interesting findings is that bulimic patients in a remitted state may be chemically hypothyroid due to a hypothalamic abnormality in the TRH neuron and that during binge-purge activity there may be activation of the HPT axis causing an apparent normalization of thyroid indices. These parameters need to be studied further in bulimic patients as they pass from the actively symptomatic state to a remitted state to a fully recovered state in order to fully assess the effects of nutrition, mood, and weight on thyroid function.

4.2 Hypothalamic-Pituitary-Thyroid (HPT) Axis

The HPT axis has been investigated in patients with bulimia nervosa (Table 9–1). Most of the nine published studies report on small numbers of subjects who were actively symptomatic. Results of these studies are somewhat contradictory, but do point to generally normal TSH response to TRH in patients with bulimia nervosa.

Table 9–1. Thyroid-stimulating hormone (TSH) response to thyrotropin-releasing hormone in bulimia nervosa

Study	N subjects	Depression status	Controls subjects	Findings[a]
Gwirtsman et al. 1983 (41)	10	D and ND	No	8 blunted (80%)
Mitchell and Bantle 1983 (36)	6	D and ND	No	1 blunted (16%)
Gwirtsman et al. 1984 (43)	3 (males)	D and ND	No	1 blunted (33%); D and ND no difference
Norris et al. 1985 (44)	10	ND	Yes	3 blunted (30%); 2 control subjects blunted (20%)
Kiriike et al. 1987 (26)	10	D and ND	No	0 blunted; D and ND no difference
Kiyohara et al. 1988 (27)	9	ND	No	1 blunted (11%)
Levy et al. 1988 (45)	9	ND	No	0 blunted
Fichter et al. 1988 (33)	24	D and ND	Yes	Bulimia nervosa reduced response compared with control subjects, ND reduced response compared with D
Kaplan et al. 1989 (46)	18	D and ND	Yes	0 blunted; D and ND no difference

Note. D = depressed; ND = nondepressed.
[a]Blunted response = Δ_{max} TSH < 5 μU/ml.

Gwirtsman et al. (41) studied 10 bulimia nervosa patients who were between 83% and 110% of ideal body weight. These patients were part of a larger sample of 18 bulimic subjects, 15 of whom were monitored as inpatients 1 week before investigations. It was unclear how many of the 10 patients studied were in this group of 15 monitored patients. These investigators found an 80% rate of blunting on the TSH response to TRH as defined by a maximal change from baseline to peak TSH (Δ_{max} TSH) of less than 5 µU/ml in response to TRH 500 µg iv (42). There was no control group in this study, and the blunting seen was not related to other variables such as weight, menstrual status, history of anorexia nervosa, positive family history of depression, or failure to suppress on the dexamethasone suppression test. One-half of the tested group demonstrated a delay in peak TSH response to TRH, as has been reported in patients with anorexia nervosa (15).

The same group of investigators (43) also reported on the TSH response to TRH in three male bulimia nervosa patients. One of the three men demonstrated a blunted response as determined by previously established criteria (42). All three patients had normal baseline levels of TSH. Noteworthy was that the blunted response was seen in a patient who was significantly thinner than his premorbidly heaviest weight, whereas the two patients with normal responses were closer to their premorbidly heaviest weight.

Another group of investigators (36) reported on the TSH response to TRH in six bulimia nervosa patients who were within 10% of matched-population weights. These patients were hospitalized for an unreported period of time but were actively symptomatic during testing. Five of the patients had normal baseline TSH levels and demonstrated normal responses to TRH. One patient demonstrated a blunted response to TRH, possibly explainable by an elevated baseline level of TSH prior to perturbation. The above studies did not specifically exclude patients who were concurrently depressed.

Norris et al. (44) reported on the TRH-stimulation test in 10 patients with bulimia nervosa who were not concurrently depressed but who may have been depressed previously, as well as in 11 healthy control subjects and 9 patients with anorexia nervosa. They found normal responses in the patients with bulimia nervosa with no differences with regard to the timing or degree of peak TSH response compared with the healthy control subjects. Noteworthy and significant is the fact that 3 of the 10 bulimia nervosa patients did produce a blunted response as previously defined (42), but this was no different from the control group in which 2 of the 10 healthy control subjects also produced peak responses that were exactly 5 μU/ml increased from baseline. There were no significant correlations with weight for basal TSH level, peak TSH level, peak incremental TSH response, area under the response curve, or peak-to-basal ratio. Patients with bulimia nervosa weighed from 95% to 120% of matched population mean weight, but there was no mention of their present weight compared with their premorbid weight. The anorexia nervosa patients demonstrated substantially delayed peak TSH levels compared with the control subjects, the bulimia nervosa patients, or themselves after weight restoration. One of the 9 patients with anorexia nervosa demonstrated a blunted response.

Kiriike et al. (26) studied serum TSH, prolactin, and growth hormone responses to TRH in 10 patients with bulimia nervosa at normal weight, many of whom were concurrently depressed, as well as in 7 patients with the restricting form of anorexia nervosa and 6 with bulimia nervosa and anorexia nervosa. The mean basal levels of TSH, prolactin, and growth hormone did not differ among the three groups. A delayed TSH response to TRH was found in 86% of the patients with the restricting form of anorexia nervosa, 80% of the patients with bulimia nervosa and anorexia nervosa, and only 22% of the patients with bulimia nervosa (with no blunted responses in this latter group). Other significant neuroendocrine abnormalities included elevated basal growth hormone levels (in 29% of the restricting anorexic patients, 32% of the bulimic anorexic patients, and 33% of the bulimic patients) and an abnormal growth hormone increase after TRH stimulation (in 50% of the restricting anorexic patients, 20% of the bulimic anorexic patients, and 13% of the bulimic patients). Generally speaking, abnormal TSH responses to TRH were observed more frequently in the low-weight restricting group than in the bulimia nervosa patients at normal weight. Abnormalities in TSH response in the bulimia nervosa patients were not related to measures of depression, weight, or reported eating behavior.

Kiyohara et al. (27) reported on responses of TSH to TRH in nine patients with bulimia nervosa, none of whom had ever had major depression but who at the time of testing endorsed significant depressive symptoms. Of the nine patients tested, the TSH response to TRH was normal in five, delayed in three, and blunted in one. The maximum increase in serum TSH and TSH net secretory response were not significantly different from those of control subjects. The patients with bulimia nervosa had maintained their body weight within 10% of matched-population mean weight for at least 2 years before the study.

Levy et al. (45) studied the TSH, growth hormone, and prolactin response to TRH in nine normal-weight female bulimic patients who were relatively depression free and compared their responses to eight female control subjects. Four of the bulimic patients had delayed peak TSH responses, but none demonstrated a blunted TSH response. The bulimic patients had an elevated mean serum growth hormone level and an inappropriate growth hormone release following TRH. In addition, their mean serum prolactin level was lower than that of the control subjects and demonstrated a significantly greater response ($P < .05$) than that of the control subjects. The authors correctly pointed out that the neuroendocrine abnormalities found in this study generally do not resemble those found in depression, specifically stating that delayed TSH response to TRH, high basal growth hormone, and exaggerated prolactin responses to TRH are not typical of depressed patients. Further, they found that none of the hormonal abnormalities were correlated with self-report or observer-rated measures of depression. The abnormalities are more likely related to a state of semistarvation in bulimia nervosa.

Fichter et al. (33) studied the TSH response to TRH in healthy subjects and in patients with bulimia nervosa. Their findings add to the evidence that neuroendocrine changes found in bulimia nervosa relate to nutritional status. The average peak TSH plasma levels following TRH perturbation were lower in bulimic subjects than in 12 healthy control subjects. They found that this difference was specifically due to a subgroup of bulimic patients who had a low percentage of carbohydrate intake compared with that of the healthy control subjects and bulimic patients with high-carbohydrate intake. They also found that older bulimic patients with a longer duration of illness had significantly reduced TSH response ($P < .03$) compared with younger bulimic patients who had been ill for less time. Moreover, reduced TSH responses were seen in bulimic patients with reduced caloric intake and in bulimic patients with high β-hydroxybutyric acid blood levels. Surprisingly, bulimic patients with a low degree of depression on the Hamilton Rating Scale for Depression showed a reduced peak TSH response compared with healthy control subjects and bulimic patients who were more depressed. There was a positive correlation between the percentage of carbohydrate intake and the plasma TSH levels after stimulation with TRH, indicating that a low-carbohydrate intake may be followed by a blunted TSH response to TRH in bulimia nervosa. The reduced prolactin response to TRH was specifically seen in those bulimic patients with a low-carbohydrate intake. The investigators interpreted their findings to indicate that temporarily restricted food intake and macronutrient composition in bulimic subjects are very important variables that can explain these findings.

Finally, Kaplan et al. (46) reported TSH response to TRH in 18 patients with bulimia nervosa at normal weight and 20 control subjects. Both groups displayed a significant response to TRH and did not differ at baseline or over time in their responses. There were no differences in peak response or in time to peak response. No bulimic or control subjects demonstrated a blunted response based on previously defined criteria (42). There was no significant difference on the TSH response to TRH between a group of bulimic patients with and a group without a concurrent diagnosis of major depression. Current weight did not correlate with TSH response to TRH in this study. Basal growth hormone and prolactin levels were normal in bulimic subjects compared with control subjects and demonstrated similar responses to TRH in both groups. These investigators also found that nonsuppression on the dexamethasone suppression test (DST) was associated with bulimic patients being thinner than patients who suppressed normally. Nonsuppression on the DST did not correlate with a less robust TSH response to TRH in this patient group.

4.3 Conclusions

No clear, consistent pattern of thyroid abnormalities has emerged in the studies of thyroid function in bulimia nervosa. The abnormalities that have been reported include delayed and blunted peak TSH response to TRH, low levels of TSH, normal levels of serum T_4 with low levels of serum T_3, and elevated levels of serum rT_3. The findings of inconsistent abnormalities in bulimia nervosa probably relate to methodological issues, most notably the clinical state of the patients being studied. Of interest is the possibility that macronutrient composition contributes to a relative state of malnutrition and secondary thyroid abnormalities. To more accurately assess the pathophysiological significance of those abnormalities, further investigations will need to control for current nutritional status, including the level of caloric intake, macronutrient composition, and weight fluctuation for a period of time prior to studying bulimic patients.

At this time, the evidence points to levels of caloric intake, macronutrient composition, and weight fluctuation as being factors in the thyroid disturbances reported in bulimia nervosa. However, these state-related variables may be superimposed on an underlying hypothalamic diathesis related to thyroid function and/or metabolism that may predispose a patient to develop an eating disorder. A recent intriguing finding (31) that bulimic patients have significantly lowered ($P < .05$) basal metabolic rates compared with control subjects and are thus calorically more efficient and that this may persist in the remitted state (47) lends support for the existence of such a trait disturbance. Further studies, assessing longitudinally the thyroid status of bulimic patients when actively symptomatic and fully recovered, may help elucidate the contribution of state- and trait-related variables to the pathophysiology of bulimia nervosa.

5. THYROID HORMONE ABUSE IN EATING DISORDERS

The abuse of thyroid hormone as a method of increasing metabolic rate to lose weight in anorexia nervosa and bulimia nervosa has been reported for many decades (48). The exact prevalence of such abuse is unknown. A retrospective review of the charts of 104 eating disorder consultations seen by us revealed a rate of 6.7% (7 of 104) for thyroid hormone abuse (49). Most such individuals obtain the medication secretly from parents or grandparents who have thyroid disorders. The duration of the abuse is thus usually short, as many patients find it difficult to obtain a regular supply of thyroid hormone. A more complicated situation arises when patients with anorexia nervosa or bulimia nervosa who have borderline low thyroid function are prescribed thyroid hormone by physicians, either because they have not revealed the presence of their eating disorder to their physician or because their physician is unaware of the connection between eating disorders and thyroid function. Such individuals can be enormously resistant to discontinuing their thyroid hormone and may eventually develop the medical complications of excessive thyroid hormone use if physicians do not refuse to continue prescribing such medication.

Another, rarer phenomenon deserves some attention. Because the physiological effects of starvation are the reverse of those of hyperthyroidism, individuals with anorexia nervosa who develop Graves' disease may have minimal symptoms for many years. Occasionally, such patients will refuse treatment of their Graves' disease because of their fear of weight gain (50). We have reported one such case (49) in which a patient with anorexia nervosa, bulimia nervosa, and Graves' disease refused treatment for her hyperthyroidism for over a year, despite twice-weekly thyroid storms that included paranoid episodes and were markedly physically debilitating.

In summary, clinicians should be aware of the effect of starvation and chaotic eating on thyroid function and avoid prescribing exogenous thyroid hormone for individuals with eating disorders until after eating and weight are normalized for an extended period of time and there is clear clinical and laboratory evidence of persisting thyroid disturbance. The prescription of thyroid hormone to patients with anorexia nervosa and bulimia nervosa without clear evidence of primary thyroid dysfunction is clinically unwise and potentially dangerous.

REFERENCES

1. Rush B: An inquiry into the functions of the spleen, liver, pancreas and thyroid gland. Medical Physics Journal 16:193–208, 1806
2. Danforth E, Burger AG: The impact of nutrition on thyroid hormone physiology and action. Annu Rev Nutr 9:201–227, 1989
3. Curran-Celeutano J, Erdman JW, Nelson RA, et al: Alterations in vitamin A and thyroid hormone status in anorexia nervosa and associated disorders. Am J Clin Nutr 42:1183–1191, 1985
4. Fichter MM, Pirke KM, Holsboer F: Weight loss causes neuroendocrine disturbances: experimental study in healthy starving subjects. Psychiatry Res 17:61–72, 1986

5. Fichter MM, Pirke KM: Hypothalamic pituitary function in starving healthy subjects, in Psychobiology of Anorexia Nervosa. Edited by Pirke KM, Ploog D. New York, Springer-Verlag, 1988, pp 124–135

6. Vinik AF, Kalk WJ, McLaren H, et al: Fasting blunts the TSH response to synthetic TRH. J Clin Endocrinol Metab 40:509–511, 1975

7. Burman KD, Vigersky RA, Loriaux DL, et al: Investigations concerning thyroxine deiodinative pathways in patients with anorexia nervosa, in Anorexia Nervosa. Edited by Vigersky R. New York, Raven, 1977, pp 225–262

8. Hurd HP, Palumbo PJ, Gharib H: Hypothalamic-endocrine dysfunction in anorexia nervosa. Mayo Clin Proc 52:711–716, 1977

9. Miyai K, Yamamoto T, Azukizawa M, et al: Serum thyroid hormones and thyrotropin in anorexia nervosa. J Clin Endocrinol Metab 40:334–338, 1975

10. Moshang T, Utiger RD: Low T3 euthyroidism in anorexia nervosa, in Anorexia Nervosa. Edited by Vigersky R. New York, Raven, 1977, pp 263–270

11. Kiyohara K, Tamai H, Takaidi Y, et al: Decreased thyroidal triiodothyroxine secretion in patients with anorexia nervosa: influence of weight recovery. Am J Clin Nutr 50:767–772, 1989

12. Croxson MS, Ibbertson K: Low serum triiodothyronine and hypothyroidism in anorexia nervosa. J Clin Endocrinol Metab 44:167–174, 1977

13. Leslie RD, Isaacs AJ, Gomer J, et al: Hypothalamic-pituitary-thyroid function in anorexia nervosa: influence of weight gain. BMJ 2:526–528, 1978

14. Pirke KM, Pahl J, Schweiger U, et al: Metabolic and endocrine indices of starvation in bulimia: a comparison with anorexia nervosa. Psychiatry Res 15:33–39, 1985

15. Wakeling A, De Sousa VA, Gore MB, et al: Amenorrhea, body weight and serum hormone concentrations, with particular reference to prolactin and thyroid hormones in anorexia nervosa. Psychol Med 9:265–272, 1979

16. Tamai H, Mori K, Matsubayashi S, et al: Hypothalamic-pituitary-thyroidal dysfunctions in anorexia nervosa. Psychother Psychosom 46:127–131, 1986

17. de Rosa G, Corsello SM, de Rosa E, et al: Endocrine study of anorexia nervosa. Exp Clin Endocrinol 82:160–172, 1983

18. Chopra IJ, Smith SR, Reza M, et al: Reciprocal changes in serum concentration of 3, 3′,5-triiodothyronine (reverse T3) and 3, 5′, 3 tri-iodothyronine (T3) in systemic illness. J Clin Endocrinol Metab 41:1043–1049, 1975

19. Vagenakis AG: Thyroid hormone metabolism in prolonged experimental starvation in man, in Anorexia Nervosa. Edited by Vigersky RV. New York, Raven, 1977, pp 243–252

20. Chopra IJ: Thyroid function in nonthyroidal illnesses. Ann Intern Med 98:946–957, 1983

21. Bannai C, Kuzuya N, Koide Y, et al: Assessment of the relationship between serum thyroid hormone levels and peripheral metabolism in patients with anorexia nervosa. Endocrinol Jpn 35:455–462, 1988

22. Brown GM, Garfinkel PE, Jeunlewic N, et al: Endocrine profiles in anorexia nervosa, in Anorexia Nervosa. Edited by Vigersky R. New York, Raven, 1977, pp 123–135

23. Casper RC, Davis JM, Pandey CN: The effect of nutritional status and weight changes on hypothalamic function tests in anorexia nervosa, in Anorexia Nervosa. Edited by Vigersky R. New York, Raven, 1977, pp 137–147

24. Beaumont PJV, George GCW, Pimstone BL, et al: Body weight and the pituitary response to hypothalamic releasing hormones in patients with anorexia nervosa. Journal of Clinical Endocrinology 43:487–496, 1976

25. Vigersky RA, Loriaux DL: Anorexia nervosa as a model of hypothalamic dysfunction, in Anorexia Nervosa. Edited by Vigersky R. New York, Raven, 1977, pp 109–122

26. Kiriike S, Nishiwaki Y, Izumiya Y, et al: Thyrotropin, prolactin and growth hormone responses to thyrotropin-releasing hormone in anorexia nervosa and bulimia. Biol Psychiatry 22:167–176, 1987

27. Kiyohara K, Tamai H, Kobayashi N, et al: Hypothalamic-pituitary-thyroidal axis alterations in bulimic patients. Am J Clin Nutr 47:805–809, 1988

28. Forbes GB, Kreipe RE, Lipinski BA, et al: Body composition changes during recovery from anorexia nervosa: a comparison of two dietary regimes. Am J Clin Nutr 40:1137–1145, 1984

29. Walker J, Roberts SL, Halmi KA, et al: Caloric requirements for weight gain in anorexia nervosa. Am J Clin Nutr 32:1396–1400, 1979

30. Stordy BJ, Marks V, Kalucy RS, et al: Weight gain, thermic effects of glucose and metabolic rate during recovery from anorexia nervosa. Am J Clin Nutr 30:138–146, 1977

31. Devlin MJ, Walsh T, Kral JG, et al: Metabolic abnormalities in bulimia nervosa. Arch Gen Psychiatry 47:144–148, 1990

32. Garfinkel PE, Moldofsky H, Garner DM, et al: The heterogeneity of anorexia nervosa: bulimia as a distinct subgroup. Arch Gen Psychiatry 37:1036–1040, 1980

33. Fichter MM, Pirke KM, Pollinger J, et al: Restricted caloric intake causes neuroendocrine disturbances in bulimia, in Psycho-biology of Bulimia Nervosa. Edited by Pirke KM, Vandereycken W, Ploog D. New York, Springer-Verlag, 1988, pp 42–56

34. Krieg JC, Backmund H, Pirke KM: Cranial computed tomography findings in bulimia. Acta Psychiatr Scand 75:144–149, 1987

35. Krieg JC, Lauer C, Pirke KM: Structural brain abnormalities in patients with bulimia nervosa. Psychiatry Res 27:39–48, 1989

36. Mitchell JE, Bantle JP: Metabolic and endocrine investigations in women of normal weight with bulimia syndrome. Biol Psychiatry 18:355–365, 1983

37. Kaplan AS: Thyroid function in bulimia, in The Psychobiology of Bulimia. Edited by Hudson JI, Pope HG. Washington, DC, American Psychiatric Press, 1987, pp 55–71

38. Laessle RG, Schweiger U, Fichter MM, et al: Eating disorders and depression: psychobiological findings in bulimia and anorexia nervosa, in Psycho-biology of Bulimia Nervosa. Edited by Pirke KM, Vandereycken W, Ploog D. New York, Springer-Verlag, 1988, pp 90–100

39. Fernstrom JDN, Wurtman RJ: Brain serotonin content: physiological regulation by plasma neutral amino acids. Science 178:414–416, 1972

40. Spalter AR, Gold PW, Demitrack MA, et al: Thyroid function in bulimia nervosa (abstract 207). Presented at the 4th International Conference on Eating Disorders, New York, April 1990

41. Gwirtsman HE, Roy-Byrne P, Yager J, et al: Neuro-endocrine abnormalities in bulimia. Am J Psychiatry 140:559–563, 1983

42. Loosen PT, Prange AJ: Serum thyrotropin response to thyrotropin-releasing hormone in psychiatric patients: a review. Am J Psychiatry 139:405–416, 1982

43. Gwirtsman HE, Roy-Byrne P, Lerner L, et al: Bulimia in men: report of three cases with neuroendocrine findings. J Clin Psychiatry 45:78–81, 1984

44. Norris PD, O'Malley BP, Palmer RL: The TRH test in bulimia and anorexia nervosa: a controlled study. J Psychiatr Res 19:215–219, 1985

45. Levy AB, Dixon KN, Malorkey WB: Pituitary responses to TRH in bulimia. Biol Psychiatry 23:476–484, 1988

46. Kaplan AS, Garfinkel PE, Brown GM: The DST and TRH test in bulimia nervosa. Br J Psychiatry 154:86–92, 1989

47. Weltzin TE, Kaye WH, Fernstrom MH, et al: The clinical significance of altered caloric utilization necessary for weight maintenance in eating disordered patients (abstract 108). Presented at the 4th International Conference on Eating Disorders, New York, April 1990

48. Binswanger L: Der Fall Ellen West. Schweiz Arch Neurol Psychiatr 54:69–117, 1944

49. Woodside DB, Walfish P, Kaplan AS, et al: Graves' disease in a woman with thyroid hormone abuse, bulimia nervosa, and a history of anorexia nervosa. International Journal of Eating Disorders 10:111–115, 1991

50. Rolla AR, El-Hajj GA, Goldstein HH: Untreated thyrotoxicosis as a manifestation of anorexia nervosa. Am J Med 81:163–165, 1986

Chapter 10

The Thyroid
and Schizophrenia

Russell T. Joffe, M.D.
Anthony J. Levitt, M.D.

CONTENTS

1. INTRODUCTION

Studies of the biological basis of schizophrenia have focused predominantly on the dopamine hypothesis of this disorder and, therefore, have largely emphasized the measurement of hormones, such as prolactin and growth hormone, that reflect dopamine function (1). There are, however, limited data on alterations of the thyroid axis in patients who have schizophrenia.

It has long been established that psychiatric symptoms accompany clinical thyroid disorders (2–10). Although disorders of affect have been most commonly described (2,3), psychotic symptoms—both delusions and hallucinations—also have been reported to occur commonly, particularly in

317

patients with hypothyroidism (5–8). Furthermore, these earlier reports suggest that successful treatment of the thyroid disease is usually associated with resolution of psychotic symptoms (4). The observations from these early clinical studies led to an extensive research effort in understanding the relationship between thyroid abnormalities and affective illness. Less attention has been paid to the potential role of thyroid hormones in the pathophysiology of psychotic disorders, particularly schizophrenia. In this chapter, we also review the limited data available on baseline thyroid function tests in schizophrenia, the effect of antipsychotics on thyroid function tests, and the effect of thyroid hormones on dopamine function.

2. BASELINE THYROID FUNCTION TESTS

2.1 Peripheral Thyroid Hormones

Few studies have examined potential abnormalities of baseline thyroid function tests in patients with schizophrenia. Early reports suggested some abnormalities of thyroid function in patients with schizophrenia, including a low basal metabolic rate in up to half of schizophrenic patients (11), reduced radioiodine uptake in schizophrenic subjects (12,13), and diminished sensitivity to the toxic effects of thyroid hormones in several schizophrenic patients (14). Taken together, these early data indicate that a substantial proportion of schizophrenic patients may have reduced thyroid function. However, conclusions from these studies are limited by several methodological difficulties, including poor definition of psychiatric diagnosis when compared with current methods and the relatively crude methods by which thyroid function was measured.

More recent studies have failed to detect a specific abnormality of basal peripheral thyroid hormone levels in schizophrenic subjects. Several (15–22), but not all (23,24), studies have reported a transient elevation in measures of thyroxine (T_4) and free thyroxine (FT_4) in acute psychiatric patients recently admitted to an inpatient unit. Although these studies included many schizophrenic patients, this observation is not specific to one psychiatric diagnostic category. This phenomenon of transient hyperthyroxinemia may occur in up to 30% of newly admitted patients and is not accompanied by any evidence of clinical thyroid disease. Furthermore, these increases in measures of T_4 usually normalize within 2 to 3 weeks after admission (15–21).

The pathophysiological significance of this finding is poorly understood. Transient hyperthyroxinemia may result from abnormalities of biogenic amines that affect thyroid function, from an alteration in peripheral metabolism of thyroid hormones, or from some more central abnormality of the hypothalamic-pituitary-thyroid axis in patients with psychiatric disorders (17). Baumgartner et al. (22) suggested that elevations in T_4 were a particular abnormality of baseline thyroid function tests that occurred in schizophrenic patients but not in affectively ill patients or healthy control subjects. However, because the schizophrenic subjects evaluated by these investigators had recently been admitted to an assessment unit, it is unclear whether this was a finding specific to schizophrenia or merely another example of transient hyperthyroxinemia documented in several previous studies (15–21). In contrast to Baumgartner et al. (22) and the previous studies (15–21), two other reports (23,24) have found no difference in baseline methods of T_4 and free thyroxine index (FT_4I) in hospitalized schizophrenic patients as compared with control subjects. Whether schizophrenic subjects are more likely to develop transient hyperthyroxinemia is not known and requires further, systematic study.

2.2 The Thyroid Axis

The thyrotropin-releasing hormone (TRH) test, the measurement of serum thyroid-stimulating hormone (TSH) (or thyrotropin) following TRH administration, is a standard endocrine test used as a dynamic measure of the function of the thyroid axis and has been widely applied to psychiatric illness over the last few years (25,26). Although most studies have evaluated the clinical utility and pathophysiological significance of the TRH test in patients with affective illness, several studies have examined the use of this test in patients with schizophrenia (27–35).

There has been wide variation in the frequency of blunting of the TSH response to TRH reported in these studies. For example, Loosen et al. (30) and Gold et al. (31) showed that none of their schizophrenic subjects had a blunted TSH response to TRH, whereas Banki et al.

(35) reported that 30% of 20 schizophrenic women showed evidence of a blunted TRH test. Furthermore, Koenig et al. (34) reported that 40% of patients with a paranoid hallucinatory syndrome had evidence of a blunted TRH test, although they did not clarify whether this psychotic syndrome was consistent with the diagnosis of schizophrenia. Taken together, these studies suggest that a blunted TRH test occurs relatively infrequently in patients with clearly diagnosed schizophrenia. This is in contrast to the extensive literature that suggests that up to one-third of patients with affective illness may show a blunted TSH response to TRH (25,26). Although this difference in frequency of blunting between schizophrenia and affective illness has been suggested as being of potential use in distinguishing acute psychotic mania from schizophrenia (36,37), other studies do not indicate that this test would be of clinical use in such a situation (38,39).

Two early reports suggested that baseline TSH levels may be elevated in patients with schizophrenia (40,41). Moreover, in the first of these studies (40), there was a significant correlation between the TSH levels and measures of paranoia. These early data raise the possibility that subclinical hypothyroidism may be associated with some cases of schizophrenia. However, more recent studies (27–35) have not found consistent abnormalities of baseline TSH levels in patients with schizophrenia. We (42) have recently reported decreased triiodothyronine (T_3) and increased TSH in psychotic versus nonpsychotic depressed patients. Further study is, therefore, required to clarify the relationship between psychotic symptoms, regardless of diagnosis and altered thyroid function. Although consistent abnormalities of basal and TRH-stimulated TSH response have not been found in schizophrenia, several studies suggest that a reduced TSH response to TRH may be associated with response to neuroleptics in some patients with psychosis. Langer et al. (43,44) found that a blunted TSH response predicted a better therapeutic effect from neuroleptics, whereas Beasley et al. (28) found that a reduced TSH response was associated with a more rapid neuroleptic treatment response.

In summary, studies to date do not show evidence of consistent alterations in thyroid function tests in patients with schizophrenia, but there may be a relationship between thyroid axis alteration and antipsychotic response.

3. EFFECT OF ANTIPSYCHOTICS ON THYROID FUNCTION

The effects of antipsychotic agents on various measures of thyroid function have been assessed in both healthy volunteers and patients with schizophrenia. With regard to T_4 and T_3, Rinieris and co-workers (23) found that 6 weeks of treatment with various neuroleptics resulted in substantial decreases in T_4 and FT_4I in 24 schizophrenic patients. However, these investigators were not able to replicate these findings in another study (24).

Several other studies using either the protein-bound iodine, an earlier measure of thyroid function, or a direct measure of T_4 or T_3 found no effect of neuroleptics on these thyroid function tests (45–47). Baumgartner et al. (22) did report substantial decreases in measures of T_4 in schizophrenic patients treated with neuroleptics; however, because the initial measure of T_4 was taken soon after admission, the changes on neuroleptics may represent a normalization of the transient elevations in T_4 seen in patients recently admitted to an inpatient unit (15–21). The study by Mason et al. (48) is of interest because they found no significant alteration in thyroid function tests in a group of schizophrenic patients treated with neuroleptics. However, within the schizophrenic group, significant increases in thyroid function tests were noted across the period of treatment, with neuroleptics in the paranoid, but not the undifferentiated, subgroup.

Although the sample sizes were small, these data suggest that close attention should be paid in future research to changes in thyroid function, even within the normal range, and various specific measures of psychopathology within diagnostic subgroups.

The data on changes in basal and TRH-stimulated TSH levels with neuroleptic treatment are variable. Treatment with antipsychotics are associated with increases (49–51), no change (47,52), and decreases (53) in basal TSH levels. Inconsistencies in these data can be explained by acute versus chronic treatment with neuroleptics, dosage differences in neuroleptics used, and differences in study groups in that both schizophrenic subjects and healthy control populations have been used. Variable effects of neuroleptics on the TRH test have also been reported (49,50,54), which may be explained by the same methodological difficulties as for measurement of basal TSH levels.

4. THE THYROID AND DOPAMINE

Although clinical studies suggest that changes in thyroid function are not a prominent feature of schizophrenia and that neuroleptics have inconsistent effects on thyroid function tests, it is well known that there is an interaction between dopamine and the hypothalamic-pituitary-thyroid axis at several levels. First, dopamine has been shown to influence the release of pituitary TSH (54). Second, several studies (55–58) indicate that thyroid hormones modify the function of dopamine receptors. Both hyper- and hypothyroidism have been shown to modify the response to dopamine agonists and antagonists in animal models (55–58). In particular, it has been consistently shown that hyperthyroidism increases and hypothyroidism decreases sensitivity to dopamine antagonists (55,57,58). Although these findings are readily demonstrated in animal models, their significance to humans and particularly to the pathophysiology or treatment response in schizophrenia remains to be clarified.

REFERENCES

1. Losonczy MF, Davidson M, Davis KL: The dopamine hypothesis of schizophrenia, in Psychopharmacology: The Third Generation of Progress. Edited by Meltzer HY. New York, Raven, 1987, pp 715–726
2. Loosen PT: Hormones on the hypothalamic-pituitary-thyroid axis: a psychoneuroendocrine perspective. Pharmacopsychiatry 19:401–415, 1986
3. Wilson WH, Jefferson JW: Thyroid disease, behaviour and psychopharmacology. Psychosomatics 26:481–492, 1985
4. Hall RCW: Psychiatric effects of thyroid hormone disturbance. Psychosomatics 24:7–18, 1983
5. Asher R: Myxoedematous madness. BMJ 2:555–562, 1949
6. Clinical Society of London: Report of a committee nominated December 14, 1883, to investigate the subject of myxedema. Transactions of the Clinical Society of London 21 (suppl), 1888
7. Jain VK: A psychiatric study of hypothyroidism. Psychiatric Clinics 5:121–130, 1972
8. Whybrow PC, Prange AJ Jr, Treadway CR: The mental changes accompanying thyroid gland dysfunction. Arch Gen Psychiatry 20:48–63, 1969
9. Robbins LR, Vinson DB: Objective psychologic assessment of the thyrotoxic patients and the response to treatment: preliminary report. Journal of Clinical Endocrinology 20:120–129, 1960
10. MacCrimmon DJ, Wallace JE, Goldberg WM, et al: Emotional disturbancing and cognitive deficits in hyperthyroidism. Psychosom Med 41:331–340, 1970

11. Bowman KM, Miller FR, Dailey ME: Thyroid function in mental disease. J Nerv Ment Dis 112:404–424, 1950
12. Cranswick EG: Tracer iodine studies on thyroid activity and thyroid responsiveness in schizophrenia. Am J Psychiatry 112:170–178, 1956
13. Simpson GM, Cranswick EH, Blair JH: Thyroid indices in chronic schizophrenia. J Nerv Ment Dis 137:582–590, 1963
14. Hoskins RG, Sleeper FH: The thyroid factor in dementia praecox. Am J Psychiatry 10:411–432, 1930
15. McLarty DG, Ratcliffe WA, Ratcliffe JG, et al: A study of thyroid function in psychiatric inpatients. Br J Psychiatry 133:211–218, 1978
16. Morley JE, Shafer RB: Thyroid function screening in new psychiatric admissions. Arch Intern Med 142:591–593, 1982
17. Spratt DI, Pont A, Miller MB, et al: Hyperthyroxinemia in patients with acute psychiatric disorders. Am J Med 73:41–48, 1982
18. Caplan RH, Pagliara AS, Wickus G, et al: Elevation of the free thyroxine index in psychiatric patients. J Psychiatr Res 17:267–274, 1982
19. Cohen KL, Swigar ME: Thyroid function screening in psychiatric patients. JAMA 242:254–257, 1979
20. Levy RP, Jensen JB, Laus VG, et al: Serum thyroid hormone abnormalities in psychiatric disease. Metabolism 30:1060–1064, 1981
21. Lambert TJ, Davidson R, McLellan GH: Euthyroid hyperthyroxinaemia in acute psychiatric admissions. Aust N Z J Psychiatry 21:608–614, 1987
22. Baumgartner A, Graf KJ, Kurten I, et al: The hypothalamic-pituitary-thyroid axis in psychiatric patients and healthy subjects, II. Psychiatry Res 24:283–305, 1988
23. Martinos A, Rinieris P, Souvatzoglou A, et al: Effects of six weeks neuroleptic treatment on the pituitary-thyroid axis in schizophrenic patients. Neuropsychobiology 16:72–77, 1986
24. Rinieris P, Christodoulou GN, Souvatzoglou A, et al: Free-thyroxine index in schizophrenic patients before and after neuroleptic treatment. Neuropsychobiology 6:29–33, 1980
25. Loosen PT: The TRH-induced TSH response in psychiatric patients: a possible neuroendocrine marker. Psychoneuroendocrinology 10:237–260, 1985
26. Loosen PT, Prange AJ Jr: Serum thyrotropin response to thyrotropin-releasing hormone in psychiatric patients: a review. Am J Psychiatry 139:405–416, 1982
27. Roy A, Wolkowitz O, Doran A, et al: TRH test in schizophrenic patients and controls. Biol Psychiatry 25:523–526, 1989
28. Beasley CM, Magnusson M, Garver DL: TSH response to TRH and haloperidol response latency in psychoses. Biol Psychiatry 24:423–431, 1988
29. Braddock L, Blake I: Neuroendocrine tests during treatment with neuroleptic drugs, II: the TRH test. Br J Psychiatry 139:404–407, 1981

30. Loosen P, Prange A, Wilson I, et al: Thyroid stimulating hormone response after thyrotropin-releasing hormone in depressed, schizophrenic and normal women. Psychoneuroendocrinology 2:137–148, 1977
31. Gold MS, Pottash ALC, Extein I, et al: The TRH test in the diagnosis of major or minor depression. Psychoneuroendocrinology 6:159–169, 1981
32. Extein I, Pottash ALC, Gold MS, et al: Using the protirelin test to distinguish mania from schizophrenia. Arch Gen Psychiatry 39:77–81, 1982
33. Ferrier IN, Johnston EL, Crow TJ, et al: Anterior pituitary hormone secretions in chronic schizophrenia: responses to administration of hypothalamic-releasing hormones. Arch Gen Psychiatry 40:755–761, 1983
34. Koenig G, Aschauer H, Langer G, et al: TSH response to TRH in patients with various psychiatric diagnoses and in normal controls. Proceedings of 15th Annual Meeting of the International Society of Psychoneuroendocrinology, Vienna, Austria, July 1984
35. Banki C, Vojnik M, Arato M, et al: Dexamethasone suppression in multiple hormonal responses (TSH, prolactin and growth hormone) to TRH in some psychiatric disorders. Eur Arch Psychiatry Neurol Sci 235:32–37, 1985
36. Extein I, Pottash A, Gold M, et al: Differentiating mania from schizophrenia by the TRH test. Am J Psychiatry 137:981–982, 1980
37. Extein I, Pottash A, Gold M, et al: Changes in TSH response to TRH in affective illness, in Neurobiology of Mood Disorders. Edited by Post R, Ballenger J. Baltimore, MD, Williams & Wilkins, 1984, pp 297–310
38. Takahashi S, Kondo H, Yashimura M, et al: Thyroid function levels and thyrotropin responses to TRH administration in manic patients receiving lithium carbonate. Folia Psychiatrica Neurologica Japonica 29:231–237, 1975
39. Baumgartner A, Hagenkamp L, Meinhold M: Effect of age and diagnosis on thyrotropin response to thyrotropin-releasing hormone in psychiatric patients. Psychiatry Res 17:285–294, 1986
40. Dewhurst KE, El Kabir DT, Exley D, et al: Blood levels of TSH, protein-bound iodine and cortisol in schizophrenia and affective states. Lancet 2:1160–1162, 1968
41. Dewhurst KE, El Kabir DT, Harris GW, et al: Observations on the blood concentration of thyrotropic hormone (TSH) in schizophrenia and affective states. Br J Psychiatry 115:1003–1011, 1969
42. Joffe RT, Levitt AJ: Thyroid function and psychotic depression. Psychiatry Res 33:321–322, 1990
43. Langer G, Rasch F, Aschauer H, et al: TSH response patterns to TRH stimulation may indicate therapeutic mechanisms of antidepressant and neuroleptic drugs. Neuropsychobiology 11:213–218, 1984
44. Langer G, Koinig G, Hutzinger R, et al: Response of thyrotropin to thyrotropin-releasing hormone as predictor of treatment outcome. Arch Gen Psychiatry 43:861–868, 1986
45. Ayd FJ: Prolonged perphenazine therapy and thyroid function. Am J Psychiatry 120:592–594, 1963

46. Brambilla F, Guerrini A, Guastalla A, et al: Neuroendocrine effects of haloperidol therapy in chronic schizophrenia. Psychopharmacologia 44:17–22,
1975
47. Naber D, Steinbock H, Greil W: Effects of short and long-term neuroleptic
treatment on thyroid function. Progress in Neuropsychopharmacology
4:199–206, 1980
48. Mason JW, Kennedy JL, Kosten TR, et al: Serum thyroxine levels in schizophrenic and affective disorder diagnostic subgroups. J Nerv Ment Dis
177:351–358, 1989
49. Kirkegaard C, Bjorum N, Cohn D, et al: Studies on the influence of biogenic
amines and psychoactive drugs on the prognostic value of the TRH stimulation test in endogenous depression. Psychoneuroendocrinology 2:131–
136, 1977
50. Kirkegaard C, Bjorum N, Cohn D, et al: Thyrotropin-releasing hormone
(TRH) stimulation test in manic-depressive illness. Arch Gen Psychiatry
35:1017–1021, 1978
51. Magliozzi JR, Gold A, Laubly JN: Effect of oral administration of haloperidol
on plasma thyrotropin concentrations in man. Psychoneuroendocrinology
14:125–130, 1989
52. Lamberg BA, Linnoila M, Fogelholm R, et al: The effect of psychotropic
drugs on TSH-response to thyroliberin (TRH). Neuroendocrinology 24:90–
97, 1977
53. Collu R, Jequier JC, Leboeuf G, et al: Endocrine effects of pimozide, a specific
dopaminergic blocker. J Clin Endocrinol Metab 44:981–984, 1977
54. Delitala G, Devilla L, Canessa A, et al: On the role of dopamine receptors in
the central regulation of human TSH. Acta Endocrinol 98:521–527, 1981
55. Crocker AD, Overstreet DH: Modification of the behavioural effects of haliperidol and of dopamine receptor regulation by altered thyroid status. Psychopharmacology 82:102–106, 1984
56. Klawans HL, Goetz CL, Winer WJ: Dopamine receptor site sensitivity in hyperthyroid and hypothyroid guinea pigs. Adv Neurol 5:495–501, 1974
57. Atterwill CK: Effect of acute and chronic triiodothyronine (T3) administration to rats on central 5-HT and dopamine-mediated behavioural responses
and related brain biochemistry. Neuropharmacology 20:131–144, 1981
58. Lake CR, Fann WE: Possible potentiation of haliperidol neurotoxicity in
acute hyperthyroidism. Br J Psychiatry 123:523–525, 1973

Index

Page numbers printed in **boldface** *type refer to tables or figures.*